ADVANCED NUTRITION:
Macronutrients
Second Edition

CRC SERIES IN MODERN NUTRITION
Edited by Ira Wolinsky and James F. Hickson, Jr.

Published Titles

Manganese in Health and Disease, Dorothy J. Klimis-Tavantzis

Nutrition and AIDS: Effects and Treatments, Ronald R. Watson

Nutrition Care for HIV-Positive Persons: A Manual for Individuals and Their Caregivers,
Saroj M. Bahl and James F. Hickson, Jr.

Calcium and Phosphorus in Health and Disease, John J.B. Anderson and
Sanford C. Garner

Edited by Ira Wolinsky

Published Titles

Handbook of Nutrition in the Aged, Ronald R. Watson

Practical Handbook of Nutrition in Clinical Practice, Donald F. Kirby
and Stanley J. Dudrick

Handbook of Dairy Foods and Nutrition, Gregory D. Miller, Judith K. Jarvis,
and Lois D. McBean

Advanced Nutrition: Macronutrients, Carolyn D. Berdanier

Childhood Nutrition, Fima Lifschitz

Nutrition and Health: Topics and Controversies, Felix Bronner

Nutrition and Cancer Prevention, Ronald R. Watson and Siraj I. Mufti

Nutritional Concerns of Women, Ira Wolinsky and Dorothy J. Klimis-Tavantzis

Nutrients and Gene Expression: Clinical Aspects, Carolyn D. Berdanier

Antioxidants and Disease Prevention, Harinda S. Garewal

Advanced Nutrition: Micronutrients, Carolyn D. Berdanier

Nutrition and Women's Cancers, Barbara Pence and Dale M. Dunn

Nutrients and Foods in AIDS, Ronald R. Watson

Nutrition: Chemistry and Biology, Second Edition, Julian E. Spallholz,
L. Mallory Boylan, and Judy A. Driskell

Melatonin in the Promotion of Health, Ronald R. Watson

Nutritional and Environmental Influences on the Eye, Allen Taylor

Laboratory Tests for the Assessment of Nutritional Status, Second Edition,
H.E. Sauberlich

Advanced Human Nutrition, Robert E.C. Wildman and Denis M. Medeiros

Handbook of Dairy Foods and Nutrition, Second Edition, Gregory D. Miller,
Judith K. Jarvis, and Lois D. McBean

Nutrition in Space Flight and Weightlessness Models, Helen W. Lane
and Dale A. Schoeller

ADVANCED NUTRITION:
Macronutrients
Second Edition

Carolyn D. Berdanier, Ph.D.
Professor, Foods and Nutrition
University of Georgia
Athens, Georgia

CRC Press
Boca Raton   London   New York   Washington, D.C.

Library of Congress Cataloging-in-Publication Data

Berdanier, Carolyn D.
    Advanced nutrition: macronutrients / Carolyn D. Berdanier.--2nd ed.
      p. cm. (Modern nutrition)
    Includes bibliographical references and index.
    ISBN 0-8493-8735-3
    1. Nutrition. 2. Diet in disease. I. Title. II. Modern nutrition (Boca Raton, Fla.)

QP141 .B52 2000
612.3′9—dc21
                                            00-037867
                                          CIP

No claim to original U.S. Government works
International Standard Book Number 0-8493-8735-3
Library of Congress Card Number 00-037867
Printed in the United States of America 1 2 3 4 5 6 7 8 9 0
Printed on acid-free paper

Series Preface for Modern Nutrition

The CRC Series in Modern Nutrition is dedicated to providing the widest possible coverage of topics in nutrition. Nutrition is an interdisciplinary, interprofessional field par excellence. It is noted by its broad range and diversity. We trust the titles and authorship in this series will reflect that range and diversity.

Published for a scholarly audience, the volumes in the CRC Series in Modern Nutrition are designed to explain, review, and explore present knowledge and recent trends, developments, and advances in nutrition. As such, they will also appeal to the educated layman. The format for the series will vary with the needs of the author and the topic, including, but not limited to, edited volumes, monographs, handbooks, and texts.

Contributors from any bona fide area of nutrition, including the controversial, are welcome.

We welcome the contribution of the book *Advanced Nutrition: Macronutrients, second edition*, by my long-time colleague Carolyn Berdanier. It can be used as a companion volume to *Advanced Nutrition: Micronutrients*, written by the same author. Together, the two volumes add luster to the series and occupy an important niche in the area of advanced nutrition.

Ira Wolinsky, Ph.D.
Series editor

Preface to the First Edition

At the turn of the century and for a few decades after, nutrition research was conducted by biochemists seeking to unlock the secrets of metabolism. The vitamins were discovered one by one and the mysteries of such endemic diseases as pellagra, beri-beri, goiter, and rickets were no more. We learned that the inclusion of the "vital amines" could be accomplished by including foods rich in these substances in our diets. The needs for certain of the fatty acids, the amino acids and the many minerals were likewise discovered during this golden age of nutrition.

Now we have another period of great discovery upon us. Today's discoveries are no less exciting, for they are showing how the genetics of the consumer affect his/her use of the food that is consumed and, in turn, how the components of the consumed food can affect the expression of the genetic heritage of the consumer. The science of nutrition and its study as an advanced topic have evolved from one in which the student learned the names of the macro- and micronutrients and their chemistry, the requirements and the deficiency symptoms. Today, the student must have a strong science background with emphasis in biochemistry, genetics, and physiology in order to integrate this knowledge with an understanding of each of the nutrients and how the body uses them. The student needs to be able to look forward to new discoveries by understanding where our gaps in knowledge exist. The basic sciences have been incorporated into the text and clinical examples have been used to illustrate the importance of particular steps in the metabolic pathways. While the primary animal of interest is the human, this text is also useful for the study of other species as well. The basic science of nutrition is all inclusive and we can learn a lot through interspecies comparisons.

This volume contains text relating only to the needs for and use of the macronutrients. It serves as the basis for the second volume, which addresses the micronutrients. The two can be integrated so that the student will gain a comprehensive view of this composite science called nutrition.

February 1994

Preface to the Second Edition

In the five years since the first edition was written, science has not stood still. Research in the problems of obesity, diabetes, and heart disease has been particularly active. The explosion of knowledge about satiety and hunger has given new meaning to our understanding of the genetics of obesity. The discovery of leptin, additional uncoupling proteins, new neuropeptides that influence feeding and, as well, new knowledge about already known compounds, has made obesity research exciting. The interest in gene expression especially as related to nutrition has also flowered. How specific dietary components can influence the phenotypic expression of the genotype has captured the imagination of nutritionists and nonnutritionists alike. As the research database for this area expands, new approaches to food-intake recommendations for the optimization of health and nutritional status will be made. Actually, we are already seeing the results of this optimization in the fact that humans are living longer than ever before, and that the productive lifespan has increased with a decrease in that phase of life that is of poor quality. Research on aging, especially as it concerns nutrition science, is a very active area. Altogether, this volume has increased in size as the newer developments have been added to the original material. Happy reading!

Carolyn D. Berdanier

Acknowledgments for the First Edition

The book would not have been possible without the encouragement and support of the faculty and graduate students in the University of Georgia Nutrition Science graduate program. Particular appreciation is extended to those who read and criticized the initial draft: Richard Lewis, Anne Dattilo, James Hargrove, Martin Hulsey, Brenda Marques, Martin Kullen, John Parente, Krystyna Kras, Shelly Nickols-Richardson, and the members of my Advanced Nutrition class, who provided constructive criticism of the content and who found innumerable errors in punctuation, spelling, grammar, and so forth. The book would not have been possible without the manuscript preparation skills of Lula Fields, Betty Brown, and Kathy Adkins. I am especially grateful for the encouragement and support of my editor at CRC Press, Harvey Kane.

Acknowledgments for the Second Edition

The author would like to thank Tonya Dalton for her careful preparation of the manuscript. Her patience with the numerous corrections is truly admirable. Thanks to Helen Everts, Roy Martin, Mary Ann Johnson, Clifton Baile, William Flatt, Malcom Watford, and Johanna Dwyer for their constructive criticisms of the initial draft. I am especially appreciative of the efforts of Linda Brady and Michael McIntosh, who reviewed the finished manuscript. Finally, the fine efforts of my editor at CRC Press, Lourdes Franco, and series editor, Ira Wolinsky, should be acknowledged. Without their encouragement and support, this book would not have been possible.

About the Author

Carolyn D. Berdanier, Ph.D., is a professor of Nutrition at the University of Georgia in Athens. She received a B.S. degree from Pennsylvania State University and M.S. and Ph.D. degrees in Nutrition from Rutgers University. After a postdoctoral fellowship year with Dr. Paul Griminger at Rutgers, she served as a Research Nutritionist with the Human Nutrition Institute, which is part of ARS, a unit of the U.S. Department of Agriculture. In 1975, Dr. Berdanier moved to the University of Nebraska College of Medicine, where she continued her research in nutrient gene interactions. In 1977, she moved to the University of Georgia, where she served as Head of the Department of Foods and Nutrition. She stepped down from this post 11 years later and devoted her full-time efforts to research and teaching in her research area. NIH, USDA, U.S. Department of Commerce, the National Livestock and Meat Board, and the Egg Board have supported her research on the diet and genetic components of diabetes.

Dr. Berdanier is a member of the American Institute of Nutrition, the American Society for Clinical Nutrition, the Society for Experimental Biology and Medicine, American Diabetes Association, and several honorary societies in science. She has served on the editorial boards of the *FASEB Journal*, *The Journal of Nutrition and Nutrition Research*, and *Biochemistry Archives*. She has also served as a contributing editor for *Nutrition Reviews* and editor of the *AIN News Notes*. Current research interests include studies on aging, the role of diet in damage to mitochondrial DNA, and the role of specific dietary ingredients in the secondary complications of diabetes.

Table of Contents

Unit 3   Energy

Unit 4   Proteins

Definitions

Throughout this text the reader may find terms or expressions that are unfamiliar. Scientists in this hybrid field of nutrition–biochemistry–physiology–genetics sometimes "speak in code." They adopt a text-shorthand that is known to them but seldom explained to the lay reader. It is for this reason that a list of definitions for these abbreviations and terms is provided. Some of the definitions are medical terms, others are biotechnology terms, and still others are those useful to people conducting population studies or studies using animals.

ACAT — acyl coenzyme A: cholesterol acyl transferase. An enzyme that catalyzes the formation of an ester linkage between a fatty acid and cholesterol

ACP — acyl carrier protein. A pantothenic acid-protein-thio-ethanolamine structure upon which fatty acid biosynthesis occurs

Active site — that part of an enzyme or carrier or other protein to which a substrate binds

Actuarial data — information used to create mortality tables and life expectancy numbers

ADH — antidiuretic hormone also called vasopressin. Acts to conserve body water by increasing water resorption by the renal distal tubule

ADP — adenosine diphosphate. Metabolite of ATP. Energy is released when ATP is split into ADP and inorganic phosphate (P_i)

Age-adjusted death rate — the number of deaths in a specific age group for a given calendar year divided by the population of that same age group and multiplied by 1000

Albumin — small molecular weight protein found in blood and sometimes in urine

Allele — any one of a series of different genes that may occupy the same location (locus) on a specific chromosome

AMP — adenosine monophosphate. Metabolite of ADP. Energy is released when ADP is split into AMP and P_i

Anabolism — the totality of reactions that account for the synthesis of the body's macromolecules

Android obesity — a form of obesity where fat distribution is mainly in the shoulders and abdominal area, sometimes referred to as the "apple" shape

Anemia — below-normal levels of red blood cells or hemoglobin

Angina pectoris — chest pain due to lack of oxygen supplied to the heart

Antecedents — events that precede or are causally linked to an event

Anthropometry — measurement of body features, i.e., weight, height, etc.

Anticoding strand — a strand of DNA that is used as a template to direct the synthesis of RNA that is complementary to it

Antigen — a compound that elicits or stimulates the production and release of antibodies

Antibody — reactive material produced by the immune system that reacts with an antigen, thus neutralizing it

Apoproteins — blood proteins that can carry lipid (or some other compound)

Apparent digested energy (DE) — energy in food consumed less energy in feces: DE = IE – FE

Apoptosis — programmed cell death

Archimedes principle — an object's volume when submerged in water equals the volume of the water it displaces. If the mass and volume are known, the density can be calculated.

ARS — autonomously replicating sequence; the origin of replication in yeast

Arteriography — a method of examining the arteries using X-rays and an infusion of a radio-opaque dye solution

Atherogenic — producing atherosclerosis

Atherosclerosis — a progressive degenerative condition occurring within the vascular tree and resulting in occlusions and loss of elasticity

ATP — adenosine triphosphate, the energy-rich compound that serves as the energy coinage in the cell

Attenuated — weakened, lessened

Autoradiography — detection of radioactive molecules (e.g., DNA, RNA, protein) by visualization of their effects on photographic film

Autosomes — all chromosomes except the sex chromosomes; a diploid cell has two copies of each autosome

Autosomal trait — a genetic characteristic carried on any pair of chromosomes except the xx or xy chromosome pair that determines the sex of the individual

B cells — cells of the immune system produced in the bone marrow

Bacteriophage — a virus that infects a bacterium

Balance method — intake, use, and excretion of a given nutrient is quantitated. When balance is positive, intake exceeds excretion; when negative, excretion exceeds intake

Base pair — a partnership of adenosine with thymidine or cytosine with guanine in a DNA double helix

Basal metabolism — the energy needed to sustain the life processes of an animal in the fasting and resting state. This energy is used to maintain vital cellular activity, respiration, and blood circulation. The rate of energy use needed to sustain these metabolic processes is referred to as the basal metabolic rate (BMR). It is expressed in terms of energy units per time units. For the measurement of BMR, the animal must be in a thermoneutral environment; a postabsorptive state; resting, but conscious; in quiescence and in sexual repose. It is difficult to determine when ruminants reach the postabsorptive state, but a common criterion is the absence of methane production. The length of the fasting period should be specified. A common benchmark of fasting metabolism is when the respiratory quotient becomes equivalent to the catabolism of fat or near 0.7. This has been achieved experimentally in 48 to 144 hours after the last meal.

BCAA — branched chain amino acids

BEE — basal energy expenditure

Beta (b) **cell** — the insulin-producing cell of the pancreas

Blunt ended DNA — two strands of a DNA duplex having ends that are flush with each other

BMI — body mass index = body weight $\div$ height^2

BMR — basal metabolic rate; the minimal amount of energy needed to sustain the body's metabolism. Frequently expressed in terms of the amount of oxygen used per unit of time

Beri beri — thiamin-deficiency disease

Bias — a measure of inaccuracy or departure from accuracy

Bioelectrical impedance — the measure of resistance to an alternating current in a body. Used to estimate percent body fat and body water

Biopsy — the removal of a very small amount of tissue from a selected site

Body cell mass — the metabolically active energy-requiring mass of the body

Body density — weight (mass) per unit volume

cAMP — cyclic 3'5' adenosine monophosphate. An activator of protein kinase; serves as a second messenger for certain hormones

CDC — Centers for Disease Control; an agency of the Department of Health and Human Services

Cancer — a group of diseases characterized by abnormal cell growth that is uncontrolled and subsumes the normal functions of vital organs and tissues

Candidate gene — a gene, if mutated, that is suspected to play a causal role in a clinical syndrome

Cap — the structure at the 5' end of eukaryotic mRNA, introduced after transcription by linking the terminal phosphate of 5' GTP to the terminal base of the mRNA. The added G (and sometimes other bases) are methylated

Cardiovascular disease — a group of diseases characterized by a diminution of heart action. The oxygen and nutrient supply to the heart may be impeded or the heart muscle degenerated

Catabolism — the totality of those reactions that reduce macromolecules to usable metabolites, carbon dioxide and water

cDNA — a single-stranded DNA molecule that is complementary to a mRNA and is synthesized from it by the action of reverse transcriptase

Cerebrovascular disease — similar to cardiovascular disease in that the vascular tree of the brain has developed atherosclerotic lesions that restrict or occlude the blood supply to this organ

Chimeric molecule — a molecule of DNA or RNA or protein containing sequences from two different species

Cholecystokinin — CCK: a hormone released from duodenal cells that stimulates the gall bladder to contract releasing bile into the duodenum

Cholesterol — a four-ringed structure in the lipid class that is an important substrate for steroid hormone synthesis

Chromatin — the complex of DNA and protein in the nucleus of the interphase cell

Chromosomes — the DNA in the cell nucleus is not one continuous strand. Rather, it breaks up into fairly predictable arrangements called chromosomes, which exist in pairs and have been numbered. Those determining the sex of the individual are labeled as x or y. If the individual has one x and one y, he is a male. If the individual has two x chromosomes, she is a female. Many characteristics have been localized to particular chromosomes. There are species differences in the number of chromosomes. There are 23 sets of chromosomes (46 total) in the human.

Chromosome walking — the sequential isolation of clones carrying overlapping sequences of DNA, allowing large regions of the chromosomes to be spanned. Walking is often performed in order to reach a particular locus of interest

Chronic disease — a disease that takes years to develop

Chylomicrons — fat–protein complex formed to carry absorbed dietary fats from the intestine to other tissues. Not normally found in the blood of a fasting individual

Clone — a large number of cells or molecules that are identical to a single parental cell or molecule

CoA — coenzyme A. Pantothenic acid-containing activator of acyl compounds

Coding strand — a strand of DNA with the same sequence as mRNA

Codon — the three nucleotides that code for a specific amino acid. An amino acid can have more than one codon

CoQ — coenzyme Q — also called ubiquinone, a carrier of hydrogens and electrons in the mitochondrial electron transport chain

Concordance — the chance that an identical mutation will occur in related family members

Consensus sequence — an idealized sequence in which each position represents the base most often found when many actual sequences are compared

Constitutive genes — genes that are expressed as a function of the interaction of RNA polymerase with the promoter, without additional regulation; sometimes also called housekeeping genes in the context of describing functions expressed in all cells at a low level

Corepressor — a small molecule that triggers repression of transcription by binding to a regulator protein

Coronary heart disease — a disease of the heart resulting from an inadequate circulation of blood to the heart muscle

Cosmid — a plasmid into which the DNA sequences from bacteriophage lambda that are necessary for the packaging of DNA (cos sites) have been inserted; this permits the plasmid DNA to be packaged *in vitro*

C-peptide — when proinsulin is activated at its target tissue, a fragment of its structure is removed. This fragment is the C-peptide

Creatine — a nitrogen-containing substance that, when phosphorylated to creatine phosphate, provides the energy needed for muscle contraction

Creatinine — the urinary-excretion product of creatine breakdown

Cytokines — small peptides that have regulatory properties or hormone-like actions

Cytotoxic agents — chemicals that destroy specific cells

Densitometry — measurement of body density

Deuterium — a hydrogen isotope having twice the mass of the common hydrogen atom

Deuterium oxide — heavy water that contains 2 molecules of deuterium and 1 of oxygen

DHHS — Department of Health and Human Services (U.S.)

Diabetes mellitus — a group of diseases characterized by an inappropriate glucose–insulin relationship. These diseases are divided into two major subgroups: Type 1 diabetes and Type 2 diabetes mellitus

DNA — deoxyribonucleic acid: dictates all of our genetically determined biochemical characteristics; each of these is coded by the sequence of purine and pyrimidine bases that are connected together in an enormous double-stranded helix found in the nucleus of the cell. Some DNA is also found in the mitochondria

DE — digestive energy: the energy of food after the energy losses of digestion are subtracted

Distal — away from the center of the body

Diurnal variation — cyclical changes in one or more features of the body over a 24-hour period

Downstream — sequences proceeding farther in the direction of expression, for example, the coding region is downstream of the initiation codon

Dual energy radiographic absorptiometry — DRA: a procedure based on x-rays that measures bone mineralization. Also known as dual x-ray absorptiometry (DXA) and dual energy absorptiometry (DEXA)

Dual photon absorptiometry — similar to DEXA but uses photons at two different energy levels to determine bone mineral content

Electrolyte — an electrically charged particle (anion or cation)

Elongation factors — proteins that associate with ribosomes cyclically during addition of each amino acid to the polypeptide chain

Endonuclease — an enzyme that cleaves internal bonds in DNA or RNA

Enhancer element — a cis-acting base sequence that binds one or more promoters. It can function in either orientation and in any location (upstream or downstream) relative to the promoter region

Enteral nutrition — the provision of nutrients as a solution infused via a naso-gastric tube

ER — endoplasmic reticulum

Erythrocyte — red blood cell (RBC)

ESADDI — estimated safe and adequate daily dietary intake

Etiology — the study of the causes of a disease

Excinclease — the excision nuclease (enzyme) that is involved in nucleotide exchange or repair of DNA

Exon — the sequence of bases used to transcribe mRNA

Exonuclease — an enzyme that cleaves nucleotides from either the 3' or 5' ends of DNA or RNA

Expression vector — a cloning vector designed so that a coding sequence inserted at a particular site will be transcribed and translated into protein

FAD — flavin adenine nucleotide: a riboflavin-containing coenzyme serving as a hydrogen and electron carrier in certain dehydrogenase reactions. FADH^{++} is its reduced form

FDA — Food and Drug Administration

Fecal Energy — (FE) — the gross energy in the feces. FE is the weight of feces times the gross energy of a unit weight of feces. FE can be partitioned into energy from undigested food (FiE) and energy from compounds of metabolic origin (FmE)

Fibrous plaque — lipids and other materials that collect on the arterial wall (atherogenesis) creating a projection into the lumen of the vessel and impeding flow

Fingerprinting — the use of restriction fragment LPs or repeat sequences of DNA to establish a unique pattern of DNA fragments for an individual

FMN — flavin mononucleotide. A nucleotide coenzyme containing riboflavin.

Footprinting — a technique for identifying the site on DNA bound by proteins that protect certain bonds from attack by nucleases

GABA — gamma amino butyric acid. A neurotransmitter formed from the decarboxylation of glutamic acid

GDP — guanosine diphosphate. A diphosphorylated form of GTP important in the activation of substances participating in the biosynthesis of proteins

Gaseous products of digestion — (GE): includes combustible gases produced in the digestive tract incident to fermentation of food by microorganisms. Methane makes up the major proportion of combustible gas normally produced in both ruminant and non-ruminant species. Hydrogen, carbon monoxide, acetone, ethane, and hydrogen sulfide are produced in trace amounts and can reach significant levels under certain dietary conditions. Present knowledge indicates that energy lost as methane in ruminants and non-ruminant herbivores is quantitatively the most significant GE loss

Gene — carrier of the genetic codes for the characteristics of the organism

Genotype — the inherited character of the individual

GIP — gastric inhibitory peptide. A peptide hormone inhibiting gastric motility and acid secretion

GI tract — gastrointestinal tract

GRP — gastrin releasing peptide. A neuroactive peptide originating in nerves of the gut and stimulating the release of gastrin from gastrin cells

GSSG — glutathionine, oxidized. A tripeptide containing glutamic acid, cysteine, and glycine. Its sulfhydryl group can undergo reversible oxidation and reduction, allowing the peptide to serve as a buffer. Its chief function is to serve as a reductant of toxic peroxides. It is designated GSH in its reduced form

Goiter — thyroid gland enlargement due to deficient iodine intake

GTP — guanosine triphosphate: a high-energy phosphate-containing compound needed for protein synthesis

Gynoid obesity — excess body fat deposited mainly on hips and thighs; sometimes referred to as the "pear" form of obesity.

Hairpin — a double helical stretch formed by base pairing between neighboring complementary strands of a single strand of DNA or RNA

HANES (NHANES I, II, III, or HHANES) — Health and Nutrition Examination Survey

Heat of Activity — (HjE) — the heat production resulting from muscular activity required in, for example, getting up, standing, moving about to obtain food, grazing, drinking, and lying down

Heat of digestion and absorption — (HdE) — the heat produced as a result of the action of digestive enzymes on the food within the digestive tract and the heat produced by the digestive tract in moving digesta through the tract as well as in moving absorbed nutrients through the wall of the digestive tract

Heat of fermentation — (HfE) — the heat produced in the digestive tract as a result of microbial action. In ruminants, HfE is a major component often included in the heat of digestion (HdE)

Heat of product formation — (HrE): the heat produced in association with the metabolic processes of product formation from absorbed metabolites. In its simplest form, HrE is the heat produced by a biosynthetic pathway

Heat of thermal regulation — (HcE): the additional heat needed to maintain body temperature when environmental temperature drops below the zone of thermal neutrality, or it is the additional heat produced as the result of an animal's efforts to maintain body temperature when environmental temperature goes above the zone of thermal neutrality

Heat of waste formation and excretion — (HwE): the additional heat production associated with the synthesis and excretion of waste products. For example, synthesis of urea from ammonia is an energy costly process in mammalian species and results in a measurable increase in total heat production

Heat Increment — (HiE): the increase in heat production following consumption of food by an animal in a thermoneutral environment. Included in HiE are heat of fermentation (HfE) and energy expenditure in the digestive process (HdE) as well as heat produced as a result of nutrient metabolism (HrE + HwE). Heat increment is usually considered to be a non-useful energy loss, but, under conditions of cold stress, HiE helps to maintain body temperature

Height-weight indices — various ratios or indices used to express weight in terms of height. Body mass index is one such expression

Hemoglobin — the iron-containing protein in the red blood cell responsible for carrying oxygen to the cells and returning carbon dioxide to the lungs

HDL — high density lipoprotein. A plasma lipid–protein complex found in the blood. Elevated HDL is associated with a decreased risk of cardiovascular disease

Heterozygote — an individual with different alleles (or copies of a particular gene) at some particular locus

Heterodimerization — the polymerization of two unlike compounds to DNA

Histones — conserved DNA-binding proteins that protect the DNA from free radical attack

HLA genes — genes that encode elements of the immune system, specifically those that dictate the formation of antibodies by the white cells (leukocytes)

HMG CoA — 3 hydroxy 3 methylglutaryl coenzyme A: a metabolic intermediate in cholesterol synthesis

HNIS — Human Nutrition Information Service, a unit of the United States Department of Agriculture (USDA)

Homozygote — an individual who has two identical copies of a gene-coding for a given characteristic

Homodimerization — the polymerization of two like compounds to DNA

Hybridization — the specific reassociation of complementary strands of nucleic acids (DNA with DNA or RNA with RNA or DNA)

Hyperlipidemia — above normal levels of lipid in the blood of a fasted individual

Hypermetabolism — above normal metabolic rate

Hypertension — blood pressure that exceeds 120/80 by 20%

IBW — Ideal body weight

Iliac crest — the crest or top of the ilium or the longest of the three bones that the pelvis comprises. Sometimes called the top of the hip bone

Impedance — the opposition to an alternating current composed of two elements: resistance and reactance

Incidence — the number of new events or cases of a disease in a population within a specified time period

Indirect calorimetry — determination of energy expenditure using the measurement of oxygen consumption

Infarct — death of local tissue fed by an obstructed artery or occluded vein

Infectious disease — any disease caused by the invasion and multiplication of an invading microorganism

Initiation factors — proteins that associate with the small subunit of the ribosome, specifically at the stage of initiation of protein synthesis

Insert — an additional length of base pairs in DNA introduced artificially

Insulitis — inflammation of the insulin-producing islet cells of the pancreas

Intake of food energy — (IE): the gross energy in the food consumed. IE is the weight of food consumed times the gross energy of a unit weight of food

Intron — the sequences of bases in a gene that are transcribed but removed during RNA editing

Inverted repeats — two copies of the same sequence of DNA repeated in opposite orientation on the same molecule; adjacent inverted repeats constitute a palindrome

IU — international unit: an amount defined by the International Conference for Unification of Formulae

Ischemia — impaired blood flow causing oxygen and nutrient deprivation resulting in pain and, if severe, death of some or all parts of the tissue

Islets of Langerhans — the particular segments of the pancreas having an endocrine function. These islets consist of several cell types, one of which is the β cell that produces the hormone insulin

ISF — interstitial fluid, fluid surrounding the extravascular cells that provides a medium for passage of nutrients to and from cells

Joule — (J) a unit of work or energy in the metric system. The amount of work done by a force of 1 newton acting over the distance of 1 meter

Kilocalorie — kcal. The amount of energy required to raise the temperature of 1 kg water 1° celsius. 1 kcal = 4.189 kJ

Kwashiorkor — protein-deficiency disorder

LDL — low-density lipoprotein

LDL receptor — molecules on the surface of the cell that have a particular affinity for LDL

Library — a collection of cloned fragments of DNA. Libraries may be either genomic DNA (in which both introns and exons are represented) or cDNA (in which only the exons are expressed in a particular cell or tissue)

Ligation — the enzyme-catalyzed reaction that results in the joining in phosphodiester linkage of two stretches of DNA or RNA into one; the respective enzymes are DNA and RNA ligases

Lines — long interspersed repeat sequences

Linkage — the tendency of genes to be inherited together as a result of their location on the same chromosome; measured by percent recombination between loci

Lipoprotein — lipid–protein complex

LHA — lateral hypothalamus

LNAA — large neutral amino acids; branched chain and aromatic amino acids

Locus — the position on a chromosome occupied by a gene or its allele

m — Greek letter prefix that indicates 10^{-6} fraction of a liter or gram

Macrophages — large mononuclear phagocytic cells that work by engulfing foreign materials and neutralizing them

Magnetic resonance imaging — a technology allowing the imaging of a body without radiation hazard

Malnutrition — inadequate or unbalanced intake of essential nutrients

MAO — monoamine oxidase; an enzyme that reduces neural transmission by inactivating amine neurotransmitters such as serotonin

Marasmus — condition of deficient energy and protein intake

MCV — mean corpuscular volume

Mean — average value for a group of values

Median — value where half the values fall below and half are above this value

Menopause — cessation of estrus cycles

Metabolizable Energy — (ME) — the energy in the food less energy lost in feces, urine, and combustible gas: ME = IE — (FE + UE + GE)

mRNA — messenger RNA: short-lived species of RNA that carries the code for the synthesis of specific compounds (peptides or proteins)

Microsatellite polymorphism — heterozygosity of a certain microsatellite marker in an individual

Microsatellite marker — a dispersed or a group of 2–5 base sequences that are repeated up to 50 times. May occur at 50–100 thousand locations in the genome. Used in linkage analysis

Morbidity — illness

Mutation — when the sequence of base pairs in the DNA is disturbed by either a deletion or substitution of one or more of the nucleotide bases, the protein coded by this sequence will not be synthesized in its normal amino acid sequence. The amino acid sequence determines the shape and function of the protein. Many mutations occur that have an effect on this sequence but have no effect on function because the substitution or deletion does not occur in the active or working part of the protein molecule

Myocardial infarction — heart attack

Myocardium — heart muscle

NAD, NADH, NADP, NADPH — niacin-containing coenzymes that function as carriers for hydrogen ions in dehydrogenase catalyzed reactions

NCHS — National Center for Health Statistics

N-corrected metabolizable energy — (MnE): ME adjusted for total nitrogen retained or lost from body tissue: MnE = ME – (k × TN). For birds or monogastric mammals, gaseous energy is usually not considered. The correction for mammals is generally k = 7.45 kcal per gram of nitrogen retained in body tissue (TN). The factor of 8.22 kcal per gram of TN is used for birds representing the energy equivalent of uric acid per gram of nitrogen. A number of different values for k have been suggested and used

NFCS — Nationwide Food Consumption Survey

NHANES — National Health and Nutrition Examination Survey

Nick translation — a technique for labeling DNA based on the ability of the DNA polymerase from E. coli to degrade a strand of DNA that has been nicked and then resynthesized; if the a radioactive nucleoside is used, the rebuilt strand becomes labeled and can be used as a radioactive probe

Northern blot — a method for transferring RNA from an agarose gel to a nitrocellulose filter on which the RNA can be detected by a suitable probe

NPU — net protein use

NDp Cal % — net protein calories percent. The percent of the total energy value of the diet provided by the protein

Nucleosome — the basic structural subunit of chromatin, consisting of ~200 bp of DNA and an octomer of histones

Null mutation — a mutation that completely eliminates the function of a gene, usually because it has been deleted

Nutrient density — the nutrient composition of food expressed in terms of nutrient quantity per 1000 kcal

Nutritional assessment — measurement of indicators of dietary status and the nutrition-related health status of individuals or populations

Obesity — excess accumulation of body fat (more than 20% of the body weight as fat)

Oligonucleotide — a short, defined sequence of nucleotides joined together in the typical phosphodiester linkage

Open reading frame — a series of triplets coding for amino acids without any termination codons; the sequence is potentially translatable into a protein

ORI — the origin of replication in prokaryotes

Osteoporosis — disease where the bone loses its mineral content

Overweight — a body weight in excess of that thought to be normal for height

Palindrome — a sequence of duplex DNA that is the same when the two strands are read in opposite directions

Parenteral nutrition — nutritional support furnished through the vascular system

Pellagra — niacin deficiency disorder

Peripheral vascular disease — atherosclerotic changes in the vessels of the limbs

PEP — phosphoenopyruvic acid, a key intermediate in glucose synthesis and degradation

PGI, PGE — prostaglandins of the I or E series of the eicosenoid group of compounds

Phenotype — a category or group to which an individual is assigned based on one or more inherited characteristics; the overt expression of the genotype

PKU — phenyketonuria — a mutation in the gene for phenylalanine hydroxylase that results in mental retardation unless diagnosed early and managed with a low-phenylalanine diet

Plasmid — a small extrachromosomal circular molecule that replicates independently of the host DNA

PLP — pyridoxal phosphate; a coenzyme required in amino acid metabolism

Polyadenylation — the addition of a sequence of polyadenylic acid to the 5' end of a eukaryotic RNA after its transcription

Polymerase chain reaction — (PCR) an enzymatic method for the repeated copying (and thus amplification) of two strands of DNA that make up a particular gene sequence

Postprandial — after a meal

Prevalence — the number of existing cases of a given characteristic in a given population at a given time; usually used in connection with a particular clinical condition of note

Primosome — the mobile complex of helicase and primase that is involved in DNA replication

Probe — a molecule used to detect the presence of a specific fragment of DNA or RNA in, i.e., a bacterial colony that is formed from a genetic library or during analysis by blot transfer techniques; common probes are cDNA molecules, synthetic oligodeoxynucleotides, or defined sequence or antibodies to specific proteins

Promoter — a region of DNA involved in binding RNA polymerase and various regulatory transcription factors to initiate transcription

Proximal — toward the center of the body

Pseudogene — an inactive segment of DNA arising by mutation of a parental active gene

PTH — parathyroid hormone: essential to the regulation of blood calcium levels

PUFA — polyunsaturated fatty acids

PVN — paraventricular nucleus in the hypothalamus. Releases hormones that affect food intake

Quantitative computed tomography — an imaging technique consisting of an array of X-ray sources and radiation detectors aligned opposite each other. As X-ray beams pass through the subject, they are weakened or attenuated by the tissues and picked up by the detectors. The signals are then compared using a computer that can construct a cross section of the body using sophisticated modeling techniques

Reading frame — one of three possible ways of reading a nucleotide sequence as a series of triplets

RBC — red blood cell; erythrocyte

Receptor — a general term applied to any protein in any part of the body that binds to a specific compound and allows that compound to do its job. Most hormones and many nutrients have specific receptors without which these hormones or nutrients would be ineffective. The term is used for specific proteins that bind both DNA and a substance that influences DNA transcription as well as for proteins in the blood, cytosol, or membranes of the cells

Recombinant DNA — altered DNA that results from the insertion of a sequence of deoxynucleotides not previously present in an existing DNA

Recovered Energy — (RE): commonly called Energy Balance, that portion of the feed energy retained as part of the body or voided as a useful product. In animals raised for meat, RE = TE, whereas in a lactating animal, RE is the sum of tissue energy, lactation energy, and energy in products of conception: RE = TE + LE + YE

Regression equation — a statistical method for calculating the relationships between an independent variable such as age and a dependent variable

Reporter gene — a coding unit whose product is easily assayed; it may be connected to any promoter of interest so that the expression of that gene can be monitored

Restriction enzyme — an endonuclease enzyme that causes cleavage of both strands of DNA at highly specific sites dictated by the base sequence

Restriction fragment length polymorphism — (RFLP): inherited differences in sites for restriction enzymes

Reverse transcription — RNA-directed synthesis of DNA catalyzed by reverse transcriptase

RBP — retinol-binding protein; a protein synthesized in the liver and used to transport retinol in the blood or in the cell

RDA — recommended dietary allowance; not to be confused with requirement

RER — rough endoplasmic reticulum. That portion of the cell that appears granular due to the profusion of ribosomes

RIA — radioimmunoassay; technique useful for determining small qualities of biologically important substances such as hormones

Rickets — bone malformation usually due to inadequate intake of vitamins and minerals

RNA — ribonucleic acid: a polynucleotide containing ribose instead of deoxyribose; the synthesis of RNA is directed by DNA

RQ — respiratory quotient. Ratio of CO_2 to O_2

SAM — s-adenosylmethionine, a principal methyl donor

Scurvy — ascorbic acid-deficiency disease

SER — smooth endoplasmic reticulum. That portion of the endoplasmic reticulum where certain lipids are synthesized and drugs are detoxified

Sex-linked trait — a genetic characteristic carried on either the x or the y chromosome of the xy pair of chromosomes

Signal — the end product observed when a specific sequence of DNA or RNA is detected by autoradiography or by some other method. Hybridization with complementary radioactive polynucleotide (e.g., by Southern or Northern blotting) is commonly used to generate the signal. This term is also applied to the transmission of intracellular reactions as in signal transmission that occurs when a hormone binds to its cognate receptor on the surface of a cell

Signal transduction — the process by which a receptor interacts with a ligand at the surface of the cell and then transmits a signal to trigger a series of reactions within that cell

Sines — short interspersed repeat sequences

Skinfold thickness — a double fold of skin and underlying tissue that can be used as a measure of the subcutaneous fat store

SnRNA — small nuclear RNA. This family of RNAs is best known for its role in splicing and other RNA-processing reactions.

SOD — superoxide dismutase

Southern blotting — a method for transferring DNA from an agarose gel to a nitrocellulose filter on which DNA can be detected by a suitable probe

Splicing — the removal of introns from RNA accompanied by the joining of exons

Splicosome — the macromolecular complex responsible for precursor mRNA splicing. The splicisome consists of at least five small nuclear RNAs (sn RNA; U1, U2, U4, U5, and U6) and many proteins

Sticky ended DNA — complementary single strands of DNA that protrude from opposite ends of a DNA duplex or from the ends of different duplex molecules

Stroke — blockage or rupture of blood vessel(s) supplying the brain, with resulting loss of consciousness, paralysis, and other symptoms

Supine — lying on one's back

Symptoms — signs or indications of disease

Tandem — describes multiple copies of the same sequence that lie adjacent to each other in the gene

Targeted mutation — (knockout): an animal that has a specific gene altered or deleted at a specific location

Terminal transferase — an enzyme that adds nucleotides of one type to the 3' end of a DNA strand

T_3 — triiodothyronine, the most active of the thyroid hormones

T_4 — thyroxine, the form of thyroid hormone released by the thyroid gland to the blood

T-cells — cells of the immune system that originated from the thymus gland. These cells recognize antigens and produce antibodies to them

TBF — total body fat

TBW — total body water

TBG — thyroxine-binding globulin: the protein that carries the thyroxine from the thyroid gland to its target tissue

TDP, TPP — thiamin-containing coenzyme required for decarboxylation reactions

Thermic effect — heat-producing response of the body to such processes as exercise or digestion and absorption. Also the response to disease or injury (fever)

Thermogenesis — heat produced by the body

Total heat production — (HE) — the energy lost from an animal system in a form other than as a combustible compound. Heat production may be measured by either direct or indirect calorimetry. In direct calorimetry, heat production is measured directly by physical methods, whereas indirect calorimetry involves some indirect measure of heat such as the measurement of oxygen uptake and carbon dioxide production using the thermal equivalent of oxygen based on respiratory quotient (RQ) and theoretical considerations. The commonly accepted equation for indirect computation of heat production from respiratory exchange is HE (kcal) = 3.866 (liters O_2) +1.200 (liters CO_2) – 1.431 (g UN) – 0.518 (liters CH_4). Heat production may also be measured by difference from the determination of total carbon and nitrogen balance or from a comparative slaughter experiment. These methods arrive at total heat production by different calculations and are subject to systematic errors of measurement

TPN — total parenteral nutrition. A method of providing all nutrient needs through a solution infused into a large blood vessel

TSH — thyroid-stimulating hormone: a pituitary hormone that stimulates the thyroid gland to produce thyroid hormone

tRNA — transfer ribonucleic acid: form of nucleic acid responsible for transferring specific amino acids to specific sites on the mRNA in the process of protein synthesis

Transcription — DNA-directed mRNA synthesis

Transgenic — an animal that has had foreign DNA introduced into its germ line

Translation — the synthesis of protein using mRNA as the template

Tritium — radioactive hydrogen

True digested energy — (TDE): the intake of energy minus fecal energy of food origin (FiE = FE – FeE – FmE) minus heat of fermentation and digestive gaseous losses: TDE = IE – FE + FeE + FmE — HfE – GE

True metabolizable energy — (TME) — the intake of true digestible energy minus urine energy of food origin: TME = TDE – UE + UeE

TXA_2 — thromboxane A_2: an eicosanoid involved in stimulating platelet aggregation

UDP, UTP — uridine di- or triphosphate: high-energy compound essential to glycogen synthesis

Upstream — sequences proceeding in the opposite direction from expression; for example, the initiation codon is upstream of the coding region

Urinary energy — (UE): the total gross energy in urine. It includes energy from non-utilized absorbed compounds from the food (UiE), end products of metabolic processes (UmE), and end products of endogenous origin (UeE)

Vector — a plasmid or bacteriophage into which foreign DNA can be introduced for the purposes of cloning

VIP — vasoactive peptide: neuropeptide originating in the neurons of the gastrointestinal system

VLDL — very-low-density lipoprotein. A lipid–protein complex involved in the transport of lipids from the liver and gut to storage sites

Western blot — a method for transferring protein to a nitrocellulose filter on which the protein can be detected by an antibody

Xeropthalmia — vitamin A deficiency: one of the world's leading causes of blindness

1 Human Health, Food, and Nutrition

CONTENTS

OVERVIEW

For centuries, man has sought the fountain of youth. The early conquistadors explored the new world hoping to find the secret to long life. What they found instead were new foods and new diseases. In the 1500s, the expected lifespan was half that of today in the advanced nations of the world. Today, despite the many advances in health care, there are still populations that are no better off with respect to lifespan than those early explorers.

We are still discovering new foods and new diseases. The discoveries of today are no less exciting, no less promising than those of yesteryear, but today's are not merely additive to those already in hand. New knowledge seems to be exponential. Each discovery leads to a multitude of related discoveries, each making possible the integration of prior knowledge. These new perspectives and discoveries allow the nutrition scientist to better understand why different animals (including humans) need certain nutrients in certain amounts to ensure a healthy, productive lifespan. While it seems obvious to the scientist that individuals could ensure a long life by consuming the appropriate amounts and kinds of foods that contain the needed nutrients, this is not so obvious to everyone.

There are many barriers that interfere with the appropriate exercise of the obvious. These include our incomplete knowledge of the need for and tolerance of specific nutrients, the social and economic status of the population, the availability of sanitary facilities and safe water, the availability and acceptance of modern medical care, the education of the consumer with respect to food choices and the availability of a wide selection of safe foods. All of these factors impinge upon the simple premise that a healthy long life can be achieved simply by consuming the "right" amounts of the "right" foods.

How do we know what the right amounts of the right foods are? What does health mean? What is long life? These are not simple questions. If they were, we would already know the answers and further study of the relationships of food choice to health and well being would be unnecessary.

One of the challenges in today's world is understanding how nutrition, or, more properly, food, can affect the health and well-being of man and animals. We must understand how the body works, its anatomy, its physiology and biochemistry, as well as how individuals interact with members of their cultural or social groups. Nutritionists are also concerned with the economic and educational status of the consumer because these will affect how much and what kinds of foods are purchased, prepared, and consumed. While nutrition researchers specialize in single aspects of these concerns, they must be aware of the larger arena in which the community of nutrition scholars performs.

Early in the history of nutrition science, a healthy diet was defined as one that contained a sufficient variety of raw and cooked foods that together provided sufficient nutrients to prevent such diseases as beri beri, pellagra, rickets, xeropthalmia, goiter, and scurvy. The prevention of such deficiency diseases was the key element in nutrient intake recommendations. While this is still true today, we have learned that one's genetic heritage might dictate both the need for and tolerance of the individual nutrients. We have begun to unravel the mystery of the role of genetics in determining nutrient need. In the future, nutrient intake recommendations based on genotype might be possible so that food choice could potentiate the expression of traits for health while suppressing those traits for disease. Throughout this text, the role of genetics in macronutrient metabolism will be discussed. Some of the many genetic diseases related to macronutrient metabolism will be listed and, where possible, nutrient-gene interactions will be indicated. However, before the macronutrients can be addressed, the reader should be aware of those aspects of nutritional status, diet, and health that justify the detailed examination of the biochemistry and physiology of these nutrients at the organismic and cellular levels. Without the recognition of the scope of nutrition-related human problems, knowledge of nutritional biochemistry is useless. Nutritional status information can be acquired in a variety of ways. Population studies as well as group and individual assessment can provide much useful information.

POPULATION STUDIES

Epidemiology is the study of disease incidence and distribution or prevalence in a defined population. The population can be defined by a few or many descriptors such as gender, age, geography, sociocultural status, and economic status. Such population studies have been responsible in large part for the discovery and description of nutrition-related diseases. Among the first of these were reports of scurvy in British sailors on long voyages and the reports of beri beri in Japanese sailors also on long sea duty. Both reports provided data on the incidence, severity, and mortality of these seafaring men and both noted the fact that their diets consisted of a limited number of foods. Only those foods that could be stored for long periods of time were found on these ships — hard tack (a sort of very stale, often maggot-infested, bread) and a meat preserved in brine were the staples of the British sailor's diet. In the Japanese navy, rice replaced the hard tack and this rice was frequently polished and milled white rice. The officers supplemented these items with fresh fruit, meat, and vegetables when these items were available and they had the money to buy them. The officers were thus less likely to develop and die from deficiency diseases. The physician-scientists who studied these sailors noted the difference in disease patterns between the officers and seamen and also noted the differences in their diets.

Although, at that time, no one knew that vitamins existed or were essential nutrients, there was recognition of a possible relationship between disease and food intake. This tradition continues today as we seek to understand the diet–disease connection. Population studies may be very detailed, with precise assessments of the foods consumed together with clinical and biochemical assessments of health status, or they may be very general.

The design of any study and its methodology are dictated by the question the scientists set out to answer. If the question relates to the incidence and severity of heart disease in 40-year-old white professional males in Chicago, the design and methods used will be very different from a study designed to answer questions about rickets in preschool children in rural Mississippi, or about the growth of children in the state of Hawaii. In each instance, the investigators have designated a specific population and a specific health concern. The information about food intake can be either very specific or very general. The amount of detailed information collected depends on many factors. These include the population size, the amount of money available for the study, and the detail needed to answer the question asked. Population studies can be labor intensive if they involve the study of representative groups within the population. However, there are ways to study disease patterns and food intake using large, computer-based data sets, without actually studying the people themselves. There are several sources for these data and each data set can provide information of use to the nutrition scientist. Each set has its limitations however, and these should be acknowledged.

MORTALITY STATISTICS

Until there was a universal recognition of the causes of infectious diseases, and, until appropriate therapeutic and preventive strategies for their control were developed, they were the leading cause of death. Death from cholera, bubonic plague, typhoid disease, smallpox, whooping cough, pneumonia, and scarlet fever were common prior to improved sanitation, clean water, the development of immunization programs, antibiotics, and the development of aseptic techniques and anesthesia that made simple surgeries safe and effective. The discovery of the essential nutrients and their role in health maintenance contributed to the extension of lifespan that characterizes technologically advanced nations. Infectious disease and malnutrition are still causing death in third-world nations where education and economics combine to effectively limit the quantity and variety of food as well as the adoption of the health-care practices that educated citizens of wealthier nations take for granted. Country comparisons of the leading causes of death show differences, depending on the nations in question. For example, a nation enduring a devastating food-production failure might have death due to starvation in the list of 10 top causes of death. A nation at war or one at the epicenter of a communicable disease such as HIV (AIDS) or cholera might have a different list from that given for the United States.

These country differences are important. Mortality statistics can be misleading if one selects only one or two diseases and tries to relate the incidence of these diseases to the food choices of the populations in these different nations. The causes of death must be taken all together — the percentages of the different causes must add up to 100%. If one nation or population reports 35% of its population dying from heart disease and another nation has only 5% dying from this cause, the reasons for death of the other 65% or 95% of the respective populations cannot be ignored. This concept is called competing causes of mortality. Perhaps the latter population has a greater problem with infectious disease or a high infant mortality. Perhaps this population has an average lifespan of only 35 years. In other words, in the final analysis, all the deaths have a cause and all causes add up to 100%.

Whether these causes are nutrition related cannot be automatically assumed merely by examining these death statistics. Nonetheless, many of the diseases have a nutrition-related secondary or contributory cause of death. For example, death from a simple communicable disease such as mumps is greater in malnourished populations than in those that are well nourished. This is because nutritional status affects the immune system. The poorly nourished individual has a less competent immune system than does the well-nourished individual. Another example is the well known increased risk of overnourished people for diabetes and heart disease. Obesity, defined as excess body fatness, is a risk factor for these degenerative diseases. Obesity, although it may be due to

TABLE 1.1

Leading Causes of Death in the United States, Death Rates and Age Adjusted Death Rates for 1996[1] and the % Change from 1995

Rank[1]	Cause of Death	% of Total Deaths	Rate/100,000 Population	Age-Adjusted Rate	Change %
1	Heart diseases	31.6	276.6	134.6	−2.7
2	Cancers	23.4	205.2	129.1	0.6
3	Stroke	6.9	60.5	26.5	0.7
4	Lung diseases	4.5	40.0	21.0	−1.3
5	Accidents[2]	4.0	35.4	30.1	1.0
6	Pneumonia and flu	3.5	31.1	12.6	−2.3
7	Diabetes mellitus	2.6	23.2	13.6	2.3
8	AIDS	1.4	12.3	11.6	−25.6
9	Suicide	1.3	12.0	10.8	−3.6
10	Liver diseases	1.1	11.6	7.5	−1.3
11	Renal diseases	1.1	9.5	4.3	0
12	Infections	0.9	9.2	4.1	0

Taken from Vol. 46, Morbidity and Mortality Weekly Report, U.S. Department Health and Human Services, October 10, 1997.

[1] Based on the total number of deaths in 1996 (2,322,421). These 12 causes account for 84.7% of the total.

[2] The preferred term is unintentional death. It includes motor vehicle related deaths.

genetic factors (See Unit 3) also has a nutrition component and this then becomes a secondary or contributing cause of death.

Chronic diseases now rank high in the leading causes of death in the United States. These are shown in Table 1.1. The reader should be aware of how the cause of death is reported. In many instances, the person who signs the death certificate may not be a physician trained in the signs and symptoms of disease. In some unsophisticated or sparsely populated regions, the person might be an elected official responsible for not only death certificates but also for marriage licenses, birth certificates, land transfers, and so forth. The deceased might not have died in a hospital, might not have been autopsied to determine the cause of death, and indeed might not have been under the care of a physician at all. For example, an individual might be at the wheel of a car and have a heart attack or stroke that would then cause the vehicle to crash. The person dies. What would the death certificate reveal as the cause of death? The crash, the heart attack, or the stroke? It all depends on the person who fills out the death certificate. In addition, there are several diseases that are interrelated. The person might die of end-stage renal disease, but this disease might have been brought on by diabetes mellitus. The latter was the primary disease, but the death certificate might show that only renal disease was the cause of death. These examples are but a few of the limitations in the use of mortality statistics, nonetheless, these data do allow health scientists to identify trends that might have a nutrition component.

YPLL-75

Some of the causes of death shown in Table 1.1 occur in the aged. The chronic diseases such as the various forms of heart disease, for example, are more frequently the cause of death for the elderly than for the young. For this reason, health statisticians use a statistical maneuver that corrects for the influence of age. The term "age-adjusted rate of death per 100,000 population" thus results. Note in Table 1.1 that the age adjustment for death due to heart disease reduces the rate by more than half. In other words, as people live longer, the causes of death will be spread out over these leading causes rather than being concentrated in the first few diseases. Another way of looking at causes of death and their impact on society is to calculate the years of potential life lost due to death from any of the above.

This statistic, years of potential life lost (YPLL), reflects the impact of deaths occurring in years preceding a cut-off age of 75 years. This number, YPLL-75, is calculated using final mortality data from the National Center for Health Statistics, U.S. Department of Health and Human Services, Centers for Disease Control and Prevention. The CDC, as it is commonly called, tracks the incidence and prevalence of all diseases and keeps records of the causes of death. The CDC also conducts a health and nutrition survey and monitors the public health not only in the United States but throughout the world. The National Health and Nutrition Survey is discussed in the next section.

The YPLL is based on the population estimate provided by the U.S. Census. While the YPLL is updated yearly based on the reports of deaths made to the CDC, the census of the U.S. population is tabulated only every 10 years. Thus, the YPLL is only an estimate, which becomes less reliable as the number of years since the most recent census increases. Nonetheless, YPLL is very useful in providing estimates of the social and economic impact of death from leading causes.

In 1980, YPLL-75 in the United States from all causes totaled 10,267.6/100,000 population. In 1996, this fell to 8,210. The age-adjusted YPLL-75 in 1980 was 9,813.5/100,000 and in 1996 this figure fell to 7,748/100,000. Over the intervening 16-year period, there have been significant reductions in the YPLL-75 as advances in medicine and disease management have extended the lifespans of affected individuals. Note the difference in the ranking of the causes of death in Table 1.2 as compared with Table 1.1. For example, although AIDS does not claim as many lives (1.4% of the total) as any of the diseases of the heart (31.6%), because its victims are often young adults, its associated crude YPLL, 5.4%, is a significant percentage of the 1996 total. This percentage is significantly less than the 7.2% that was reported for 1995. Better diagnosis, treatment, and management of the disease, together with major public health campaigns for prevention, probably explain this significant change. Cardiovascular disease, while accounting for more than 30% of all deaths, strikes much older persons, so the years of potential life lost is a much smaller number than might be expected. In 1996, the age-adjusted YPLL for all diseases of the heart accounted for 24.9% of the total YPLL-75. Therapies have been developed that attenuate the progress of cardio-vascular disease so that affected individuals have their lifespans extended. Accident-prevention programs, improved prenatal and postnatal care, plus better treatments for alcoholism and lung diseases, also account for decreases in the YPLL-75 figures for these disorders. Hopefully, this means that the public health efforts are worthwhile.

As noted, the calculation of YPLL is based on age 75. Originally, the age of 65 was used because it was considered to be the age at which retirement from full-time employment occurred. Now, mandatory retirement at age 65 is illegal in most settings. Some people continue employment beyond this age. Social Security has raised the age at which full benefits can be acquired for people born since 1960. Indeed, those wishing to retire and collect Social Security benefits will be penalized for applying for these prior to their allowed retirement age. The change in Social Security eligibility was made, in part, because of the extension in lifespan due to improved health-care and public health measures. When Social Security was first created, life expectancy was far shorter. The Social Security Act of 1935 was designed to ensure income for the retired worker. Its cost was based on the actuarial tables in use at that time. Since 1935, as noted above, these tables have had to be revised upward, as has the cost of the program. All of this discussion is by way of justifying the change in the calculation of YPLL. It used to be YPLL-65. It is now YPLL-75. Years lost from age 75 are considered to have a more significant social and economic impact on the population than years lost from the total expected lifespan.

TABLE 1.2
Years of Potential Life Lost (YPLL) in the United States Before Age 75* for Selected Causes of Death from 1980–1996

Cause of Death (All Persons)†	Crude					Age-adjusted				
	1980	1985	1990	1995	1996	1980	1985	1990	1995	1996
	Years lost before age 75 per 100,000 population under 75 years of age									
All causes	10,267.6	9,255.3	8,997.0	8,595.8	8,210.0	9,813.5	8,793.2	8,518.3	8,128.2	7,748.0
Diseases of heart	2,065.3	1,842.3	1,517.6	1,430.2	1,396.8	1,877.5	1,664.1	1,363.0	1,259.2	1,222.6
Ischemic heart disease	1,454.3	1,207.4	942.1	841.8	820.4	1,307.4	1,078.5	834.8	727.9	704.9
Cerebrovascular diseases	332.9	277.3	246.2	241.1	240.7	302.9	250.8	221.1	211.5	210.2
Malignant neoplasms	1,932.4	1,911.8	1,863.4	1,779.4	1,755.1	1,815.2	1,776.2	1,713.9	1,587.7	1,554.2
Respiratory System	521.1	536.1	538.0	495.9	490.2	479.5	488.1	486.3	432.7	424.1
Colorectal	175.8	168.8	153.4	146.8	142.2	158.5	151.0	137.3	128.3	123.5
Prostate	78.8	81.5	89.5	77.8	75.5	67.2	69.2	76.6	66.6	64.6
Breast	408.5	417.1	416.5	389.0	375.5	393.0	392.7	381.9	340.0	324.3
Chronic obstructive pulmonary diseases	164.5	182.6	182.5	188.0	187.9	141.4	156.2	156.9	161.4	161.1
Pneumonia and influenza	156.4	139.3	139.9	128.5	125.8	149.1	130.4	128.5	115.3	114.5
Chronic liver disease and cirrhosis	254.1	199.4	176.4	166.4	164.1	259.1	196.0	168.8	149.7	145.7
Diabetes mellitus	124.6	120.3	147.0	169.6	174.6	115.1	109.8	133.0	149.9	153.5
Human immunodeficiency virus infection (AIDS)	...	...	391.2	615.0	435.1	...	...	366.2	570.3	401.9
Unintentional injuries	1,688.7	1,344.6	1,221.2	1,098.1	1,079.1	1,688.3	1,365.8	1,263.0	1,155.5	1,136.5
Motor vehicle-related injuries	1,017.6	803.1	752.4	634.1	626.9	1,010.8	817.0	788.8	687.9	680.8
Suicide	401.6	407.5	404.8	395.0	380.8	402.8	404.5	405.9	405.6	387.8
Homicide and legal intervention	459.5	358.0	452.3	399.1	360.4	460.9	357.1	466.4	436.4	394.7

* YPLL-75 is calculated as 75 minus the middle age for each age group, times the number of deaths from a specific cause within that age group, added for all age groups to 75.
† International Classification of Diseases, Ninth Revision (ICD-9)

Source: Adapted from a table published by the CDC in its Monthly Mortality Weekly report, October 1997.

LIFE EXPECTANCY

The U.S. Census Bureau maintains an international database that tracks the births and deaths in a number of countries. As can be seen in Table 1.3, the largest gain in life expectancy in the United States occurred between 1900 and 1950. Recall that it was during this period that antibiotics were discovered, immunizations against a number of diseases were developed, and many public health measures were put in place. The importance of many of the micronutrients in the diet was likewise uncovered. Altogether, these discoveries and practices resulted in an improvement in the general health of the population and, as a consequence, lifespan increased. Today, as health-related research continues, health and expected lifespan can be expected to steadily increase, although not at the same dramatic rate as occurred in the first half of the 20th century. Nonetheless, a male child born today in the United States can expect to live 72.1 years, and a female, 79.6 years. In some parts of the country, even longer life expectancies have been observed. There are racial and cultural differences as well. Black males have shorter life expectancies than white males. Hispanic males fall in between the black and white males. Asian males and females generally have longer life expectancies if born in the U.S. than white or black males and females. Immigrants from third-world nations do not fare as well as non-immigrants.

TABLE 1.3
Change in Life Expectancy in the United States[a]

Year[b]	Life Expectancy at Birth	Decade Gain, %	Life Expectancy at Age 45	Decade Gain, %
1900	49.2	–	24.8	–
1910	51.5	4.7	24.5	–1.2
1920	56.4	9.5	26.3	7.3
1930	59.2	5.0	25.8	–1.9
1940	63.6	7.4	26.9	4.3
1950	68.1	7.1	28.5	5.9
1960	69.9	2.5	29.5	3.5
1970	70.8	1.3	30.1	2.0
1980	73.6	4.0	32.1	6.1
1987	75.0	1.8		
2050[c]	83.6			

From *The FASEB Journal*, Vol. 9, August 1995.
[a] Sources: J. M. McGinnis, "Recent Health Gains for Adults," *New Eng. J. Med.* Vol. 306; p. 751 (1982); National Center for Health Statistics, Prevention Profile, Health United States 1987 (Hyattsville, Maryland, Public Health Service, 1990).
[b] Except for 1910 and 1980, the numbers given are three-year composites. For example, the 1970 data reflect changes occurring from 1969 to 1971.
[c] Population profile of the United States, 1995 (published by the Census Bureau, July 31, 1995; a prediction).

During this century, gender differences in life expectancy have developed and broadened. Prior to this century, many females died in childbirth. If they survived the child-bearing years, they lived as long or longer than their male counterparts. After the implementation of better sanitary procedures for childbirth, the development of medical practices that could successfully manage and care for pregnant women, and the development of safe and effective birth control measures, female mortality associated with childbirth decreased. Thus, as more females survived childbirth, a gender gap in life expectancy began to develop. In 1900, the gender gap was 2.8 years. In 1970, females lived 7.8 years longer than males. By 1996, this gender gap fell to 6.0 years. The gender gap may continue to fall as females adopt the same behaviors as males that in turn affect their health and lifespan. The rise in smoking by females is one such change that impacts health. In the last 25 years, more females adopted the smoking practice than in the previous 25 years. Over the last 25 years, premature death (prior to age 75) from lung cancer has tripled for females. If the percentage of the female population that smokes increases further, one might anticipate a reduction in the gender gap in mortality and life expectancy. Other health behaviors likewise influence health and mortality. Among these are exercise, food choice, willingness to accept medical advice and prophylactic measures, and to change or adapt one's behavior in the face of need.

The strength of each of the many factors that influence human health and longevity is difficult to assess, given the long life of the human and the complexity of that life. Thus, health statisticians use the concept of probability in assigning the influence of specific characteristics to disease development. Probability is the language of uncertainty. It is a statement of risk with respect to a certain outcome. It actually arose from games of chance in which the player risked money on the chance of winning a game — perhaps playing poker or flipping a coin. At any rate, epidemiologists use this concept in calculating the risk of disease, given the factors known to be present in a given population. For example, obesity increases the risk of developing diabetes. This means that if a person is overly fat, that person has a much higher risk or probability of developing diabetes. Such probability is not a statement of causality but merely a statement of risk assessment based on population studies of these conditions. A causality statement is one that defines the outcome, not in terms of risk, but in terms of certainty. There is a cause and there is a result and the two are directly related.

While population surveys and health and mortality statistics can suggest a relationship between one or more characteristics and the incidence of one or more diseases, causality cannot be shown. An example of a causal statement might be as follows: if an individual steps in front of a moving train, that individual will be injured. The moving train and the stepping in front of it has the outcome of injury. A probability statement on the other hand might be as follows: if an individual consumes a fat-rich, cholesterol-rich diet, that individual has a greater risk of death from cardiovascular disease. This statement is not necessarily true. A lot depends on how that individual's body handles this type of diet and what kind of medical care the individual receives and whether the individual is overweight or is physically active. All the statement says is that the risk of coronary disease is increased. It does not say that the disease is developing or has developed.

In health and population assessments, there are very few absolutes when it comes to assessing the strength of a given behavioral attribute and disease development. Scientists are more certain about causal factors in infectious disease than in the chronic diseases that compose the majority of reasons for death in the United States. As noted, many of the chronic diseases take years to develop and the initial symptoms are quite elusive. Furthermore, scientists cannot conduct cause-and-effect studies on humans. It would be unethical to intentionally cause a mortal disease. In addition, the time frame of degenerative diseases such as heart disease in humans is so long that the researcher may not live long enough to see the results of his or her work. Because of these considerations, population studies are very valuable. They can suggest relationships between external variables such as diet choice and internal responses such as a disease process. These relationships or correlations are then converted into risk factors, and thus, risk factors are a statistical expression used in public health to indicate the correlation between a given characteristic and the presence of a given disease or death from a given disease.

Risk factors give the individual an indication of whether a certain characteristic has a strong chance of influencing health outcome. Again, risk factors are not synonymous with causal factors. They are statements of chance. For example, consuming food heavily infested with active salmonella will result in signs of food poisoning. Diarrhea, vomiting, and enteric distress will result. In this example, the disease is a food-borne illness and the cause is the salmonella. In contrast, consider the risk factor of obesity. As men increase in body fatness, their risk of having a major coronary event doubles. This does not mean that excess body fat *causes* coronary disease, but rather that the two problems are related or associated. The cause of this relationship or association may not be known. Furthermore, it is also possible that an obese man may die of some other disease. Obesity, no doubt, is mathematically related to mortality. There is indeed a positive mathematical expression for this relationship, but a mathematical expression of risk is just that. It is not synonymous with a biological cause.

Shown in Table 1.4 are some of the risk factors that have been identified for heart disease, cancer, and stroke. Of course, other factors have been or will be identified. More risk factors have been identified for diseases of the heart than for cancer and stroke. Actually, stroke and the heart diseases are related disorders in that the vascular system that supports these organs loses its elasticity and may either become blocked or rupture. In the brain, this results in a stroke. In the heart, this results in myocardial infarction or heart attack. Not all diseases of the heart involve the vascular system, nor do all diseases of the brain, but there is this similarity with respect to risk-factor analysis. Note that all three of the leading causes of death have smoking and family history as risk factors. One's family history may determine, to a large extent, the diseases to which a person is most susceptible. A family history of heart disease or cancer is strongly suggestive of a need to adopt behaviors that will forestall a repeat of this family history. While science has not developed sufficiently to provide tests that will definitively identify people whose genetics place them at risk, physicians are quite aware of the importance of the family's medical history and will frequently inquire about this history so as to be alerted to potential health problems.

TABLE 1.4
Risk Factors for Heart Disease, Cancer, and Stroke

Heart Disease	Cancer	Stroke
Excess body weight as fat	Excess body weight	Excess body weight
Hypertension	Family history	Hypertension
Hyperglycemia	Abdominal obesity	Diabetes Mellitus
Diabetes mellitus	Smoking	Family history
Family history	Age	Age
Physical inactivity		Elevated blood cholesterol
Smoking		Racial background
Elevated blood cholesterol		Smoking
Elevated blood triglycerides		
Gender		
Age		
Abdominal obesity		

In Table 1.4, diseases of the heart include congenital structural defects, damage to the heart secondary to infections, and degenerative changes in both the heart muscle and its vascular system. All forms of cancer are lumped together, and stroke due to vascular aneurysm (rupture of blood vessel followed by hemorrhage) and ischemia (decreased blood supply due to athero-sclerotic change in the brain's vascular system) are combined. These factors were developed using epidemiologic study techniques as well as the mortality statistics. Note in this table that age is a risk factor for all of the diseases. This relates, in part, to the earlier discussion of mortality in different countries of the world. Obviously, if one escapes death from infectious disease, malnutrition, or childbirth, one lives long enough to die from heart disease, stroke, or cancer. The older the individual, the greater the risk of developing one of these diseases or one or more other diseases (diabetes or hypertension or renal disease) which, in turn, increases the risk for death due to heart disease and stroke. Some investigators have used factor analysis to age adjust these risk factors. In other words, they acknowledge that as one survives the more devastating infectious diseases and other life-threatening conditions, one is more likely to die of heart disease or cancer or stroke.

Over the past decade, age-adjusted mortality from heart disease has decreased in the developed nations of the world. While nutritionists would like to take credit for this decrease due to their efforts to educate the public about the value of low-fat diets, weight reduction, and exercise, in reality, it is probably due to a number of medical and nonmedical interventions that include advice and guidance on food choices and physical activity, medical management of elevated blood lipid levels, early diagnosis followed by appropriate medical management of hypertension, and early diagnosis and treatment of vascular problems and of diabetes. Alto-gether, these proactive practices retard disease development and lengthen life. This, in turn, means that mortality from diseases of the heart occur at a later age. The same can also be said for cancer and stroke. Proactive diagnosis, treatment, and management of these diseases extend the lifespan and delay death.

Human studies using small groups of subjects with or without a definitive disease diagnosis have provided support for the risk factors given for each of groups of diseases listed in Table 1.4. However, as indicated earlier in this text, cause-and-effect human studies cannot be con-ducted. Nonetheless, scientists conducting diet, exercise, or family-history studies have shown improvements or relationships between their treatments and changes in the relative risks for these diseases. For example, human subjects have been provided low-fat diets for periods up to a year or, in some instances, longer. The investigators have been able to show that, as a result of these diets, serum lipids decreased. Similarly, other investigators have reduced the total energy value of the diet and have reported a decrease in body fat and serum lipids. These results do not mean that heart disease, if it existed in these subjects, was "cured" or reversed, or that the obesity had been corrected. What was shown was that certain features of the human that appear to be associated with heart disease can be attenuated through the use of special diets or exercise or other treatments.

AGING

As mentioned above, citizens of western, technologically advanced nations are living longer than their ancestors. In the U.S., the segment of the population over the age of 65 has grown rapidly. For example, between 1960 and 1990, the total U.S. population increased by 39%. The segment of that population over the age of 65 grew by 89%. The segment of the population over the age of 84 grew by 232%. Figure 1.1 shows the increase in the number of people in the United States over the age of 100. This population segment is rising rapidly.

Due to the increase in the over-65 segment, scientists are beginning to pay much more attention to the nutrition-related health problems facing these people. As well, more nutrition scientists are examining the nutrition needs of this population. Obviously, the health care system will need to be expanded as the elderly segment of the population expands. The costs of elder care and its delivery will need continual reexamination.

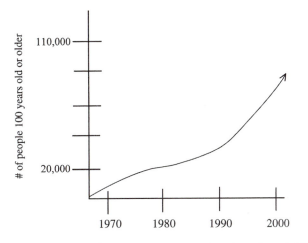

FIGURE 1.1   The number of centenarians in the United States has risen from 4,447 in 1960 to 35,808 in 1990. This group of people is steadily increasing in number.

As people age, many aspects of their lives change. Upon retirement, their income may be reduced and their health care expenses may increase. Age-related changes in the muscular-skeletal systems of the elderly will probably mean less mobility. Older sensory systems may be less acute. Diminished senses of balance, hearing, smell, sight, and the overall perception of self in society have an impact on health and well being, as well as on aging individuals' ability to care for themselves. The development of senile dementia of the Alzheimer's Type (SDAT) with subsequent losses in both mental and physical function occurs more frequently as the population ages. Shown in Table 1.5 are the predicted age-specific prevalence rates for SDAT. With the significant gain in average life expectancy, a parallel rise in these age-related failures in brain function must be anticipated.

However, as the study by Johnson and colleagues has shown, some deteriorated mental function might not be strictly age related. It might be due to malnutrition. Older adults may show signs of inadequate protein, mineral, and vitamin nutriture that impact on mental function. Lack of Vitamin B_{12}, folacin, and protein, as well as other problems, have been identified. If these inadequacies can be addressed and nutritional status improved, some of the so-called age-related impaired mental function can be reversed. Some malnutrition can also be attributed to the loss of ability to purchase the needed food — either for economic reasons or because elders may not be able to get to the grocery store to select the foods they need. Their diminished sensory faculties may mean that they can no longer drive and thus must depend on their families and communities for their food supply. They may also be unable to prepare the food or store it appropriately, due to their diminished sensory function. If dentition is poor, the choice of foods might be limited to those items that are easy to swallow with minimal mastication. The absence of dentures or the presence of poorly fitted dentures can be a major impediment to the consumption of the wide variety of foods needed to assure good nutritional status.

How can these problems be identified and corrected? This is not an easy question to answer. The nutrition screening of people over the age of 65 can present some special problems and hurdles. For a variety of reasons, many elders may not be able to read. Thus, acquiring information about their usual food intake has this additional complication. Short-term memory loss may cause some elderly to be unable to recall the food they consumed yesterday or the day before. If elders are blind or have failing vision, they may not be able to complete a diet-recall form or to compile a food-intake diary. A number of innovative techniques must be developed to address this problem. Some researchers have used a picture-sort approach where the subject selects pictures of foods and recalls to the interviewer how frequently that food is consumed. Other researchers have used

TABLE 1.5
Predicted Age-Specific
Prevalence Rates (%) for
DSM-III Senile Dementia
and SDAT

Age	DSM-III Dementia	SDAT
62.5	0.9	0.2
67.5	1.6	0.4
72.5	2.8	0.9
77.5	4.9	2.1
82.5	8.7	4.7
87.5	15.5	10.8
91.5	24.5	21.0
95.0	36.7	37.4

Senile dementia of the Alzheimer's Type (SDAT): Epidemiology and Public Health Issues. Karen Ritchie. Taken from: *Facts and Research in Gerontology 1994* (Supplement on Dementia and Cognitive Impairment). Vol. 4:2.

interview techniques that involve the use of food group patterns as well as individual food-recall methods. Having an observer record the actual food consumed is a possibility, but this method is labor intensive and time consuming unless the elderly are in a group setting such as in an assisted-care facility. Individual observation may not be practical if the elderly person is living independently. In addition, the line between screening and diagnostic testing is blurred. In areas where there is good, widely available geriatric care, the need for such testing is reduced. In other words, where the elderly are well served by the medical community, the need for screening is much less than where they are poorly served. Early indications of health's being impacted by malnutrition are usually observed in the former situation and ignored in the latter. Thus, anemia due to mineral or vitamin deficiency might be corrected as elderly people are routinely cared for by their physicians. Osteoporosis, arthritis, and other degenerative diseases that have a nutrition component likewise will be identified and effectively treated.

Good geriatric care also includes the recognition that some of the medications used in managing such chronic diseases as hypertension or diabetes mellitus may interact with certain nutrients, thus placing the patient at risk for malnutrition. Thiazide diuretics, for example, are widely prescribed for the management of hypertension. They are excellent medications for this purpose, however, they increase the loss of potassium and frequently the elderly need to supplement their diets with potassium-rich foods (citrus fruits, bananas, etc.) or take a potassium supplement. The elderly may develop chemical imbalances in the brain that affect their emotional state. It is not unusual for physicians to prescribe antidepressants. Those drugs that are anticholinergics can have the side effects of dry mouth, altered taste perception, nausea, vomiting, constipation, and reduced appetite. All of these side effects can affect nutritional status because of their influence on food consumption. Similarly, nutritional status can be affected by the use of antacids and laxatives. Some of the elderly believe that a daily large bowel movement is essential. Despite day-to-day variation in the kinds and amounts of foods consumed, there is this belief that a daily movement is a feature of good health. Thus, many elderly are chronic laxative users. This use may disturb gastrointestinal function and promote diarrhea as well as the possibility of an electrolyte imbalance. In turn, this will reduce gut passage time and thus absorptive cell exposure time for nutrients. Again, this can result in impaired nutritional status.

Diseases of the joints and connective tissue are frequently managed with the use of anti-inflammatories. Both steroids and nonsteroids are used to reduce the inflammation and associated pain. Aspirin and indomethacin are among the non-steroidal, over-the-counter medications frequently used. If used daily in large doses, both can result in iron-deficiency anemia. High aspirin intake can deplete the hepatic iron stores because it interferes with normal blood coagulation. The elderly can have bruises and small "bleeds" that result in blood loss and anemia. A number of other drugs can influence nutritional status. However, many drugs have not been studied at all with respect to their effect on nutritional status especially in the elderly. Nonetheless, interest in drug–nutrient interactions is building as we learn more about the gradual losses in body function that characterize aging.

DIET AND DISEASE RELATIONSHIPS

The preceding tables on the causes of death do not include the many health problems that have a diet component. They give only the causes of death, not disability. Among the health disorders are the nutrient deficiency disorders, excess intake disorders, and a variety of degenerative and incapacitating disorders. Listed in Table 1.6 are diseases that fit into these categories.

Most of these disorders have a genetic component as well. The individual's genetic background dictates how much of each vitamin, mineral, or macronutrient is needed for optimal health. There can be considerable variation in these needs, as will be discussed later. The details of some of the macronutrient influences on the degenerative disorders can be found in the units on energy, protein, carbohydrate, and lipid in this volume. These details would not have been sought and elucidated had not epidemiologists suggested that such relationships existed, i.e., the risk factors described in the preceding section.

TABLE 1.6
Nutrition-Related Disorders

Deficient Intake	Excess Intake	Degenerative Disorders
Rickets	Alcoholism[1]	Coronary vessel disease
Anemia	Mineral toxicities	Diabetes mellitus
Pellegra	Hypervitaminoses	Cirrhosis
Beri beri	Obesity	Hypertension
Scurvy		Cancer
		Renal disease

[1] Alcohol in excess can compromise food intake when alcohol is consumed instead of food.

Diabetes is one such degenerative disease that has a profound influence on heart, renal, and neurological diseases. Heart-disease death rates of people with diabetes are two–four times as high as those of adults without diabetes. Persons with diabetes have five times the risk of having a major coronary event as do persons without diabetes. More than 40% of all persons undergoing dialysis for renal disease are people with diabetes mellitus. Because of the discovery of insulin as the replacement hormone and with the development of effective management of the disorder, people with diabetes mellitus are living longer than ever before. Thus, the number of people with diabetes mellitus in the total population has increased dramatically. Estimates of the number of people with diabetes vary from 1 in 14 to 1 in 20 in the general population. The CDC estimates that 5.9% of the total population in the United States have diabetes. Certain populations have even larger numbers of affected individuals.

Despite the problems associated with studying humans, considerable progress has been made in understanding human disease processes. This progress has been possible because investigators have found similar problems in small laboratory animals. Especially valuable are small rodents that have short reproductive cycles and, compared with man, a short lifespan. This is very important to the study of genetic diseases in which the expression of the disease does not occur until midlife or late adulthood. Diseases that are degenerative in nature or that take several decades to become clinically observable in the human are extremely difficult to understand. Observations of subcell and cellular changes that precede tissue and organ changes that in turn develop into a clinical condition of note are needed. With diseases such as cardiovascular disease, cancer, diabetes mellitus, or renal disease, diagnosis in the human is possible only after the biomarkers or the clinical signs and symptoms appear.

Scientists seeking to understand how the disease developed and the sequence of biological changes that led to the clinical state must study animals whose disease time frame is considerably shorter than that of the human. Several types of animals can be used. Some are the products of today's biotechnology, while others have appeared spontaneously in breeding populations. The use of animals called "knockouts" or "transgenic" animals has facilitated the testing of hypotheses about the genetic factors important in the disease process. Knockout mice, for example, have had one or more genetic messages removed from the nuclear DNA. Transgenic animals, on the other hand, have had one or more genetic messages inserted. In each instance, the researcher is hypothesizing that these messages play a critical role in cell or organ function. Use of these genetically modified animals has shed new light on how specific disease processes occur and how specific nutrients work in cell metabolism. These new techniques are gradually providing very useful animal models for nutrition research. In addition to these are animals that have spontaneously developed humanlike conditions. Table 1.7 presents a partial list of such animals. In this list, subdivided by clinical disorder, the reader will note some duplication of animal models between the clinical conditions. This illustrates the crossover effect of one condition on another. For example, obesity can affect the development of diabetes. Thus, the reader will note that the ob/ob mouse, an animal that becomes obese, also can be used to study type 2 diabetes. While the majority of the models used are those that spontaneously develop the specified clinical condition, some of the models are "man made." That is, the trait develops as a consequence of a chemical or a gene introduced into the animal. This trait was not spontaneous. Type 1 diabetes, for example, can be induced with the treatment of the animal with either streptozotocin or alloxan. The chemicals attack the insulin-producing cells of the pancreas and destroy them, thus inducing diabetes.

Over the last century, considerable effort has been expended by animal breeders to provide scientists with a uniform animal for laboratory use. In an effort to provide this uniform animal, breeders have developed strains of rats, mice, chickens, rabbits, guinea pigs, and so forth that meet a well-defined standard of identity. Growth rate, hair color, health status, and nutrient needs are fairly similar within a given breeding group within a given strain and species. This is particularly true for mice and rats. For many breeders, the genetic history of every animal produced can be traced back many generations to a particular set of breeding animals.

TABLE 1.7
Small Animal Analogs of Human Degenerative Diseases*

Type 1 Diabetes Mellitus (IDDM)

Streptozotocin or alloxan treated animals of most species
Pancreatectomy will also produce IDDM
BB rat, NOD mouse (Both of these develop diabetes as an
  autoimmune disease and both mimic Type I diabetes
  mellitus as found in humans.)
db/db mouse
FAT mouse
NZO mouse
TUBBY mouse
Adipose mouse
Chinese hamster (*Cricetulus griseus*)
South African hamster (*Mystromys alb*)
Tuco-Tuco (*Clenomys tabarum*)

Type 2 Diabetes Mellitus

ob/ob mouse
KK, yellow KK mouse
A^{vy}, A^y yellow mouse
P, PB 13/Ld mouse
db PAS mouse
BHE/Cdb rat
Zucker diabetic rat
SHR/N-cp rat
Spiny mouse
HUS rat
LA/N-cp rat
Wistar Kyoto rat

Obesity

Zucker rat
SHR/N-cp rat
LA/N-cp rat
ob/ob mouse
Ventral hypothalamus lesioned animals
Osborne-Mendel rats fed high fat diets

Hypertension

SHR rats	WKY rats
JCR:LA rats	Transgenic rats

Gallstones

(The rat does not have a gall bladder nor does it
  have stones.)
Gerbil fed a cholesterol-rich, cholic acid-rich diet
Hamster, prairie dog, squirrel monkey, or tree
  shrew fed a cholesterol-rich diet

Lipemia

Zucker fatty rat
BHE/Cdb rat
NZW mouse
Transgenic mice given gene for atherosclerosis

Atherosclerosis

Transgenic mice given gene for atherosclerosis
NZW mouse
JCR:LA cp/cp rat

* There are several compilations of animal models for human disease. See the series of books edited by Shafrir
having the general title *Lessons from Animal Diabetes* published by Smith Gordon, London. See also the NIH
Guide for Animal Resources, updated annually, and the Jackson Laboratory catalog, Bar Harbor, Maine.

To produce homogeneity within a breeding group, breeders select the traits they wish to preserve
(and those they wish to delete) and plan their breeding accordingly using brother–sister matings
or backcrosses to strengthen the desired trait. If full sib matings of mice, for example, are used for
21 sequential generations, the colony of animals is considered inbred and should be homozygous
at every gene locus. Producing an inbred animal is not without risk, however, since an unknown
trait that is lethal might appear. If enough animals possess this trait, the colony dies. Hence, many
breeders do not strive for full homozygosity at every locus. Instead, they are satisfied with homozygosity at only one, two, or three loci. The use of inbreeding to attain a specific trait(s) without full
homozygosity has made possible the detection of several mutations that result in animals that
spontaneously become obese or develop diabetes mellitus and some of its secondary complications,
or become hypertensive or lipemic. Not all of these mutations develop the same form of the disease
as found in the human. In this respect, these animals represent the variety of disease seen in man.
Some of these animals inherit the mutant gene that is responsible for their disease in a dominant
mode. That is, the animal needs only one copy of the mutant gene to develop the disorder. The

majority of these animals, however, inherit their particular mutant gene in a recessive manner. That is, they must inherit two copies of the mutant gene (one from each parent) to express the genetic trait or disease. This is probably also true for those genes that result in diseases in humans. A few may be transmitted via a dominant mode, but most are usually thought to be inherited via a recessive mode of transmission. In addition, many of these mutant genes might not be expressed unless the environmental conditions are such that their expression is stimulated. For example, an individual might carry a mutant gene for obesity but, unless presented with an unlimited supply of food, might not develop obesity.

With respect to diseases of nutritional importance to man, almost every micro and macronutrient need has been established using small animals. Almost every nutrient-related degenerative disease that afflicts man likewise can be found in one or another form in one or more small animals. The choice of animals to be used for research depends wholly on the objective of the research. It would be folly to study heart disease development, for example, in a strain of rat that is not genetically susceptible to this problem or that is too young to develop it. The researcher must carefully define the problem before selecting the most appropriate animal model.

Once the species and strain have been selected, the researcher must then design an appropriate diet for this test animal. For example, the BHE/Cdb rat has a mitochondrial defect and develops impaired glucose tolerance as well as renal disease. If one were to study this disease process, one should be aware of its greater than normal need for vitamins A and E. Thus, the diet would have to supply these micronutrients so that an inadvertent variable was not added to the design of the experiment. Other animal analogs might also have deviations in their needs for specific nutrients and these would need to be investigated as well. The National Research Council provides tables of nutrient needs for a variety of species and these tables should be consulted prior to the onset of an experiment. Further, the American Society of Nutritional Sciences (ASNS) has a recommended basal diet that should meet the nutritional needs of most rodents. This is sold as the AIN-93 diet. There is both a maintenance diet (AIN-93M) and a growth diet (AIN-93G). The former should adequately nourish adult nonpregnant animals while the latter should be used for pregnant, lactating, or growing animals. This diet is reviewed periodically for its adequacy and, from time to time, adjustments in its composition are made. Table 1.8 provides the composition of these diets.

TABLE 1.8
Composition of the AIN-93 Maintenance (M) and Growth (G) Diets

Ingredient	AIN-93M g/kg	AIN-93G g/kg
Casein	140	200
Cornstarch	465.692	397.486
Dextrose	155	132
Sucrose	100	100
Cellulose	50	50
Soybean oil	40	70
Mineral mix	35	35
Vitamin mix	10	10
L-cystine	1.8	3
Choline bitartrate	2.5	2.5
t-Butylhydroquinone	0.008	0.014
Energy	~3.8 kcal or ~16 kJ/g	~3.9 kcal or ~16.4 kJ/g

From: *Journal of Nutrition* 123:1941-44, 1993.

FOOD INTAKE STUDIES IN HUMANS

As part of an epidemiological survey, the researcher might ask about the food consumed by the population being studied. These data can be acquired in several ways. Food-disappearance data are frequently used to assess the use of food by very large population groups. In the United States, the Department of Agriculture has monitored the disappearance of foods from the marketplace since 1909. Knowing the population number (data from the Census Bureau), agricultural production, the processed-food production by the food industry, the amount of food exported, the food not intended for human use directly, i.e., animal feed, and the year-end inventory of food stocks, U.S. Department of Agriculture (USDA) experts can estimate the disappearance of food from the marketplace on a per capita basis. Specific nutrients and their availability or disappearance are calculated using published values on the nutrient composition of food. Because these data are calculated, they are not direct measurements of individual food consumption. They are, instead, estimates of the food (and the nutrients this food contains) that is available and that disappears from the marketplace. As such, these data reveal overall trends in consumption, but make no corrections for food loss in preparation, food not consumed, or for uses of food for non-food purposes. Shown in Figure 1.2 are moving averages for the per capita total energy, fat, protein, and carbohydrate that have disappeared from the marketplace over the last eight decades. Note that since World War II there have been very small changes in the estimate of the per capita disappearance (assumed consumption) of total energy. The overall energy intake over the last 90 years varies little. There have been changes in the distribution of the energy sources. For example, the disappearance of protein in the food supply decreased during the Depression and World War II but has steadily increased since that time. The disappearance of fat has steadily risen from 1950 to the current high, which is 25% higher than that estimated for 1909. The increase in food fat disappearance together with decreases in physical activity or energy expenditure may be related to the increase in obesity that characterizes our nation. However, once again, the reader is reminded that food-disappearance data are not very specific. These data show trends rather than actual food use. Thus, they are useful adjuncts to discrete studies of small population groups where detailed diet analysis or traditional food consumption patterns are studied.

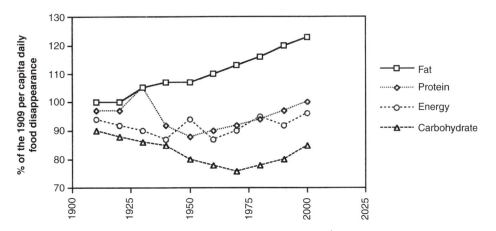

FIGURE 1.2   Percent of the 1909 value for the per capita daily intake of the macronutrients. These values are derived for food-disappearance data.

USDA, in addition to computing food disappearance based on the large data sets as described above, also collects data on the food consumed by households. This survey has also been conducted on a regular basis since the early 1900s. Representative householders participate in the survey by completing a questionnaire about the amounts of foods purchased and their cost. The early surveys used a food inventory method that requested that the person responsible for food preparation inventory their food supply over a set period of time. Corrections for initial and final food stocks were made. This method of assessing food consumption proved cumbersome. The participants in the survey lost interest and some provided records that were incomplete or not useful for other reasons. Realizing these problems, the food-inventory sheets were replaced by a check list of foods used. This frequency-of-use system was subsequently replaced by individual sequential 24-hour food-intake records. Results of the 1997-98 USDA Food Consumption Survey are shown in Table 1.9.

TABLE 1.9
Results of the 1997–1998 National Food Consumption Survey Conducted by the USDA-Human Nutrition Information Service. These are daily intake estimates.

Nutrient	Males	Females
Energy (kcal) (kJoules)	2154(9012)	1497(6263)
Protein (g)	87.8	61.9
Fat (g)	90.7	61.1
Carbohydrates (g)	239.4	175.2
Vitamin A (IU)	6639	5690
Vitamin C (mg)	99	84
Thiamin (mg)	1.59	1.14
Riboflavin (mg)	1.98	1.46
Niacin (mg)	23.4	16.6
Vitamin B6 (mg)	1.82	1.31
Vitamin B12 ((g)	5.95	5.02
Calcium (mg)	821	602
Magnesium (mg)	281	209
Iron (mg)	14.9	10.9

Source: HNIS, USDA, Hyattsville, MD.

Several techniques are available for obtaining individual food-consumption data. The dietary-recall method asks participants to remember the amounts of all the food they have consumed over the last 24 hours or the last three days. Sometimes a participant is very good at recalling the food consumed and sometimes not very good at all. Recall data are not very reliable, for example, when obtained from children or the aged. Unreliability is also a problem if the participant believes that the choice of food will be criticized or if there is something to be gained or lost through truthful (or untruthful) answers. Some people honestly cannot remember what they ate or how much. Another approach to this recall method is to ask the participant to indicate how often (daily, weekly, yearly) food items in a list are consumed. This food-frequency check list, in conjunction with an interview of the respondent, is often used by investigators interested in health problems as related to food consumption. The interview provides an opportunity for more in-depth questioning about the frequency of use of particular food items. When coupled with a health- or nutritional-status assessment, this approach is very useful. The investigator using the food-frequency method should be careful to include food consumed outside the home. In using the food-frequency approach, the investigator should also question subjects with respect to their personal food likes and dislikes and intake patterns. The frequency of consumption, together with simple measures of height and weight, and questions about age and perhaps health status and medication use, can provide much useful information. When coupled with a physical examination and perhaps selected biochemical and physiological measurements, the nutritional status of the individual can be assessed. Because this kind of intake assessment is far more time consuming, it is more expensive to use than the simple recall method. However, it has the advantage of providing a more reliable assessment of food intake and nutritional status. Reliability can be further increased (with a consequence of further time and dollar expense) if the participant can be convinced to keep a food diary in which every morsel of every food consumed is described and quantified. The participant must be trained in this record keeping so that the correct serving size is reported. The record is then used as the basis for computing the intake of nutrients using a table of food composition that gives the amounts of the major nutrients in most foods.

These tables are available in computer format so that the foods can be entered by code and the operator can quickly assess the daily nutrient intakes of the participant. Which method a researcher or a government agency uses to obtain food-intake data depends on the particular use for that data and the goals of the study. If all that is desired is an assessment of the food supply, individual consumption patterns are not needed. However, if the goal is to assess the health of a discrete population group in relation to the foods consumed, a different technique will be needed.

The most comprehensive survey of nutrient intakes and health status is the National Health and Nutrition Examination Survey (NHANES). The first survey (NHANES I) was conducted in the early 70s (1971–1975) by the National Center for Health Statistics, a branch of the Centers for Disease Control (CDC) of the U.S. Department of Health and Human Services. NHANES I consisted of dietary intake measures (24-hour food-intake recall and food frequency), anthropometric measurements, clinical assessment for signs of nutrient deficiency(s), and a biochemical assessment of key blood and urine nutrients and metabolites. This was a cross-sectional survey that examined representative age groups and racial groups, both male and female. Approximately 29,000 (age 1 to 74 years) noninstitutionalized individuals from all parts of the country were examined. NHANES II followed NHANES I and examined a similar number of people. The lowest age group was 6 months. Ninety-one percent of the subjects were interviewed as in NHANES I and 73% were clinically evaluated via a variety of biochemical tests, a glucose-tolerance test, blood pressure measurement, electrocardiography and radiography of the chest and spine. A survey with particular attention to Hispanics was conducted using these same methods during 1982–84. This was called the HHANES. NHANES III was carried out from 1988–94. Each study used a variety of biochemical and physiological assessment techniques and were not fully identical. Nonetheless, these surveys provide important estimates of the nation's health, especially as it relates to nutritional status. In the most recent survey (as yet not complete with respect to data analysis and reporting), the elderly segment of the population (age 75 and older) was studied in detail. Six age groups in all were included: 2 months to 5 years, 6–19 years, 20–39 years, 40–59 years, 60–74 years, and 75 years and older. All of the subjects were interviewed to ascertain living group composition, individual and family food-intake patterns, occupation, and general economic status, educational attainment, and family characteristics. Subjects 17 years and older were questioned about chronic health conditions such as hypertension, diabetes, lipemia, and cardiovascular disease and were asked about their vision, hearing, dental care and status, tobacco and alcohol use, exercise or activity patterns, their occupations, and whether they routinely used nutritional supplements. In addition to these interviews, information about food intake was collected. The three-day recall method as well as the food-frequency method followed by an interview was used. In some instances where the subjects were not able to read, the methodology was amended to acquire the needed information. This was especially important when the subjects were illiterate or non-English speaking. Picture presentations of food and an intense interview assisted in the collection of food-intake data. Estimates of compromised nutritional status, trends of nutrition-related diseases, prevalence of obesity, and data on growth and development of children are available on disc for computer analysis. Shown in Table 1.10 are the various measurements made.

TABLE 1.10
Measurements Made by NHANES

Hematology:

Sedimentation rate
Differential white cell count
Hemoglobin, carboxyhemoglobin, glycosylated hemoglobin
Red cell number and distribution width
Neutrophil hypersegmentation
Mean cell volume
Fibrinogen

Nutrition Profile:

Red cell folate, vitamins C, D, A, B_{12}, E, selenium, cholesterol, lipoprotein
  profile, calcium, zinc, copper, iron binding capacity, ferritin, chloride,
  phosphorus, sodium, potassium, lead, protoporphyrin, methyl malonic acid

Biochemistry Profile:

Total carbon dioxide, blood urea nitrogen, total bilirubin, Apolipoprotein A,
  B, alkaline phosphatase, transaminase activities, lactate, lactate
  dehydrogenase activity, total protein, albumin, creatinine, glucose,
  lipoprotein (a), triglycerides, HDL cholesterol, total cholesterol

Disease Exposure Profile:

Carotenes, nicotine, bile salts, pesticides, syphilis serology, hepatitis A, B,
  C, E serology, tetanus, diptheria, rubella, polio serology, herpes simplex I
  and II, IgE, HIV, c-reactive protein, rheumatoid factor, homocysteine,
  varicella

Hormone Profile:

Follicle stimulating hormone, luteinizing hormone, thyroxine (T4), thyroid
  stimulating hormone, insulin, C-peptide, toxoplasmosis, antithyroglobulin
  antibodies, antimicrosomal antibodies, her

Urinalysis:

Pesticides, vitamin metabolites, creatinine, albumin

Note in Table 1.10 that blood measurements of vitamins and minerals were made. These blood values give only the amounts of these nutrients in transit, not the amount in storage. Tissue samples such as a liver biopsy or a bone biopsy would be required for the true assessment of stores and hence status. Biopsies are quite risky as well as being time and resource consuming. Unless there is a specific reason for harvesting such tissue samples, this is not done. In particular, tissue sampling was not done in any of the NHANES studies. The anthropometric measurements included weight; sitting, standing and recumbent height; skinfold thickness at preselected sites; grip strength; bioelectrical impedance (an indirect measure of body fat mass); head, chest, waist, hip, and thigh circumference; thickness at wrist and elbow; shoulder breadth; and breadth of hips. While participants of all ages were evaluated, not all the subjects had all of the measures taken. Adults were more rigorously examined than infants and children. The laboratory methods have been carefully described in the NHANES manuals and, as well, can be found in *Nutritional Assessment,* by Lee and Nieman.

While federal agencies such as USDA and the U.S. Public Health Service are concerned with the nutritional status of the general population, there are numerous smaller studies either already published or in progress. These studies may involve only a few subjects by comparison with NHANES and they may be very highly focused to answer one or two discrete questions. Many of these have been used as a basis for dietary recommendations for specific target groups. The book *Diet and Health,* published in 1989 by the National Academy Press, is a compilation and summation of a number of these studies.

DIETARY REFERENCE TABLES

RECOMMENDED DIETARY ALLOWANCES (RDA)

Soon after it became apparent that certain components in the diet were necessary to prevent or cure endemic diseases such as scurvy, goiter, blindness, pellagra, and so forth, nutrition scientists set about determining how much of each of these nutrients humans required to prevent the deficient state. Feeding studies using human subjects were conducted. These feeding studies were very time consuming, very expensive, and labor intensive. The preliminary work that established sensitive criteria for detecting the earliest possible indication of deficiency was conducted using small laboratory animals. Rats, mice, guinea pigs, chickens, and rabbits were frequently used. The species selected was critical, since animals do differ in their nutrient needs. Most species synthesize ascorbic acid. The human and the guinea pig do not. Therefore, the study of scurvy, if not in man, had to be conducted with the guinea pig, not the rat or mouse or rabbit. Choosing an appropriate animal with nutrient needs analogous to that of the human requires some knowledge about the species differences as well as the acknowledgment that human metabolism cannot always be duplicated in a single laboratory species.

Once sensitive criteria were developed, the feeding studies were conducted one by one by various investigators in the United States and elsewhere. They published the results of their work in the scientific literature. These results were then used as the basis for the RDAs for each nutrient. When the RDA table was first assembled in 1940, the database was very small. In some instances, the members of the Food and Nutrition Board of the National Academy of Sciences (the group charged with setting the RDAs) had little or no data to use for specific age groups. Adolescents and preadolescents were the least studied, yet the Board was charged with making recommendations for all age groups from infants to the elderly.

Because the Board recognized that considerable variation in need can exist among individuals of the same age and gender, a safety factor was incorporated into the recommendation. The Board took the highest reported value for each nutrient need and doubled it for safety. Thus, if the highest reported daily need for riboflavin was 0.6 mg, the Board doubled it and recommended an intake of 1.2 mg. As the database expanded through additional reports in the literature, the Board adjusted its recommendations. Hence, the RDA for protein has declined from 100 g per day for the adult man to 70 g to 63 g per day. The recommended intake for vitamin C likewise has been adjusted downward from 75 mg to 60 mg per day for the adult. Shown in Tables 1.11 and 1.12 are the current RDAs published in 1997 and 1998. In these tables, several new columns have been added. We now have recommended dietary allowances for fluoride, pantothenic acid, biotin, and choline that were absent in earlier tables.

TABLE 1.11
Food and Nutrition Board, National Academy of Sciences—National Research Council Recommended Dietary Allowances,[a] Revised 1998 (Abridged) Designed for the Maintenance of Good Nutrition of Practically All Healthy People in the United States

Category	Age (years) or Condition	Weight[b] (kg)	Weight[b] (lb)	Height[b] (cm)	Height[b] (in)	Protein (g)	Vitamin A (µg RE)[c]	Vitamin E (mg α-TE)[d]	Vitamin K (µg)	Vitamin C (mg)	Iron (mg)	Zinc (mg)	Iodine (µg)	Selenium (µg)
Infants	0.0–0.5	6	13	60	24	13	375	3	5	30	6	5	40	10
	0.5–1.0	9	20	71	28	14	375	4	10	35	10	5	50	15
Children	1–3	13	29	90	35	16	400	6	15	40	10	10	70	20
	4–6	20	44	112	44	24	500	7	20	45	10	10	90	20
	7–10	28	62	132	52	28	700	7	30	45	10	10	120	30
Males	11–14	45	99	157	62	45	1,000	10	45	50	12	15	150	40
	15–18	66	145	176	69	59	1,000	10	65	60	12	15	150	50
	19–24	72	160	177	70	58	1,000	10	70	60	10	15	150	70
	25–50	79	174	176	70	63	1,000	10	80	60	10	15	150	70
	51+	77	170	173	68	63	1,000	10	80	60	10	15	150	70
Females	11–14	46	101	157	62	46	800	8	45	50	15	12	150	45
	15–18	55	120	163	64	44	800	8	55	60	15	12	150	50
	19–24	58	128	164	65	46	800	8	60	60	15	12	150	55
	25–50	63	138	163	64	50	800	8	65	60	15	12	150	55
	51+	65	143	160	63	50	800	8	65	60	10	12	150	55
Pregnant						60	800	10	65	70	30	15	175	65
Lactating	1st 6 months					65	1,300	12	65	95	15	19	200	75
	2nd 6 months					62	1,200	11	65	90	15	16	200	75

Note: This table does not include nutrients from which Dietary Reference Intakes have recently been established (see Dietary Reference Intakes for Calcium, Phosphorus, Magnesium, Vitamin D, and Fluoride [1997] and Dietary Reference Intakes for Thiamin, Riboflavin, Niacin, Vitamin B6, Folate, Vitamin B12, Pantothenic Acid, Biotin, and Choline [1998]).

[a] The allowances, expressed as average daily intakes over time, are intended to provide for individual variations among most normal persons as they live in the United States under usual environmental stresses. Diets should be based on a variety of common foods in order to provide other nutrients for which human requirements have been less well defined.

[b] Weights and heights of Reference Adults are actual medians for the U.S. population of the designated age, as reported by NHANES II. The median weights and heights of those under 19 years of age were taken from Hamill et al. (1979). The use of the these figures does not imply that the height-to-weight ratios are ideal.

[c] Retinol equivalents. 1 retinol equivalent = 1 μg retinol or 6 μg ß-carotene.

[d] α-Tocopherol equivalents. 1 mg d-α tocopherol = 1 α-TE.

Reprinted with permission from Food and Nutrition Board, National Academy of Sciences—Institute of Medicine. Copyright 1998 and 1997, respectively, by the National Academy of Sciences. All rights reserved. Courtesy of the National Academy Press, Washington, D.C.

TABLE 1.12
Food and Nutrition Board, Institute of Medicine—National Academy of Sciences Dietary Reference Intakes: Recommended Intakes for Individuals (1998)

Life-Stage Group	Calcium (mg/d)	Phosphorus (mg/d)	Magnesium (mg/d)	Vitamin D (µg/d)[a,b]	Fluoride (mg/d)	Thiamin (mg/d)	Riboflavin (mg/d)	Niacin (mg/d)[c]	Vitamin B_6 (mg/d)	Folate (µg/d)[d]	Vitamin B_{12} (µg/d)	Pantothenic Acid (mg/d)	Biotin (µg/d)	Choline[e] (mg/d)
Infants														
0–6 mo	210*	100*	30*	5*	0.01*	0.2*	0.3*	2*	0.1*	65*	0.4*	1.7*	5*	125*
7–12 mo	270*	275*	75*	5*	0.5*	0.3*	0.4*	4*	0.3*	80*	0.5*	1.8*	6*	150*
Children														
1–3 yr	500*	460	80	5*	0.7*	0.5	0.5	6	0.5	150	0.9	2*	8*	200*
4–8 yr	800*	500	130	5*	1*	0.6	0.6	8	0.6	200	1.2	3*	12*	250*
Males														
9–13 yr	1,300*	1,250	240	5*	2*	0.9	0.9	12	1.0	300	1.8	4*	20*	375*
14–18 yr	1,300*	1,250	410	5*	3*	1.2	1.3	16	1.3	400	2.4	5*	25*	550*
19–30 yr	1,000*	700	400	5*	4*	1.2	1.3	16	1.3	400	2.4	5*	30*	550*
31–50 yr	1,000*	700	420	5*	4*	1.2	1.3	16	1.3	400	2.4	5*	30*	550*
51–70 yr	1,200*	700	420	10*	4*	1.2	1.3	16	1.7	400	2.4f	5*	30*	550*
>70 yr	1,200*	700	420	15*	4*	1.2	1.3	16	1.7	400	2.4f	5*	30*	550*
Females														
9–13 yr	1,300*	1,250	240	5*	2*	0.9	0.9	12	1.0	300	1.8	4*	20*	375*
14–18 yr	1,300*	1,250	360	5*	3*	1.0	1.0	14	1.2	400g	2.4	5*	25*	400*
19–30 yr	1,000*	700	310	5*	3*	1.1	1.1	14	1.3	400g	2.4	5*	30*	425*
31–50 yr	1,000*	700	320	5*	3*	1.1	1.1	14	1.3	400g	2.4	5*	30*	425*
51–70 yr	1,200*	700	320	10*	3*	1.1	1.1	14	1.5	400	2.4f	5*	30*	425*
>70 yr	1,200*	700	320	15*	3*	1.1	1.1	14	1.5	400	2.4f	5*	30*	425*
Pregnancy														
≤18 yr	1,300*	1,250	400	5*	3*	1.4	1.4	18	1.9	600h	2.6	6*	30*	450*
19–30 yr	1,000*	700	350	5*	3*	1.4	1.4	18	1.9	600h	2.6	6*	30*	450*
31–50 yr	1,000*	700	360	5*	3*	1.4	1.4	18	1.9	600h	2.6	6*	30*	450*
Lactation														
≤18 yr	1,300*	1,250	360	5*	3*	1.5	1.6	17	2.0	500	2.8	7*	35*	550*
19–30 yr	1,000*	700	310	5*	3*	1.5	1.6	17	2.0	500	2.8	7*	35*	550*
31–50 yr	1,000*	700	320	5*	3*	1.5	1.6	17	2.0	500	2.8	7*	35*	550*

Note: This table presents Recommended Dietary Allowances (RDAs) and Adequate Intakes (AIs) followed by an asterisk (*). RDAs and AIs may both be used as goals for individual intake.

RDAs are set to meet the needs of almost all (97 to 98 percent) individuals in a group. For healthy breastfed infants, the AI is the mean intake. The AI for other life-stage and gender groups is believed to cover needs of all individuals in the group, but lack of data or uncertainty in the data prevent being able to specify with confidence the percentage of individuals covered by this intake.

[a] As cholecalciferol. 1 μg cholecalciferol = 40 IU vitamin D.

[b] In the absence of adequate exposure to sunlight.

[c] As niacin equivalents (NE). 1 mg of niacin = 60 mg of tryptophan; 0–6 months = preformed niacin (not NE).

[d] As dietary folate equivalents (DFE). 1 DFE = 1 μg food folate = 0.6 μg of folic acid (from fortified food or supplement) consumed with food = 0.5 μg of synthetic (supplemental) folic acid taken on an empty stomach.

[e] Although AIs have been set for choline, there are few data to assess whether a dietary supply of choline is needed at all stages of the life cycle, and it may be that the choline requirement can be met by endogenous synthesis at some of these stages.

[f] Because 10 to 30 percent of older people may malabsorb food-bound B12, it is advisable for those older than 50 years to meet their RDA mainly by consuming foods fortified with B_{12} or a supplement containing B_{12}.

[g] In view of evidence linking folate intake with neural tube defects in the fetus, it is recommended that all women capable of becoming pregnant consume 400 μg of synthetic folic acid from fortified foods and/or supplements in addition to intake of food folate from a varied diet.

[h] It is assumed that women will continue consuming 400 μg of folic acid until their pregnancy is confirmed and they enter prenatal care, which ordinarily occurs after the end of the periconceptional period—the critical time for formation of the neural tube.

From: National Food and Nutrition Board, National Academy of Sciences—Institute of Medicine, Academy of Sciences, Washington, D.C. with permission.

The RDAs should not be confused with the requirements for nutrients. They were originally devised as a means for planning adequate food supplies (nutrition) for the civilian population in the United States. Recall that in 1941 the nation was involved in World War II and food rationing was being implemented. The nation's food planners had to have a guide in hand so that rationing could be implemented on as scientific a basis as was possible given the level of knowledge at that time. Although the RDAs were developed in 1941, they were not officially published and publicly available until 1943. Every five years the database is reviewed and, if needed, the RDAs are revised. The latest edition includes recommendations for 23 different nutrients, whereas the first edition included only 10. There is no energy-intake recommendation because humans are so variable in energy need that this recommendation is not at present possible.

Other countries also have developed similar tables. The recommendations are not always the same. The reasons for this may vary. The country's nutrition experts may use different criteria for adequacy of intake. The choice of criteria can range from absence of physical signs of deficiency to blood and tissue saturation by the nutrient in question. There may be political and economic pressures on the review panel that influence the choice of adequacy criteria. They may decide to set the value at a level sure to meet the needs of 75% of the people rather than the 97–98% called for in the U.S. This figure reflects the concept of a Gaussian distribution (the typical bell-shaped curve of the statistician). The mean value of all the published data on the requirements for a particular nutrient plus two standard deviations is used to set the RDA for that nutrient. The mean plus two deviations is thus 97–98% of the total population. Of course, the more data available to calculate the mean and its deviation, the better the estimate of real need and the closer one can predict an intake figure that will meet that need. Intercountry variation also could be due to interpopulation differences. Suffice it to say that no one country is "wrong" or "right" in their nutrient intake recommendations, simply that these guides are just that — guides. About 40 different nations in the world now have RDAs for their people.

Estimates of nutrient intakes for items not on the RDA table have also been made. This group of nutrients falls into the category of items for which there are insufficient data to make a recommended daily allowance but for which there are sufficient data to estimate a range of intake. Some of the minerals — copper, manganese, chromium, and molybdenum — fall into this category. The Food and Nutrition Board gives a figure that is an estimate of an amount generally considered safe and adequate. For the minerals, this definition is especially important because an intake in excess of this recommendation could be toxic. The range of safety with some of the minerals is relatively small. A two- to threefold increase in intake could elicit a toxic response.

The RDAs are not requirements, yet there is the tendency to view them as such when populations are studied with respect to nutrition and health. Individuals differ so much that identifying persons at risk for nutrient deficiency using the RDA as the standard of comparison is invalid. Rather, before such risk can be established, clinically established biochemical/physiological criteria of adequacy must be used. The usual nutrient intake can be estimated using the computed nutrient composition of food consumed, but whether that food sufficiently nourishes the individual can only be determined on the detailed assessment of that individual. Furthermore, although one can now easily evaluate the nutrient intake of the person's usual food consumption, the investigator should realize that a) people typically underestimate the quantities of food consumed and b) the handbooks of food composition may not be completely accurate. Just as individuals differ in their needs for and use of the foods they consume because of their genetic makeup, so too do the foods differ in the nutrients they contain. While the differences may not be large, they nonetheless exist.

Efforts to circumvent the concept that the RDA is synonymous with the requirement has led to the development of additional terms. The Food and Drug Agency (FDA) developed the term minimum daily requirement (MDA), a misnomer that implied knowledge about an individual's absolute need for a given nutrient. The MDA later was called the USRDA (Table 1.13). This term was developed for use in regulating the labeling of the nutrient content of food. It was based on the RDA. Note the differences between this table and Tables 1.11 and 1.12. The FDA has included those nutrients for which an RDA has not been set. The rationale for FDA to do this is to protect the consumer from overdosing on potentially toxic nutrients. The other main difference between the tables is the compression of the categories of consumers. The FDA recognized infants, children, adults, and pregnant or lactating women, whereas the Food and Nutrition Board subdivided these categories into age groups. Note also the differences in units. This table uses IU for the fat soluble vitamins A, D, and E, whereas the RDA table uses µg.

TABLE 1.13
U.S. Recommended Daily Allowances (U.S. RDAs)

	Infant	Children 4 and Under	Adults	Pregnant/lactating Women
Vitamin A, IU	1500	2500	5000	8000
Vitamin D, IU	400	400	400	400
Vitamin E, IU	5	10	30	30
Ascorbic acid, mg	35	40	60	60
Folacin, mg	0.1	0.2	0.4	0.8
Thiamine, mg	0.5	0.7	1.5	1.7
Riboflavin, mg	0.6	0.8	1.7	2.0
Niacin, mg	8	9	20	20
Pyridoxine, mg	0.4	0.7	2	2.5
Vitamin B12, µg	2	3	6	8
Biotin, mg	0.05	0.15	0.30	0.30
Pantothenic acid	3	5	10	10
Calcium, g	0.6	0.8	1	1
Phosphorous, g	0.6	0.8	1	1
Iodine, g	45	70	150	150
Iron, mg	15	10	18	18
Magnesium, mg	70	200	400	450
Copper, mg	0.6	1	2	2
Zinc, mg	5	8	15	15

In 1992, the FDA established further labeling regulations for processed foods. It established reference values that were based not only on RDA but also on the Surgeon General's Report on Nutrition and Health and on the recommendations for Diet and Health made by the Food and Nutrition Board of the National Research Council. Two terms were devised: the Reference Daily Intake (RDI) and the Daily Reference Values (DRV). These values are to be used as the basis for the nutrient labeling of packaged foods. The typical food label format is one that gives information about the nutrients that most concern the consumer. This information is presented as a percentage of the total recommended intake and assumes that the average consumer would consume 2000 kcal (8368 kJoules)/day. On the label the consumer might see that the product contained 10% of the recommended day's intake of protein. The consumer could read the label and learn that product A provided 10% of the day's allowance for protein, while product B provided 15%.

The consumer can then make a judgment about the relative nutritional value of the two products vis à vis protein. Again, just as the RDA does not provide individual values, neither do the DRV and the RDI. However, by using these percentages, the FDA attempted to provide the consumer with a way of comparing the nutritional value of products.

Devices to help the consumer understand how to select foods that provide appropriate amounts of different nutrients likewise have been based on the RDA. The USDA Nutrition Information Service has put forth the Food Pyramid. The American Dietetics Association has developed a food-exchange system that has many applications in planning meals for both normal persons and those needing to control their intakes of certain nutrients such as sodium or protein or fat or total energy. All of these devices are directed toward consumers to educate them about food choices that will assist them in maintaining good health.

SUPPLEMENTAL READINGS

Articles

Houston, D.K., Johnson, M.A., Poon, L.W. (1994) Individual foods and food group patterns of the oldest old. *J. Nutr. for the Elderly* 13:5-23.
Kumanyika, S., Tell, G.S., Fried, L., Martel, J.K., Chinchilli, V.M. (1996) Picture-sort method for administering a food frequency questionnaire to older adults. *JADA* 96:137-144.
Kinsella, K.G. (1992) Changes in life expectancy. *Am. J. Clin. Nutr.* 55:1196S-1202S.
Kirkwood, T.B.L. (1992) Comparative lifespans of species: Why do species have the lifespans they do? *Am. J. Clin. Nutr.* 55:1191S-1195S.
Ritchie, K. (1994) Senile dementia of the Alzheimer's Type (SDAT) epidemiology and public health issues. *Facts and Research in Gerontology* 4:2.
Rush, D. (1997) Nutrition screening in old people: Its place in a coherent practice of preventive health care. *Ann. Rev. Nutr.* 17:101-25.

Books

Berg, F. M. (1993) *Health Risks of Obesity.* Healthy Living Institute, 402 South 14th Street, Hettinger, ND 58639.
____ (1989) *Diet and Health.* Implications for Reducing Chronic Disease Risk. National Research Council. National Academy of Sciences, Washington, DC.
Lee, R.D. and Nieman, D. C. (1993) *Nutritional Assessment.* W.C.B. Brown and Benchmark, Madison, Wisconsin, 407 pages.
Shafrir, E. (1984,1988, 1990,1991) *Lessons in Animal Diabetes* (several volumes). John Libby/Smith Gordon Publishers.
Watson, R.R. (Ed.) (1994) *Handbook of Nutrition in the Aged, 2nd Edition,* CRC Press, Boca Raton, 445 pages.

Government Publications (U.S. Government Printing Office)

Putnam, J.J., Allshouse, J.E. (1997) Food Consumption, Prices, and Expenditures, 1970-95.
____Morbidity and Mortality Weekly Reports. U.S. Department of Health and Human Services.
____U.S. Recommended Daily Allowances, Federal Register, July 19, 1990 55:29477.

Journals that Specialize in Reporting on Gerontology Research

The International Journal of Aging and Human Development
Journal of Nutrition for the Elderly
Journal of Gerontology
Journal of Nutrition, Health and Aging
The Gerontologist

Other Publications

Holtsberg, P. (Ed.) (1994). *Georgia's Centenarians: The Quintessential Positive Models of Aging?* University of Georgia Gerontology Center Technical Report (IGAGC-94-01S), Athens, Georgia.

____*Gerontology Newsletter*, 11200 Montgomery Blvd. NE, Suite 8, El Dorado Square, Albuquerque, NM 87111.

____Dairy Council Digest 69:19-24, 1998.

2 Water

CONTENTS

OVERVIEW

Of the macronutrients mammals need, water is by far the most important. Deprived of water, man can live only three to four days. He can, however, survive much longer than this if deprived only of food. If deprived of food and water, the sensation of hunger abates after a short time, whereas the sensation of thirst tenaciously persists.

Water, as a nutrient, is essential because of its unique function as a solvent and as an important component of the temperature regulation system. Water is present throughout the body, yet is in constant flux between the various body compartments and between the internal and external environment. Water flux is so closely controlled that the total water content in the fat-free body remains constant in normal adults. In this unit, water as an essential nutrient will be discussed.

CHEMICAL AND PHYSICAL PROPERTIES OF WATER

The functions of water in the body relate directly to its unique chemical and physical properties. When compared with other common solvents such as ethanol, ether, acetone, methanol, or toluene, water has a higher freezing point, a higher boiling point, a higher specific heat of vaporization, a higher heat of fusion, and considerable surface tension. These unique properties are related to the great internal cohesion of the water molecules, which are due to the presence of relatively strong intermolecular forces. These forces are the result of an unequal sharing of electrons by the oxygen and hydrogen ions that compose the water molecule. Oxygen has a stronger affinity for electrons than does hydrogen (oxygen is more electron-negative) and thus, hydrogen tends to develop a partial positive charge while oxygen develops a partial negative charge. Just as oppositely charged magnets strongly attract each other, the hydrogen and oxygen atoms in different water molecules attract each other to create strong intermolecular forces. This electrostatic attraction, which keeps the oxygen and hydrogen from separate molecules in proximity, is called the hydrogen bond.

The electrons are arranged around oxygen in a nearly tetrahedral array. As a result, each water molecule is able to bond to four neighboring water molecules (see Figure 2.1). Through this kind of interaction among many water molecules, a lattice is formed. Hydrogen bonding exists in ice, liquid water, and water vapor. As the phase changes from solid to liquid to vapor, the average number of water molecules that associate decrease and the distance through which a hydrogen bond can be formed increases. This means a decrease in the intermolecular forces of attraction as heat is applied and, thus, the water changes its physical state. Water is a solid at temperatures below 0°C and vaporizes at temperatures above 100°C. Water must be heated to 600°C to completely dissipate the intermolecular forces described above. While the intermolecular forces are great, the hydrogen bonds themselves are not very stable. They form and reform with great ease and speed. The half life of the hydrogen bond in water is about 10^{-10} to 10^{-11} seconds. For this reason, water can be viewed as both fluid and rigid. The lattice-like structure of water, because it is constantly changing, has been aptly described as a "flickering cluster."

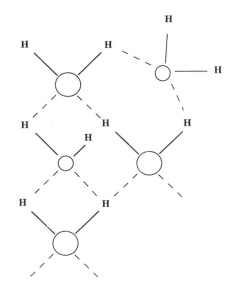

FIGURE 2.1   Schematic representation of water showing transient hydrogen bonding.

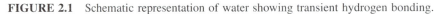

As a result of its dipolar nature, water dissolves or disperses many substances. It will form ionic solutions with salts such as sodium chloride, and it will form solutions with such polar compounds as ketones, sugars, and alcohols. It can dissolve these latter compounds because it will form hydrogen bonds with the polar groups of these substances. It will not form true solutions with large molecules such as proteins; instead, small particles of these proteins (1–100 nm) form colloidal solutions. Finally, as discussed in the unit on lipids, water is involved in the formation of emulsions. Emulsions are suspensions of particles in water with diameters in the range of 1–100 μm. Homogenized milk is an example of an emulsion of fat globules, protein particles, and other solutes in an aqueous medium. It is not a true solution.

FUNCTIONS OF WATER

Water serves many functions in the body. Due to its low thermal conductivity and high specific heat, it participates in the heat economy of the animal. Metabolic reactions in the cell produce heat, which can be absorbed by the water in the cell with no appreciable rise in temperature. The heat can then be transferred to the body surface and, through the vaporization process, can cool the body. Because of water's high heat of vaporization (586 cal/g water evaporated at 0°C), evaporative water losses can account for 25% of the total heat emission of the adult under nonstress conditions. This principle has been used to calculate the basal heat loss of animals (see Unit 3). Under the stress of an environment incapable of receiving heat from the animal by radiation, convection, or conduction, the total heat produced by the adult human may dissipate entirely as the latent heat from the vaporization of water. This is especially true if profuse sweating occurs and the relative humidity of the environment is low. Thus, the properties of water — high specific heat and high heat of vaporization — help maintain a relatively constant body temperature even though the environmental temperature may vary over a wide range. If body temperature were not to remain at or near 37°C (98.6°F), such processes as enzymatic reactions would be seriously impaired.

Because of its dipolar nature, water is an excellent solvent. Both true and colloidal solutions are formed, thus making possible the transport of large and small molecules throughout the body. Truly, it is said, water is the "medium of exchange in the body." Water is an essential constituent of all tissues. Many (but not all) enzymes are soluble in or suspended in water and most enzymes function best in an aqueous medium.

The high dielectric constant of water promotes the ionization of solutes, particularly the inorganic salts, thus facilitating their function as cofactors in a variety of metabolic processes. In metabolism, water participates in a number of reactions. It enters into compounds undergoing hydrolysis (addition of water) and is removed (dehydration) when other compounds are made. An example of the latter is the removal of one molecule of water when a peptide bond is formed during protein synthesis or when two monosaccharides are joined to form a disaccharide. Water also participates in the regulation of acid–base balance.

Another important function of water is that of a lubricant. Water in conjunction with a variety of proteins lubricates the joints and protects, through its lubricating action, a variety of important organs such as the heart, the intestines, the eyes, and the lungs. Water is the major component of the pericardial sac, the peritoneum, and the conjunctive and pleural sacs. The secretions of the salivary glands, the respiratory tract, and the gastrointestinal tract are primarily water, and among the functions of these secretions is that of lubrication.

BODY WATER

Water is ubiquitous and abundant in all living things. A living cell is approximately 80% water. Frequently, the amount of water in the body is given in terms of the lean body mass. Lean body mass refers to the weight of the body less its fat content. It includes muscle, bone, the internal organs, and essential structural lipids. Fat-free body mass, on the other hand, is not equivalent to lean body mass; it refers to the weight of the body less its fat content, including structural lipids. Because of the differences in the definition of lipid, i.e., the inclusion of structural lipids, the percentage of the total body weight that is lean body mass is slightly higher than that for fat-free body mass.

While body protein and body mineral content are fairly constant as a percentage of the body weight, body lipid and body water fluctuate in an inverse relationship to each other; i.e., as the percent body lipid increases, the percent body water decreases and vice versa. However, if the lipid content were to be excluded and only the lean body weight referred to, then the percentage of water remains relatively constant. For the normal adult, approximately two-thirds of the lean body weight is water. As a constituent of the body, it is the most abundant. The constancy of the body protein, minerals, and water in the lean body mass allows investigators to express values that relate to these components on a lean-body-weight basis. For example, the protein intake required for maintenance can be expressed as g protein required per g lean body weight under the assumption that the maintenance of the fat depots is a function of the energy intake and requires little or no protein. Expressing protein intake requirements in this fashion allows the comparison of protein nutritive need of animals of different body sizes or weights.

WATER COMPARTMENTS

Total body water (TBW) is distributed into two main compartments or spaces, the intracellular and the extracellular spaces. There are gender and age differences in TBW distribution. The water contained in the intracellular space — the intracellular water (ICW) — is that portion of the TBW that is contained within the cells. In normal healthy adults, about 55% of the TBW is found in the cells. However, differences do occur. Females tend to have equal quantities of water within and around the cells, whereas trained young male athletes, who have a relatively large skeletal muscle mass, have more TBW in the intracellular compartment than in the extracellular space.

Extracellular water (ECW) is distributed into several subcompartments (plasma, interstitial, and lymph fluids; fluids of the connective tissue, cartilage and bone; and transcellular fluids) that are not clearly defined. About 45% of TBW is found in the extracellular compartments.

Plasma is the fluid within the heart and blood vessels. It is the fluid in which the blood cells are suspended. The interstitial and lymph fluids are similar to plasma. There is an active exchange of water between the cells and the fluid surrounding them and between this fluid and the plasma. Dense connective tissue, cartilage and bone, and the transcellular fluids, however, do not participate to any great extent in this exchange. The transcellular water includes such fluids as the spinal and ocular fluids; the synovial fluid that lubricates joints; the fluids in the mucous secretions of the linings of the gastrointestinal, respiratory tract, and genitourinary tracts; and the fluids found in the pancreas, liver and biliary tree, thyroid and skin.

Accurate determination of ECW is difficult. Ideally, it requires a substance that does not penetrate into the cell, that is nontoxic in the required dose, that does not participate appreciably in metabolic reactions, and is distributed rapidly and evenly in all of the extracellular fluid. A tracer substance such as this has not been found. Certain saccharides, manitol and inulin, give a reasonable estimate of the interstitial and lymph fluid. Plasma volume can be measured by injection of Evans blue dye into the bloodstream. Knowing the volume and concentration of the injected dye allows for the calculation of the volume of distribution, i.e., the plasma volume, by determining the concentration of the dye in a blood sample drawn at a fixed time after dye injection. The equation $C_1V_1 = C_2V_2$ is used for this calculation. Estimates of the volume of the remaining components of the extracellular fluid can be obtained in experimental animals from direct chemical analysis of representative samples of individual tissues. This is not usually done in humans. The transcellular water volume is usually not determined experimentally. It is assumed to be the difference between the TBW and the measurable ECW and ICW.

COMPOSITION OF EXTRACELLULAR AND INTRACELLULAR FLUIDS

An important difference exists between the chemical composition of the fluids within the cells and those of the extracellular compartment. Intracellular fluid contains primarily potassium cations with phosphate, protein, and bicarbonate anions. Extracellular fluid is primarily a solution of sodium chloride. The composition of plasma is more precisely known than is that of interstitial or intracellular water. Table 2.1 shows the approximate composition of the plasma and the intracellular fluid in terms of concentration and charge. The number of solute molecules are similar in both compartments and so too are the number of charged particles. The serum has an osmolarity of about 312 and the cell fluid 307. Actually, this is only an estimate, because osmolarity can vary depending on the metabolic and nutritional state of the individual. For example, just after a meal, the blood will increase its content of the absorbed nutrients as these solutes (glucose, amino acids, etc.) are distributed to all parts of the body. Thus, the osmolarity of the serum will rise. The difference in the number of charged solutes between the serum and cell fluid is less variable. The serum has 322 meq/L while the cell fluid has 333. Ions or charged particles can move across the cell membrane and, in fact, do so as part of the active transport systems used to facilitate the entry of nutrients into the cell. These ion exchange systems are also used for the export of cell constituents. For example, the release of insulin by the pancreatic β cell involves the exchange of sodium, potassium, and calcium ions, the latter of which return to the islet cell to maintain its osmolarity and ion composition.

TABLE 2.1
Composition of Serum and Cell Fluid in Normal Human Blood

	Serum		Cell Fluid	
	mM/kg	mEq/L	mM/kg	mEq/L
Urea	7	—	7	—
Glucose	4	—	4	—
Other organic compounds	Variable	—	Variable	—
Sodium	150	150	27	27
Potassium	4	4	135	135
Calcium	3	5	0	0
Magnesium	1	2	3	5
Chloride	111	111	74	74
Bicarbonate	28	28	27	27
Inorganic Phosphate	2	3	2	3
Organic Phosphate	Trace	—	21	—
Sulfate	1	1	—	—
Protein	1	18	7	62
Total milliosmoles	312		307	
Total mEq/L		322		333

Water exchanges rapidly between the plasma, lymph, and interstitial fluids and between the interstitial and intracellular fluids. For instance, the water found in the capillaries will exchange with that found in the interstitial space several times a second. Diffusion, osmotic pressure, and hydrostatic pressure regulate the direction and rate of exchange.

Diffusion is the result of random motion of the molecules. Because of this motion, water molecules pass from one fluid compartment to another. Osmosis is the passage of water across a semipermeable membrane from an area of low solute–high solvent to an area of high solute–low solvent. By this process, the concentrations of the solutes and ions on each side of the semipermeable membrane are maintained. The osmotic pressure is the pressure that must be applied to prevent the flow of solvent. It can be calculated using the same equation as is used to calculate gas pressure: $P = 0.082 \, TC$ where P is the pressure, T the absolute temperature, and C the concentration of the solutes in mols/L. The figure 0.082 is a constant. Using this equation, the osmotic pressure of blood plasma at 37°C should be $0.082 \times 310 \times 0.31$ or about 7.9 atmospheres. This is not the actual pressure because, as mentioned above, the plasma membrane is semipermeable and some of the solutes do pass through it. Thus, the figure 7.9 is only an approximation, not true osmotic pressure as defined by the physical chemist. Only those particles that do not pass through the semipermeable membrane contribute to osmotic pressure. Thus, the proteins contribute to this pressure because they do not pass through the membrane unassisted. The osmotic pressure does not depend on the nature of the solvent particles; it depends, instead, on their number. A solution of NaCl, which completely dissociates to sodium ions and chloride ions, will have twice the osmotic pressure of an equimolar solution of glucose, which does not dissociate.

A specialized form of osmotic pressure is oncotic, or colloid osmotic pressure. The proteins of the plasma do not pass through the capillary membrane, the point at which most of the water exchange between plasma and the interstitial space occurs; hence, a concentration gradient and its associated osmotic pressure exist at this membrane. The term colloidal pressure is applied to this type of osmotic pressure because the solutes are large protein molecules that are held in the solution (plasma) as colloids.

Hydrostatic pressure is the pressure that is caused by the weight of a column of water. In a large chamber of water, the pressure on the surface of the water is equal to atmospheric pressure. For each 13.6 mm below the surface of the water, there is a corresponding pressure increase of 1 mm mercury. Hydrostatic pressure also occurs in the vascular system of the human being; the pressure of the fluids in the arteries descending to the feet is greater than that in the neck. Hydrostatic pressure will push fluid out of the capillaries into the interstitial space and hence into the intercellular fluids. The various pressures — osmotic, hydrostatic, and that exerted by the pumping action of the heart — serve to regulate the volume of the water in each of the water compartments. Should any of these regulatory mechanisms become compromised, water will not move as easily between the compartments, and will accumulate. When water accumulates, the clinical condition known as edema develops.

The transport of substances against a concentration gradient requires energy. This is called osmotic work. A number of metabolically important substances are transported this way. Energy-driven transport, also called active transport, is essential to living systems. For example, nutrients released through the enzymatic breakdown of the consumed food are in many instances actively transported against a concentration gradient into the enterocyte or absorptive cell. Osmotic work can be calculated using the same equation format we use to determine metabolic energy flux. Osmotic work is equivalent to the free energy change (ΔF) associated with the process. Thus, the equation

$$-\Delta F = nRT \ln \frac{C_1}{C_2}$$

where ΔF = change in free energy in calories
      n = number of mols of a substance transported
      R = gas constant = 1.987 cal/°C
      T = temperature in °K
      C_1 = lower concentration from which substance is transported
      C_2 = higher concentration to which substance is transported

The absorption of nutrients by the enterocyte thus uses energy and later when the energy losses from the food consumed is discussed (Unit 3), this use of energy is subtracted from the gross energy of the food. All this because of the need to actively transport needed nutrients from the gut lumen into the body.

The kidney is another organ that uses a lot of energy as it serves its function in the excretion of waste products. Urea, in particular, requires considerable energy for its excretion. In fact, it has been estimated that the kidneys account for a large portion (10–35%) of the total basal body energy expenditure simply because this tissue must export a variety of metabolic end products using active transport systems. The osmotic work of the kidney, especially in people consuming large excesses of protein, can be quite substantial.

CELL STRUCTURE AND FUNCTION

The typical cell (Figure 2.2) consists of a nucleus, mitochondria, lysosomes, endoplasmic reticulum, golgi apparatus, and microsomes surrounded by the cell sap or cytosol. Membranes surround each of these organelles as well as the cell itself. Each segment or organelle has a particular function and is characterized by specific reactions and metabolic pathways. These are listed in Table 2.2.

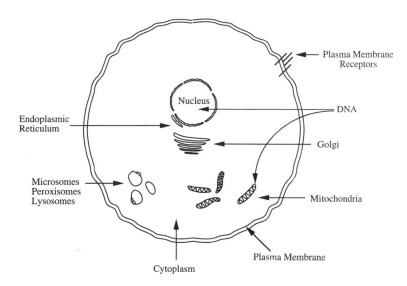

FIGURE 2.2 Typical eukaryotic cell showing representative intracellular structures.

Receptors

Among the specific structures in the cell are a group of proteins called receptors. There are both plasma and intracellular membrane receptors. Plasma membrane receptors typically bind peptides or proteins. These are called ligands. In many instances these compounds are hormones, or growth factors. Upon binding, one of two processes occurs. In one, the binding of the peptide or protein (ligand) to its cognate receptor is followed by an internalization of this ligand–receptor complex. In the other, the receptor is not internalized, but when ligand bound, generates a signal that alters cell metabolism and function. Internalization allows for the entry of the ligand or its activated fragment into the cell where it may target specific intracellular components. The ligand can either transfer to another receptor or move to its target site in the cell by itself as it dissociates from its plasma membrane receptor. The receptor in turn is either recycled back to the plasma membrane or it is degraded. Figure 2.3 illustrates this plasma membrane–hormone binding.

There are actually four types of membrane-spanning receptors: 1) simple receptors that have a single membrane-spanning unit; 2) receptors with a single membrane-spanning unit that also involves a tyrosine kinase component on the interior aspect of the plasma membrane; 3) receptors with several membrane-spanning helical segments of their protein structures that are coupled to a separate G-protein on the interior aspect of the plasma membrane; and 4) receptors that not only have membrane-spanning units but also have a membrane-spanning ion channel. Examples of each of these are shown in Table 2.3.

Immunoglobulins typically are moved into the cell via the single membrane-spanning receptor, as are nerve growth factor and several other growth factors. The receptors for these proteins are usually rich in cysteine. The cysteine-rich region projects out from the plasma membrane and is important for the binding of its ligand through disulfide bonds. Insulin and thyroid-stimulating

TABLE 2.2
Functions of the Organelles/Cell Fractions that the Typical Eukaryotic Cell Comprises

Organelle/Cell Fraction	Role in Cell	Processes Found
Plasma membrane	Cell boundary holds receptors for a variety of hormones; signal systems begin here	Processes, exports and imports substrates, ions, etc., binds hormones to their respective receptors
Cytosol	Medium for a variety of enzymes, substrates, products, ions, transporters, and signal systems	Glycolysis, glycogenesis, glycogenolysis, lipogenesis, pentose shunt, urea synthesis (part, protein synthesis (part)
Nucleus	Contains DNA, RNA, and many proteins that influence gene expression	Protein synthesis starts here with DNA transcription
Endoplasmic Reticulum	Ca^{++} stored here for use in signal tranduction; glucose transporters accumulate here until needed	Has role in many synthetic processes
Golgi apparatus	Sequesters, processes and releases proteins	Export mechanism for release of macromolecules
Mitochondria	Powerhouse of cell; contains DNA that encodes 13 components of oxidative phosphorylation	Krebs cycle, respiratory chain, ATP synthesis, fatty acid oxidation, first step of urea synthesis
Ribosomes	Site for completion of protein synthesis	Protein synthesis
Lysosomes	Intracellular digestion	Protein and macromolecule degradation
Peroxisomes	Suppression of oxygen free radicals	Antioxidant enzymes
Microsomes	Drug detoxification	Detoxification, fatty acid elongation

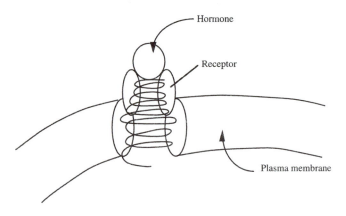

FIGURE 2.3   Schematic representation of a hormone bound to its cognate receptor in the plasma membrane.

hormone are moved into the cell via a single membrane-spanning unit that has tyrosine kinase activity. There is considerable homology between the first type and this type of receptor in the portion of the receptor that binds the ligand. Where the receptors differ is in the portion that extends into and projects through the interior aspect of the plasma membrane. On the interior aspect of these single-membrane-spanning receptors is a tyrosine kinase domain.

The tyrosine kinase portion of the receptor is involved in the intracellular signaling systems. These can be very complex cascades, as illustrated in Figure 2.4. In this illustration, an ion (Ca^+) channel is also depicted, as are the two major intracellular signaling systems, the phosphatidylinositol (PIP) and the adenylate cyclase signaling systems.

TABLE 2.3
Types of Plasma Membrane Receptors and Examples of Ligands

a) Single membrane spanning unit, no tyrosine kinase
    Ligands: Immunoglobulins
                        T-cell antibodies
                        Insulin like growth factor (IGF)
                        Nerve growth factor (NGF)
                        Growth hormone (GH)
b) Single membrane spanning unit with tyrosine kinase activity
    Ligands: Thyroid stimulating hormone (TSH)
                        Insulin
                        Platelet derived growth factor (PDGF)
c) Multiple membrane spanning unit coupled with G protein
    Ligands: Calcitonin
                        Parathormone
                        Luteinizing hormone
                        Rhodopsin
                        Acetylcholine
                        Thyrotropin releasing hormone
d) Multiple membrane spanning unit coupled with G protein and an ion channel
    Ligand: γ aminobutyric acid (GABA)

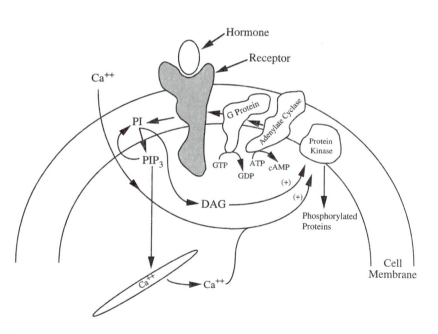

FIGURE 2.4   Hormone-receptor reaction that involves G proteins, adenylate cyclease, proteins, the PIP cycle and cAMP. When the hormone binds to the receptor, a cascade of events follows. The G protein (a protein that binds GTP) moves over the receptor protein and binds GTP. Adenylate cyclase moves over and binds to the G protein and, in the process, energy is released. The cAMP level then rises and through the action of phosphodiesterase is converted to 5′ AMP. ATP is regenerated by the mitochondrial oxidative phosphorylation system or through substrate phosphorylation. The ATP furnishes the phosphate group and the energy for the subsequent phosphorylation of intracellular proteins via the membrane-bound protein, kinase. This enzyme is also stimulated by the calcium ion and diacylglycerol, one of the products of the PIP signaling system.

Once the ligand has entered the cell, one of two events occurs. If the ligand is a hormone that has its primary effect at the plasma membrane, then its "job" is done. It will then be taken into the cell and degraded via the enzymes of the lysosomes. If the ligand has an intracellular function, it will move to its target within the cell. One of these targets may be DNA. The ligand may be transferred to an intracellular transport protein and/or to another receptor protein that has DNA-binding capacity or may bind directly to the DNA affecting its transcription. These binding proteins make up another group of receptor proteins, the intracellular receptors. These intracellular receptors function in the movement of ligands from the plasma membrane to their respective targets. In this instance, the ligands may be lipid-soluble materials, or minerals or vitamins, or carbohydrates, peptides, or proteins. There is no evidence that these receptors participate in the intracellular signaling cascades except as recipients of their ligands.

Intracellular receptors bind such compounds as the retinoids, vitamin D, certain minerals, steroid hormones, thyroxine, and some of the small amino acid derivatives that regulate metabolism. As such, they serve to move these materials from their site of entry to their site of action. In many instances, these receptors bind DNA and thereby function in the mode of action of their ligand. The steroid receptors, for example, each bind a specific steroid. These receptor proteins are grouped together and referred to as the steroid hormone super family of receptors. This is something of a misnomer, because not all of the ring-structured compounds they bind are steroids or steroid hormones. For example, these receptors bind thyroxine, retinoic acid, and the peroxisome prolif-erators (PPARs). In some instances, the receptor protein binds the DNA and more than one of these ring structures at the same time. Figure 2.5 illustrates a generic steroid hormone receptor. In this receptor there are six basic domains that have functional importance with respect to its action in transcription. Of interest is the homology that exists among the various members of this super family of receptors. 60–95% of the amino acid sequence of the zinc finger domain is homologous; 65–75% of the heat shock domain (HSP) is homologous; and 30–60% of the ligand-binding domain is homologous.

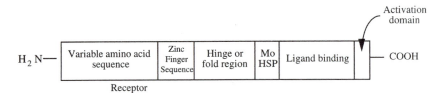

FIGURE 2.5 Generic structure of a receptor having a single polypeptide chain with six basic domains. The first is a variable amino acid sequence that confers immunologic identity to the receptor. The second is the zinc finger domain, which is rich in histidine and cysteine. Next is the hinge or fold region, which provides flexibility to the polypeptide chain. This is followed by the ligand-binding domain and the activation domain.

The regions where nonhomology exists determine which of the many ligands will be bound. The first hypervariable region allows researchers to separate these receptors based on their immu-noreactivity. This has use in the study of gene expression, especially in the area where investigators are trying to understand how specific nutrients affect the expression of specific genes. Other members of the receptor class of cellular components bind specific ligands and in turn may also bind to DNA at specific base sequences called elements. There are specific proteins that bind copper or zinc or one or more of the vitamins or one of the many amino acids, fatty acids, carbohydrates, or metabolites. In addition, there are intracellular receptors that bind one or more of these substances but do not bind to DNA. Instead, these binding proteins serve as transporters of their ligands from their point of entry to their point of use. Altogether, the proteins called receptors are important structural components of living cells.

Signal Systems

Once hormones are bound to their cognate receptors, changes in cell function occur. How are these changes brought about? As mentioned in the section on plasma membrane receptors, a number of hormones, particularly the protein and peptide hormones, affect cellular metabolism via a signaling system. There are several of these. Some couple to adenylate cyclase, others to guanylate cyclase, and still others involve the phosphatidylinositol pathway. Some use the calcium ion as a second messenger and others use ion channels. Some hormones use elements of all of these in signaling the cell to respond appropriately. Table 2.4 lists some of the hormones and the signaling systems they use. A hormone that uses the G protein as part of its signaling system does so when bound to its cognate receptor. G proteins are proteins that are bound by the nucleotide guanosine diphosphate (GDP). When the hormone binds to the receptor, a conformational change occurs that causes the G protein to exchange guanosine triphosphate (GTP) for GDP. This activates the G protein. The activated G protein modulates the catalytic subunit of the membrane-bound adenylate cyclase, which in turn catalyzes the conversion of ATP to cyclic AMP. Cyclic AMP stimulates protein kinase A, which phosphorylates a number of proteins, usually enzymes, thereby amplifying the original signal elicited by the binding of the hormone to the receptor.

TABLE 2.4
Some Hormones and their Signaling Systems

Hormone	System
Atrial natriuretic hormone (ANH)	Cyclic GMP
Bradykinin, $\alpha2$ adrenergic norepinephrine somatostatin	Cyclic AMP (decreases cAMP)
ACTH	Cyclic AMP and PIP pathway
Acetylcholine	Ion channel
Calcitonin, FSH, Glucagon PTH, Vasopressin, β adrenergic norepinephrine	Cyclic AMP (increases cAMP)

Some G proteins are coupled to the PIP_3 phospholipase C pathway. Phospholipase C catalyzes the hydrolysis of the membrane phospholipid, phosphatidylinositol releasing two second messengers, diacylglycerol (DAG) and phosphatidylinositol 4,5 phosphate (PIP_2), which is phosphorylated to the 1,4,5 phosphate form (PIP_3). Each of these second messengers has its own targets. PIP_3 migrates to the endoplasmic reticulum and, when bound to its receptor on this organelle, opens up a calcium channel. The calcium ions sequestered in the endoplasmic reticulum are then free to migrate out into the cytoplasm, whereupon they serve as cofactors in several reactions or are bound to calmodulin or stimulate exocytosis. This latter function is important to the insulin-producing β cell of the pancreatic islets. Insulin is exocytosed and this exocytosis is calcium stimulated.

DAG, the other second messenger released through the action of phospholipase C, binds to an allosteric binding site on protein kinase C which, in the presence of phosphatidylserine and the calcium ion, becomes activated so that still another group of proteins become phosphorylated.

G proteins also regulate the ion channels in both the plasma membrane and the sarcoplasmic reticulum. There are two types of channels, one that is voltage gated (depolarization/repolarization) and those that are coupled to specific membrane receptors via G proteins. Altogether then, hormones that bind to membrane-bound receptor proteins elicit their effects on cell function via an integrated set of intracellular signals. These signal cascades are both simple and complex and involve a number of different proteins, each having a specific role in this signal transduction.

CELL DIFFERENTIATION

Although all nucleated cells possess the same DNA, some of the specific DNA regions (genes) are not transcribed or translated. If translated, some gene products are not very active. Thus, not all cells have the same processes with the same degree of activity. Cellular differentiation has taken place so that muscle cells differ from fat cells, which differ from brain cells, and so forth. In each cell type there are processes and metabolic pathways that may be unique to that cell type. An example is the great lipid storage capacity of the adipocyte, a feature not found in a bone or brain or muscle cell, although each of these cells does contain some lipid. Similarly, the capacity to form and retain a mineral appetite (a mixture of different minerals) is characteristic of a bone cell; the synthesis of contractile proteins by muscle cells is also an example of cell uniqueness. Cells differ in their choice of metabolic fuel. Hepatic and muscle cells make, store, and use significant amounts of glycogen. Adipocytes and hepatocytes make, store, and sometimes use triacyglycerols. All of these special features have an impact on the composition of specific organs and tissues in the body that collectively contribute to body composition. Analysis of the composition of specific organs and tissues does not necessarily reflect the whole body composition. One must consider the function of each organ and tissue in the context of the whole body. Similarly, the determination of the activity of a single process in a single cell type or organ may not necessarily predict the activity (and cumulative result) of that process in the whole body. However, some processes are unique to certain tissues so some exceptions to the above role are possible. For example, one can measure glycogenesis in samples of liver and muscle and be fairly confident that these measures will represent whole body glycogen synthesis.

With respect to cell function and its contribution to the body's metabolic processes, mention should be made of the differing rates of cell renewal or cell half-life. Cells differ in their lifespan depending on their location and function. Skin cells (epithelial cells) are short lived compared with brain cells. The turnover time for an epithelial cell in man is of the order of seven days. Brain cells are not regenerated and renewal of neural tissue is fragmented. That is, there is turnover of individual cellular components such as the lipid component but the cell once formed is not replaced as an entity, as are the epithelial cells. Shown in Table 2.5 are some estimates of the lifespan of several sources of epithelial cells in man and in rats. While the average lifespan of man is on the order of 70 years, that of the rat is between 2 and 3 years. Despite this species difference in whole-body lifespan, the lifespan of epithelial cells is surprisingly similar.

TABLE 2.5
Lifespan of Epithelial Cells From Different Organs in Man and Rat

Cell Type	(Days)	
	Human	Rat
Cells lining the gastrointestinal tract	2–8	1.4–1.6
Cells lining the cervix	5.7	5.5
Skin cells	13–100	19.1
Corneal epithelial cells	7	6.9

The half-life of a cell can be calculated using measurements of the appearance and/or disappearance of a labeled material such as thymidine. Thymidine is taken up by the nuclear DNA as the cell prepares to divide or renew itself. It then disappears as the cell dies. By definition, the half-life of the cell (or of any biologically active material) is defined as the amount of time required for half of the number of cells or amount of active material to disappear or be eliminated. Careful measurements of both time and the number of labeled cells or biologic material must be made.

The fractional elimination constant (which is the same as the fractional appearance rate) can then be calculated and the half-life of the item in question derived. Suppose the number of cells initially equals Co. Over a period of time (t), this number is reduced to half (the half-life).

The equation $\dfrac{dC}{dt} = k_e C_o$ can be written and solved as follows:

$C = C_o e^{-kt}$
$\ln C = \ln C_o - k_e t$
Rearranging gives us $\ln (C_o/C) = k_e t$
At one half-life, $C = 0.5 C_o$
Therefore, $\ln (2.0) = k_e t_{1/2}$
$0.693 = k_e t_{1/2}$
$t^{1/2} = 0.693/k_e$

Note that 0.693 is always equal to the natural log of 2. This concept of half-life is part of the overall concept of steady state. Steady state, a feature of living systems, is that state where no net change occurs yet there is a steady flow of materials through the system. There are no net losses or gains, merely maintenance of the status quo. This probably characterizes the steady ebbs and flows of the adult non-pregnant, non-growing adult. In this individual, there is no body weight gain or loss, no change in skeletal or muscle mass, no measurable changes in body function. Perturbation of steady state occurs from birth to death under well-defined conditions but in the adult the steady state is the maintenance state.

APOPTOSIS

The half-life of cells varies throughout the body. It depends on a variety of factors including age, nutritional status, health status, genetics, as well as factors not yet identified. Age is important. Growing individuals are in a phase of life in which cell number is increasing exponentially. Once growth and development are complete, this increase in cell number slows down. In contrast, senescence is characterized by a gradual loss in total cell number as well as losses in discrete cell types. In part, these changes in cell number are analogous to the observations of cell biologists, who have reported on the growth of cells in culture. These cells go through a rapid growth phase doubling in number for 50–100 generations. Eventually, the cells reach a "turning point" and grow poorly or not at all, despite the continual provision of new media. Finally, the culture ceases to thrive and the number of cells begins to decline. At this time, the cells begin to die off slowly through a process called apoptosis or programmed cell death. Cell cultures that do not become apoptotic are called immortal; i.e., they do not have the mechanism for programmed cell death. These cells have been genetically altered so that they can sustain themselves indefinitely. This alteration in the genetic control of the life of a cell is called transformation. Transformed cells are powerful research tools and allow for the study of these cells in culture so as to learn about their metabolism. In particular, cell growth has been studied and a number of growth factors have been identified that have relevance to our understanding of how mammalian growth and development occurs. Now, interest is building in learning how cells senesce and die through the process of apoptosis. This is relevant to our understanding of how cell turnover is controlled.

Cell turnover has two parts: cell replacement and cell death. Cell death is either a concerted, all-at-once event or a programmed, gradual process. If the former, cell death is called necrosis. This occurs if a tissue sustains an injury, small or large. A small cut in the skin results in necrosis of the injured cells in and around the cut. A ruptured coronary vessel results in the death of the heart muscle supplied by that vessel. If only a small capillary ruptures, the necrosis of the myocardium will be small. If a larger vessel ruptures, damage to the heart can be quite large and indeed may be a mortal event. Necrotic cell death is preceded by cell enlargement and a swelling of all the organelles within the cell. The DNA disintegrates and its nucleotides are degraded.

In contrast, programmed cell death or apoptosis involves a shrinkage of the cell and enzyme-catalyzed DNA fragmentation. This fragmentation can be detected as a laddering when the DNA is extracted from the cell and separated by electrophoresis. Apoptosis is a process that is an integral part of living systems. It is part of the growth process as well as the maintenance of cell and tissue function. It is also part of wound healing and recovery from traumatic injury. Adipose tissue remodeling, immune function, epithelial cell turnover, and the periodic shedding of the uterine lining are but a few examples of this process. Apoptosis is viewed as a defense mechanism to remove unwanted and potentially dangerous cells such as virally infected cells or tumor cells. The process involves the mitochondria as the "central executioner." The mitochondria produce reactive oxygen (free radicals) as well as other materials that participate in apoptosis. Alterations in mitochondrial function have been observed to occur prior to any other feature of apoptosis. A decrease in mitochondrial membrane potential that, in turn, affects membrane permeability, is an early event. The increase in permeability is followed by a release of cytochrome c that in turn regulates the caspases, which are cysteine proteases. These caspases stimulate the proteolysis of key cell proteins in various parts of the cell. Altogether, the fragmentation of the DNA and the destruction of cell proteins result in the death of the cell via a very orderly process.

TABLE 2.6
Contributory Factors in the Regulation of Apoptosis

Factor	Effect Suppress	Effect Stimulate
Age		√
Apaf-1 protein		√
P53 protein		√
Bcl 2 protein	√	
Bcl-x_3 protein		√
Bcl-x_L protein	√	
Bax protein		√
Bak protein		√
WAF-1		√
ced 3 and 4		√
Glucocorticoids		√
ced 9	√	
High zinc	√	
Low zinc		√
Low retinoic acid	√	
High retinoic acid		√
Interleukin 1β		√
Leptin		√
TNFα		√
Insulin	√	
Low manganese		√
IGF$_1$	√	
Low SOD activity		√
Peroxidized lipid		√

Apoptosis is the mechanism used in the thymus to eliminate thymocytes that are self reactive. By doing so, the development of autoimmune disease is suppressed. Indeed, this mechanism is being examined as an explanation of autoimmune insulin-dependent diabetes mellitus. Apoptosis is being carefully studied to learn about the signals that initiate or suppress it. Figure 2.6 illustrates the process of apoptosis and Table 2.6 lists some of the signals and regulatory compounds that influence this process.

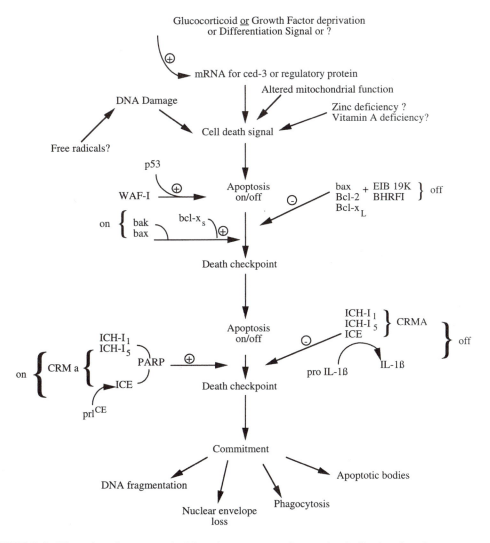

FIGURE 2.6   Flow chart for apoptosis. Note the many question marks, indicating that there are as many unknown factors in this process as there are known.

Many cells can be stimulated to become apoptotic. The p53 protein, for example, can induce apoptosis as one of its modes of protecting the body against tumor cells. The p53 protein is a DNA-binding protein. Mutations in tumor cells that inactivate p53 have been found. The result of such mutation is that tumor cells grow and multiply. The gene for p53 likewise can mutate and this mutation has been associated with tumor development and growth. Apparently, this gene has several "hot spots" (likely places for mutation to occur), which explains its role in carcinogenesis and its loss in normal function. The bcl-2 protein, a membrane-bound cytoplasmic protein, is another player in this regulation of apoptosis. It is a member of the family of proteins called protooncogenes.

Its normal function is to protect valuable cells against apoptosis. It is down regulated when cells are stimulated to die. Inappropriately high bcl-2 protein levels can provoke cell overgrowth. The cell regulates bcl-2 protein so as to maintain a normal homeostatic state. Bcl-2 and its homologue, Bcl-xL, blocks apoptosis. Both Bcl-2 and Bcl-xL can heterodimerize with Bax or Bcl-xs and, when Bcl-2 or Bcl-xL is overexpressed, an enhancement of oxidative stress mutagenesis can be observed. This occurs because these proteins suppress the apototic process, allowing more exposure of the cell to DNA damage by mutagens.

Nutrients play a role in apoptosis. High levels of zinc (500 μm) have been found to block apoptosis in cultured thymocytes. The zinc blocks the action of glucocorticoids in stimulating apoptosis. Zinc also interferes with tumor necrosis factor (TNF)-induced apoptosis as well as heat-induced death. In contrast, low levels of zinc (0.3 to 200 μm) have the reverse effect. That is, at low levels of zinc, apoptosis could be stimulated by TNF, glucocorticoid and heat exposure. The mechanism whereby zinc has these effects must be multifaceted. Zinc has an important role in transcription control as part of the zinc fingers but it is not known how this relates to apoptosis.

Manganese, another essential nutrient, also is involved as a cofactor for superoxide dismutase (SOD). In instances where SOD is less active than normal, apoptosis is stimulated coincident with an increase in C_2-ceramide, TNFα, and hydrogen peroxide. Peroxides form from unsaturated fatty acids as well as certain of the amino acids. There may be a link, therefore, between the fatty acid intake of the individual and apoptosis of certain cell types. In one study of genetically obese diabetic rats, an increase in fatty acid intake was associated with an increase in β cell apoptosis.

Retinoic acid (and dietary vitamin A) deficiency stimulates apoptosis. The well-known feature of vitamin A deficiency (suppressed immune function) suggests that vitamin A and its metabolite, retinoic acid, serve to influence the sequence of events leading to cell death. This link is made because it is known that T cell apoptosis is an important defense mechanism and T cells are part of the immune system. Vitamin A is also an antiproliferative agent, so its effect on abnormal cell growth is two pronged — it stimulates apoptosis and suppresses proliferation.

Genetic regulation of apoptosis involves not only the transcription factors mentioned above but also specific genes. Already described are the p53 and bcl-2 DNA-binding proteins that, like zinc, retinoic acid, and fatty acids, affect gene expression. Add to this list the mitogen-activated protein kinases (p42/44) Erk1 and Erk2. When phosphorylated, these proteins suppress apoptosis in brown adipocytes. Apoptosis is also suppressed by certain of the cytokines (IL6, IL3, interferon (γ) and stimulated by others (leptin). Finally, the gene Nedd 2 encodes a protein similar to the nematode cell death gene ced 3 and the mammalian interleukin 1β-converting enzyme. Overexpression of this gene induces apoptosis.

With the understanding of apoptosis comes the understanding of how and why the body changes in its composition as it ages from conception to death. The young animal has little fat, while the older one has gained fat sometimes at the expense of body protein. Clearly, the body is continually being remodeled, and quite clearly this remodeling is the result of a combination of many factors including the apoptotic process.

BODY COMPOSITION

Of the four major body constituents — fat, protein, water, and ash (minerals) — water is by far the most abundant. Normal bodies usually consist of 16–20% protein, 3–5% ash (mineral matter), 10–12% fat, and 60–70% water. Age, diet, genetic background, physical activity, hormonal status, and gender can affect not only the proximate composition of the whole body — that is, the magnitude of each of these components — but also their distribution.

Regardless of the methods used to estimate lean body mass, total body water, and percent body lipid, it is generally agreed that the composition of the human body, as well as the bodies of other species, can vary. Age, sex, degree of physical activity, and diet have all been shown to affect body composition. For example, a 175-g fetus contains 154 g of water (88%); a 3.5-kg baby contains 2.4 kg of water (69%); and a 70-kg man contains 42 kg of water (60%). As the human progresses from conception to birth to maturity, the percentage of water decreases and, as mentioned previously, the percentage of fat increases. Actively growing tissue has a high water content and very little fat.

Differences in water content on the basis of sex have also been observed in adults. Females tend to have less water and more fat than do males. These differences can be attributed in part to the effects of the female sex hormones on fat synthesis and deposition and, in part, to the tendency of young adult males to engage in more-strenuous physical activities that increase their muscle mass and hence their bodies' water content.

Diet, particularly energy-rich diets that increase fat deposition, affects body composition. For example, Brozek and Keys found that in overfed men who gained weight, 14% of the weight gain was due to an increase in extracellular fluid, 24% was an increase in cellular components, and 62% was an increase in fat. When humans are fed energy-poor diets, changes in body composition can also be observed. One such subject was followed for 60 days and, as might be anticipated, showed a loss in body weight, body fat, and body water. The pattern of loss is shown in Figure 2.7. Weight loss and regain (weight cycling) alter body composition, particularly the distribution of the body fat. There is a tendency to accumulate subcutaneous fat at the expense of visceral fat by obese people who lose weight and then regain it, yet their total body fat following regain is not different from that prior to weight loss.

While each cell type has a unique composition and organization, altogether they contribute to the composition of the whole body. Frequently, nutritionists wish to know whether dietary and non-dietary factors affect body composition. Researchers might want to know, for example, whether changes in dietary protein can affect the protein content of the whole body or whether a certain exercise routine affects the body fat content, or how age affects bone mineral content. In small animals, body composition can be determined directly. The fat content is the difference in body weight before and after extraction with a fat solvent. Typically a 2:1 mixture of chloroform:methanol is used.

$$\% \text{ Fat} = \frac{\text{body weight} - \text{extracted body weight}}{\text{body weight}}$$

Similarly, % body water can be determined as the difference in body weight before and after drying.

$$\% \text{ body water} = \frac{\text{body weight} - \text{dried body weight}}{\text{body weight}}$$

The percent of the body that is mineral (ash) is determined as the difference in body weight before and after all the organic matter is oxidized using a muffle furnace. This furnace can achieve heat up to 3000° and will oxidize everything except the mineral matter.

$$\% \text{ body ash} = \frac{\text{body weight after complete oxidation}}{\text{body weight}}$$

Finally, the protein content of the body is determined by measuring the nitrogen content and multiplying by 6.25 to convert to protein and then calculating percentage as above:

$$\% \text{ body protein} = \frac{\text{nitrogen content} \times 6.25}{\text{body weight}}$$

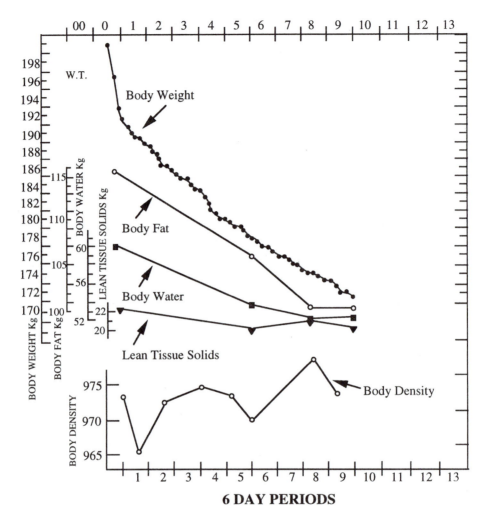

FIGURE 2.7   Changes in body weight, total body water, and body density, and calculated fat and lean tissue solids in a subject consuming 800 calories per day. (From Berlin et al., *Metab.* 11:302, 1962.)

Body composition is not measured directly using the whole body but rather using a sample taken from a homogenate of the whole body. In this manner, all components (water, ash, fat, protein) in the same body can be determined using a small sample size.

A limited amount of data are available (Table 2.7) on the body composition of the adult human as determined through direct measurements; however, most of the data in the literature on humans are based on indirect or derived values for each of the major body components. Sequential estimates of body fat, bone density, body water, or protein content are possible using sophisticated instrumentation together with established methods for estimating the magnitude of the fat store and the lean body mass.

The data in Table 2.7 were collected in the early 50s from persons who had donated their bodies for scientific research. Ages and causes of death varied widely. Four of the ten patients had died from heart disease, two were accident victims. The others died from a variety of degenerative diseases. The values were obtained from many very small samples of tissues taken as representative of each tissue type.

It is not always practical, however, to determine the body composition directly. The animal under study may be too large for convenient handling, or one may wish to make sequential

TABLE 2.7
**Proximate Composition
of Adult Humans**

% water	50–70
% fat	4–27
% protein	14–23
% ash	4.9–6

measurements in the same body, i.e., to study changes in body composition in response to dietary or nondietary (e.g., exercise) treatments, or one may wish to work with humans. In the latter instance, direct measurements would be out of the question. Indirect methods must be used.

Lean body mass can be calculated if one assumes that the fat-free body has a constant water content (72%) and that the neutral fat is stored dry. Thus, the formula

$$\text{LBM (kg)} = \frac{\text{Total body water (kg)}}{0.72}$$

can be used. The figure 72% is an average figure derived from careful direct measurements of the water content of lean tissue. It may not be applicable to all situations. To confirm the usefulness of the 0.72 figure, a biopsy of the lean tissue must be obtained and its water content determined. This may not be practical, so 0.72 is generally assumed to be usable. TBW and body fat must also be determined. TBW can be measured by infusing heavy water (deuterium), allowing this to equilibrate within the body and then withdrawing a sample of blood. This method is called the Water Dilution Method. Knowing the concentration of the deuterated water, the volume that was infused, and the concentration in the blood sample withdrawn, one can calculate the volume of dilution of the infused labeled water. This will provide a value for TBW.

The calculation of TBW is as follows: $C_1V_1 = C_2V_2$ where V_2 is the volume in which the solute is distributed or the TBW. Dividing TBW by 0.72 (as per the above equation) gives an estimate of the lean body mass (LBM). LBM is also equal to the total body mass minus its fat content.

Lean body mass can also be predicted from skeletal measurements and from bone weight. Sophisticated techniques using ultrasound, neutron activation analysis, infrared interactance, dual energy x-ray absorptiometry, computer-assisted tomography, magnetic resonance imaging, or bio-electrical impedance are available, and, as the instrumentation improves, these methods may become practical in the clinical setting. Presently, considerable effort is being expended to validate these methods because they are noninvasive and allow for the sequential determination of changes in one or more of the major body components as a result of a change in diet, activity, age, or endocrine status. In addition, these noninvasive methods could be useful in assessing population groups in relation to fat mass, bone density, or adipose tissue distribution. For example, Sohlström et al. used magnetic resonance imaging (MRI). They compared these estimates with those obtained from underwater weighing and from body water dilution studies. The three methods gave similar results with MRI and body weight dilution providing 1.4 ± 2.9% less and 4.7 ± 4.0% more, respectively, than underwater weighing for total body fat. However, because MRI can provide information about where this fat is found, this method is superior to the others. In MRI, images are created by a combination of electromagnetic radiation and a magnetic field. Individual body segments such as shoulders, chest, hips, thighs, etc., can be examined as discrete entities. Thus, the amount and distribution of fat can be detailed.

Dual energy x-ray absorptiometry (DEXA) is another of the newer methods being developed. It has been used to estimate bone density and soft-tissue composition. The advantage of this method is that it eliminates the need to use the assumption that the body exists as a two-pool system. The one pool is the fat and the other is the fat-free mass (or lean body mass). Bone density as a fraction of the fat-free mass can be distinguished and quantitated using DEXA. The result is that bone mass and density can be quantitated, as can the fat mass, and the remaining tissue is more legitimately the lean body mass. One can then distinguish and quantitate the muscle mass using its creatine content.

If the major component of the lean is assumed to be the muscle, muscle mass can be determined using the dilution of radioactive creatine or creatine labeled with a heavy nonradioactive isotope. This has been used successfully in rats and may be applicable to humans because creatine is almost exclusively located in the muscle. Labeled creatine must be infused and, after a set interval, a muscle biopsy obtained. The total muscle mass can be calculated using the $\dfrac{C_1}{C_2} = \dfrac{V_2}{V_1}$ equation as follows:

$$\frac{\text{Total } {}^{14}\text{C creatine infused}}{\left[{}^{14}\text{C creatine}\right] \text{ in sample}} = \frac{\text{Muscle sample size}}{\text{Total muscle mass}}$$

On the assumption that lean body mass has a constant potassium content and that neutral fat does not bind the electrolyte, lean body mass can be estimated by measuring the body content of the heavy potassium isotope ${}^{40}\text{K}$ or by measuring the dilution of ${}^{42}\text{K}$ (the radioactive isotope) in the body cells. The former requires a whole-body scintillation counter, whereas the latter can be determined in a small tissue (muscle biopsy) sample. The formula for calculating lean body mass is as follows:

$$\text{LBM} = \frac{\text{Total K content}}{\text{Concentration of K/kg tissue}}$$

Either of these methods may underestimate the lean body mass because of the lack of correction for the small amounts of potassium in the extracellular fluids.

Lean body mass and percent fat can be estimated using measures of body density or specific gravity of the individual. The fat-free body will have a specific gravity of 1.1000. This will decrease as the body increases its fat content since fat has a lower (~0.92) specific gravity than the fat-free body mass. Thus, the fatter the subject, the lower the specific gravity or density. The body density can be determined in the adult using Archimedes' principle. The subject is weighed in air and again when immersed in water. The difference in the two body weights is the weight of the body that is water. Since water has a density of 1 (1 ml of water weighs 1 g), the volume of the water displaced represents both the volume of the body immersed and its density. The immersion weight/unit volume of water displaced then is diluted by the air weight/unit volume of water displaced, which in turn is the specific gravity of the subject. Corrections for the residual air in the lungs and intestines must be made. There are a number of reports on body density and body fat using this technique. Age affects body density and percent body fat. In one study of women of different ages, it was found that young (16–40 years of age) women had body densities of 1.0342 g/ml to 1.0343 g/ml and percent body fats of 28.69 to 28.75. Older women (50–70 years of age) had body densities that ranged from 1.0095 g/ml to 1.0050 g/ml and percent body fats of 41.88 to 44.56. Body fat can be estimated using the Siri et al. equation:

$$\text{fat \%} = \frac{2.118 - 1.354 - 0.78}{\text{density}} \cdot \left(\frac{\text{\% TBW}}{\text{body weight}} \right)$$

where 2.118, 1.354, and 0.78 are constants and the density (g/cc), body weight (Kg), and TBW (Kg) are determined.

Other prediction equations for percent fat from specific gravity are available. Another Siri et al. equation allows one to calculate % fat $= 100 \dfrac{(5.548 - 5.044)}{\text{specific gravity}}$. The Pace-Rathbun method calculates % fat $= 100 - \dfrac{\text{TBW}}{0.732}$. The Pace-Rathbun method is based on TBW only and compensates for the structural lipids (those in cell membranes, etc., as contrasted to the depot lipids) by adding 3%. This gives a lean body mass that is somewhat different from that of Siri et al.

Underwater weighing as described above is based on the difference in density of the different body components. Estimating fat stores in this way is cumbersome or not feasible in many clinical settings or under conditions of field surveys. Researchers using this method have made some correlations between this estimate and estimates of body fatness using the measurements of skinfold thicknesses at key locations, i.e., places where subcutaneous fat can be assessed using calipers to estimate the skinfold thickness. The fold below the upper arm (triceps fold) and the fold at the iliac crest are frequently used locations. Other locations include the abdominal fold and the thigh fold. Equations (Table 2.8) have been derived to calculate body fatness using these measurements.

TABLE 2.8
General Formulas for Calculating Body Fatness From Skinfold Measurements

Males:

$\quad$ % Body Fat $= 29.288 \times 10^{-2}(\times) - 5 \times 10^{-4}(\times)^2 + 15.845 \times 10^{-2}(\text{Age})$

Females:

$\quad$ % Body Fat $= 29.699 \times 10^{-2}(\times) - 43 \times 10^{-5}(\times)2 + 29.63 \times 10^{-3}(\text{Age}) + 1.4072$

$\quad$ where $\times$ = sum of abdomen, suprailiac, triceps and thigh skinfolds, and age is in years.

Source: Jackson, A.S. and Pollack, M. L. 1985. Practical Assessment of Body Composition. *Phys. and Sports Med.* 13:76–90.

For population surveys where close estimates of body fat, protein, lean body mass, etc., are not critical, simpler estimates of body fatness are frequently used. Using the patient's body weight and height one can compare these values with those considered desirable for men and women. The first such tables were developed by the Metropolitan Life Insurance Company, which made the assumption that young (age 20–30) people applying for life insurance (and found insurable) were healthy. They then took the body weights of these people and arranged them according to height for both males and females. They called these weights "desirable" weights because they were associated with the lowest mortality due to disease. Because the weight range for each height was so large, they later subdivided each weight-for-height range into thirds and presented these thirds as being representative of small, medium, and large frame sizes. This table has been found useful by many in estimating desirable body weight, but the user must remember that this table was not based on actual measurements of skeletal size. The table is based only on heights and weights of individuals in the third decade of life who wanted (and could afford) life insurance. In this respect, there is a bias in the table. Minority groups were largely underrepresented in the database used for these tables.

A broader database using subjects of all ages, economic status, both sexes, and from minority and majority cultural/ethnic groups was obtained by the National Health and Nutrition Examination Survey (NHANES), which has been conducted at intervals by the Centers for Disease Control of the U.S. Department of Health and Human Services. These surveys have collected data not only from young adult men and women but also from children and aging adults. These weights and heights have been used to create tables giving weight ranges for males and females. In addition, NHANES made more detailed measurements of skinfold thickness, skeletal size and density, and a variety of biochemical and physiological features using a representative subset of the population assessed. The NHANES tables therefore have a broader database than the Metropolitan Life Insurance tables. Despite the difference in databases used to construct the tables, both are useful in evaluating humans in terms of desirable body weight.

Perhaps more popular now is the use of body mass index (BMI). This is useful in that it is an index of the body weight (kg) divided by the height (meters) squared (wt/ht²). BMI correlates with body fatness and with the risk of obesity-related disease or diseases for which obesity is a compounding factor. Overweight is defined as BMI between 25 and 30 and obesity is a BMI over 30. The BMI varies with age. A desirable BMI for people age 19–24 is between 19 and 24, while that for people age 55–64 is between 23 and 28. While simple in concept, this term does not assess body composition per se. It provides a basis only for assessing the health risks associated or presumed to be associated with excess body fatness. BMI applies only to normal individuals, not the super athlete or the body builder, who may be quite heavy yet have little body fat.

While total body fatness is an important risk factor for several degenerative diseases, the distribution of the stored fat may impact upon these disease states as well. Males and females differ in the pattern of body-fat stores. Males tend to deposit fat in the abdominal area, while females tend to deposit fat in the gluteal area. Measuring the waist and hip circumference allows computation of the waist-to-hip ratio (WHR). As this ratio increases, so does the risk for cardiovascular disease, diabetes mellitus, and hypertension. In men, if the WHR is greater than 0.90 and in women greater than 0.80, the risk for cardiovascular disease increases significantly.

WATER BALANCE

The existence of several body compartments and the knowledge of the importance of water in the body, as well as the fact that water has an average half-life of 3.3 days in the body, gives a clear indication that both water intake and excretion must be closely regulated. Numerous investigators have been involved in the study of thirst regulation and the regulation of water excretion.

The quantitative features of water balance are presented in Table 2.9. As can be seen, water is obtained through the beverages consumed, as a component of food, and as an end product of metabolism. Foods vary in their water content: lettuce, for example, is 96% water; beef steak, 60%; and table sugar, 0.5%. Typically, a mixed diet providing 2000 kcal (8364 KJ) will provide 500–800 g of water. The water consumed as such, the percentage available from food, and that lost in the urine, feces, and by evaporation can be determined directly. Metabolic water, preformed water, insensible water, and respirative losses must be estimated. The term metabolic water refers to that amount of water liberated through the metabolism of carbohydrates, lipids, and proteins. In addition to metabolic water, when polysaccharides, triglycerides, or proteins are formed, one molecule of water is produced when each interglycosidic linkage, each ester bond, and each peptide bond is formed. This water is referred to as the preformed water and is sometimes separated from the water that is produced when fats, carbohydrates, and proteins are oxidized.

The amount of metabolic water available to the subject can be calculated if the amount of carbohydrate, fat, and protein consumed and the respiratory quotient (RQ) are known. The respiratory quotient is the ratio of carbon dioxide released to oxygen consumed. The typical RQ of an individual consuming a mixed diet is 0.85. The water produced by the combustion of carbohydrate, fat, and protein is 0.60, 1.07, and 0.41 g/g nutrient, respectively, or 15.8, 11.5, and 10.3 g of water per 100 g of the nutrient mix. This assumes that the individual is in energy and protein balance. If the individual is gaining weight, then a correction for the gain in weight as fat must be made. If the weight gain results in a positive nitrogen balance, then a correction for the gain in protein

TABLE 2.9
Typical Water Balance in Adult Humans

Sources of Water	gm	Water Losses	gm
Liquid*	1100–1200	Urine	1000–1300
Solid Food	500–800	Feces	80–100
Metabolic Water	300–500	Evaporative losses	550–600
		Lungs	375–400
TOTAL	1900–2500	TOTAL	2000–2400

*water, beverages, soup, etc.

must also be made. Similar corrections must be made if the subject is losing weight, since more fat and protein will be oxidized than can be accounted for by these respective components in the diet. This oxidation will contribute additional water to the metabolic water category. For example, Newburgh studied a human who consumed 69 g protein, 83 g fat, and 267 g carbohydrate. Newburgh calculated that this subject had an average heat production of 1907 kcal (7979 KJ) per day, and, based on nitrogen balance data, a daily destruction of 11.9 g of tissue protein. If 1907 kcal (the heat produced by the subject) is subtracted from the kcal of the diet plus the available kcal of the tissue protein (11.9 x 4), it is determined that 232 kcal were stored. This means that 26 g (232 ÷ 9) of fat were stored. Applying all the correction factors, Newburgh's subject is found to be oxidizing 80.9 g (69 + 11.9) of protein, 267 g of carbohydrate (assuming all the carbohydrate was oxidized), and 57 g (83–26) of fat. Newburgh separated the preformed water from the metabolic water. He assumed that the destruction of 11.9 g of tissue protein would release approximately 36 g of water since tissue protein is associated with about three times its weight in water. This 36 g was corrected for the storage of 26 g of fat, which he estimated would hold about 3 g of water. Thus, 33 g of preformed water was available to this subject.

Heat production by an animal represents the energy lost from the body as heat. This energy loss is the result of its metabolism (see Unit 3). It can be calculated from the insensible water loss (IWL), which is defined as the loss in body weight attributable to the vaporization of water from the body surface. This is not to be confused with the water and heat loss due to profuse sweating. IWL is just that: the insensible water lost by the body when it is at equilibrium with its environment in its zone of thermic neutrality, i.e., an environmental temperature and humidity that induces neither shivering nor sweating. The IWL can be determined by careful weighing of the fasting (but not starving) subject during short periods of time. The difference in the body weights corrected for any loss in weight through the urine and feces is then the insensible weight loss (IW). In the fed subject, a correction for the weight of the food and drink consumed must be made. Thus, IW is equal to the difference between the initial weight (Wi) corrected for intake (I) and the final weight (Wf) corrected for loss of excreta (E).

$$IW = (Wi - I) - (Wf - E)$$

IW must then be converted to IWL. This is possible if the weight of the carbon dioxide exhaled and the oxygen consumed is known. Thus, IWL can be calculated using the equation, $IWL = IW - (CO_2 - O_2)$. If, for example, the IW was 1213 g and the difference between the carbon dioxide produced and oxygen consumed was 111 g, then the insensible water loss would be 1213–111 or 1102 grams. The heat produced by the IWL, which is the heat production by the animal as a result of its metabolism, can be calculated if one assumes that one g of water will absorb 0.58 kcal of heat at skin temperature. For example, heat production (HP) of a human consuming a low-carbohydrate diet will equal the IWL times 0.58 divided by the vapor heat ratio (100/24.5).

$$HP = IWL \times 0.58 \times (100/24.5)$$

The vapor heat ratio can vary depending on diet, clothing, and environmental temperature. Likewise, the IWL can vary depending on the environment and on age. As humans approach old age, there is an impairment in ability to regulate the evaporative heat loss from the skin. The reasons for this decrease in ability to regulate evaporative heat loss are not fully understood; however, older persons frequently do not tolerate cold or very hot environments as well as younger persons.

There are other methods available for the calculation of metabolic water. One, devised by Morrison, uses the respiratory exchange, the urinary nitrogen production, and the energy production. This formula is as follows:

$$W = \frac{[K(0.1998 + 0.4692R) - N(3.3352 + 0.2443R)]}{(3.840 + 1.195R)}$$

where W = metabolic water in grams
          K = energy production in kcal or kcal × 4.2 (Kjoules)
          N = total urinary production in grams
          R = respiratory quotient

This method is useful if the composition of the diet consumed is not known, but both respiratory quotient and urinary nitrogen can be measured. As indicated earlier, heat production can be calculated, measured directly, or estimated using indirect methods.

As for the other components of the water balance sheet (Table 2.9), the water in food, beverages, urine, and feces can be determined directly. The water lost through respiration can be estimated. Respired air is fully water saturated and, if the volume of air expired and the number of respirations can be measured, the grams of water lost in this manner can be estimated. Newburgh, in his calculations of water balance, did not correct for water loss by this route; however, others generally agree that man loses 350–400 g of water/day through the lungs. Newburgh and others lump the respiratory water loss in with the IWL because it is an unavoidable loss and meets the criteria of being insensible.

As mentioned earlier, urine and fecal water losses can be determined directly. Typically, the urine is 97% water; normal excretion is 1 to 2 L per day. Fluid is filtered through the kidney tubule at an average rate of 125 ml per minute. An amount sufficient to maintain blood volume is resorbed; the rest is excreted. If the fluid intake is low, more of the water is resorbed and a more-concentrated urine is excreted. If fluid intake is high, the urine is less concentrated. The regulation of water resorption by the kidney is under the control of antidiuretic hormone (ADH, also called vasopressin). When ADH is high, water resorption is high; when ADH is low, water resorption is low. The loss of water via the feces is low under normal conditions. Although there is a continuous secretion of water in the form of digestive juices into the alimentary canal, little of this is excreted in the feces. As much as 7–10 L per day can be cycled through the intestinal tract. The majority of this liquid is resorbed along with the water from food and drink; about 100–200 ml is excreted in the feces.

REGULATION OF WATER BALANCE

Thirst, like hunger, is a basic physiological drive. The urge to drink as a factor in the overall control of body fluid homeostasis has been studied by both psychologists and physiologists alike. In contrast to a number of species, man's urge to drink is not directly related to water requirement. While thirst is a factor in the overall control of body fluid requirements, other factors play important roles as well. The concentration of the Na^+ in the extracellular fluid, ADH, and the angiotensin-renin-aldosterone system are all involved in the regulation of water balance.

VASOPRESSIN (ADH)

Vasopressin is synthesized by the supraoptic and paraventricular neurons of the posterior pituitary. The synthesis of ADH occurs in the ribosomes and proceeds via the formation of a macromolecular precursor or prohormone. This precursor or propressophysin has a molecular weight of about 20,000 Da. The prohormone contains several subunits, each of which has a biological function. One of these, ADH, is preceded by a signal peptide. When the osmoreceptors located in the anterolateral hypothalamus perceive a change in the osmolarity of the blood (normal range: 275–290 mOsm/kg), this signal peptide is alerted and ADH is released. It binds to receptors in the glomerulus and renal convoluted tubules with the result that water is reabsorbed. The exact mechanism by which this system operates is not known. However, it is known that the sensitivity of the system can be affected by the physiological status of the individual. For example, the phase of the menstrual cycle in females affects the sensitivity to the action of ADH so that water balance (water retention) varies through the cycle.

The osmoregulatory mechanism is not equally sensitive to all plasma solutes. Sodium and its anions (which contribute roughly 95% of the osmotic pressure of the plasma) are the most potent solutes with respect to the stimulation of the osmoreceptors. Certain sugars such as sucrose and manitol have been shown to stimulate these receptors *in vitro*, but these sugars do not normally appear in the plasma. Urea concentrations above 2 pg/ml stimulate ADH release, as does sustained hyperglycemia. Uncontrolled diabetes and end-stage renal disease both are characterized by abnormal water balance. Uncontrolled diabetics are polyuric (excess urine production) and very thirsty. In severe hyperglycemia, the solute load in the blood is increased. This triggers both thirst and ADH release. Both serve to dilute the excess solute load. The body then responds by increasing urine production and release. This excess urination gets rid of the excess solute and the excess consumed water. In principle, the same thing happens in the early phase of renal disease. In this instance, the solutes are not excreted because of the diseased state of the kidney. ADH functions to retain water so as to dilute these solutes. Later, in the end stage of this disease, patients are thirsty and polyuric because their disease renders them less able to reabsorb water via the convoluted tubules. They may have the signals to release ADH but the target tissue (the renal convoluted tubules) is not able to respond. Other stimuli for ADH release include emesis (vomiting), changes in blood volume or pressure, excessive sweating, hemorrhage, diarrhea, drugs that act as diuretics or that are antihypertensive agents, hyperinsulinemia, and other hormones related to water balance, i.e., angiotensin.

ATRIAL NATRIURETIC HORMONE

The action of ADH in retaining water is counteracted by the peptide hormone, atrial natriuretic hormone (ANH). This hormone induces water, sodium, and potassium loss, decreases blood pressure, and increases glomerular filtration rate. ANH interferes with the renin-angiotension system by decreasing the release of renin and aldosterone. It also antagonizes the action of such vasoconstrictors as angiotensin II and norepinephrine.

RENIN, ANGIOTENSIN II, ALDOSTERONE

In addition to the effects of ADH and ANH on water balance, there is another system, shown in Figure 2.8, that is composed of renin, angiotensin, and aldosterone. This system exerts effects not only on water balance but also on blood pressure. It involves a cascade of reactions to produce

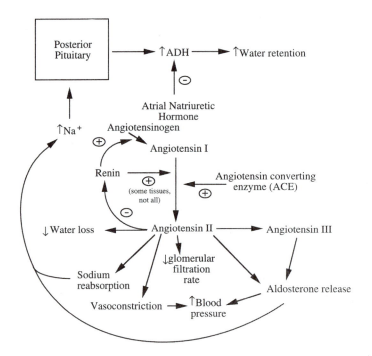

FIGURE 2.8 Hormones that affect water balance.

angiotensin II, the active form of this hormone. Angiotensinogen is converted to angiotensin I, which is in turn converted to angiotensin II. The conversion of angiotensin I (the inactive hormone) to angiotensin II is catalyzed by the angiotensin-converting enzyme (ACE). Angiotensin II stimulates water and sodium resorption and vasoconstriction. Angiotension II affects a wide variety of physiological processes but the one of importance in this discussion is its effect on water excretion. Through its effects on sodium balance, it affects ADH release. At low serum sodium levels, it conserves sodium by increasing its reabsorption. At high sodium levels, it has the reverse effect. Through its effect on vasoconstriction, it reduces glomerular filtration rate and decreases water loss. Lastly, through effects on aldosterone, an adrenal cortical steroid hormone responsible for electrolyte conservation, it also indirectly affects serum sodium levels, ADH release, and water retention. A number of antihypertensive drugs serve to inhibit ACE activity and by doing so decrease the production of angiotensin II. By controlling the amount of angiotensin II production, these ACE inhibitors can lower blood pressure. ACE inhibitors, thiazides, and calcium blockers all have antihypertensive effects, but each has a different mode of action. The cascade used for angiotensin II production is influenced by renin, an acid protease. Renin arises from prorenin and is produced by the juxtaglomerular cells of the kidney. It is also produced by other cells. Its release is controlled by neurons in the sympathetic nervous system, negative feedback by angiotension II, prostaglandin E, calcium, potassium, arginine vasopressin, and a number of other factors whose effects are not well understood. If any aspect of this intricate system for controlling water balance is disturbed, excessive thirst and/or excessive urination will result.

Infusion of epinephrine, acetylcholine, or other monoamines into the third ventricular cavity has been shown to elicit thirst and ADH release in the goat and rat. These effects have generally been regarded as being due to their transmitter action at the various synapses in the ventricular cavity. In so doing, they act directly on the juxtaventricular receptors involved in the control of water balance. Angiotensin II, norepinephrine, and prostaglandin E have all been found to elicit ADH and thirst and, in addition, have been shown to activate the Na^+-K^+ ATPase in cerebral as well as other tissues. This activation would then allow one to relate Na^+ concentration to thirst (since Na^+ activates this ATPase) and suggests that this enzyme may be essential to receptor excitation. This suggestion is not new. Several years ago it was shown that an inhibitor of trans-membrane Na^+ transport, hydrochlorothiazide, markedly reduced drinking in sodium-loaded, nephrectomized rats. Inhibition of drinking can also be shown with ouabain, an inhibitor of Na^+-K^+ ATPase, and with glycerol. Glycerol also suppresses the thirst induced by dehydration.

SATIATION OF THIRST

It is evident that thirst does not become satiated until enough water has been absorbed to offset those factors responding to Na^+ concentration, osmolarity, and volume changes in the body fluids. The mechanism for this satiation is unknown. In fact, more is known about the initiation of drinking than about its cessation. Work with monkeys has provided evidence for the existence of pre- and postabsorptive signals elicited from the intestine that play important roles in the cessation of drinking. When water was drained from the stomach via a gastric cannula, the monkeys drank several times their normal intake of water. When a duodenal cannula was used, water intake was increased above normal but was not as great as when the stomach was drained. If water was reintroduced into the intestine, the monkeys that had gastric drainage ceased drinking. Whatever the ultimate mechanism is that counterbalances the initiation of water intake, water consumption is closely regulated, so that under wide variations in activity, diet, and environmental conditions, normal man is able to maintain himself in fluid balance.

WATER NEEDS

Human need for water varies with the kinds of foods consumed, the level of physical activity, environmental temperature, and age. Water need is dictated by water loss, as can be seen in Table 2.9. Obviously, the variability is great. While there is no minimum requirement for adults, it has been recommended that infants be given 1.5 ml water/kcal of food. As discussed in an earlier section in this unit, if excess protein is oxidized for fuel, this will increase water needs since water assists in the elimination of the nitrogenous end products of protein catabolism. This increase has been termed the protein overload effect on water needs.

ABNORMALITIES IN WATER BALANCE

As indicated in the preceding sections, the regulation of both water intake and excretion is extremely important to the regulation of water balance and, indeed, to survival itself. A variety of clinical conditions have been described that have as one of their characteristics a change in the normal pattern of intake and/or excretion of water. Only rarely does the primary disorder reside with the regulation of water balance itself. The disorder *diabetes insipidus* develops in the absence of ADH. The disease is characterized by extreme urinary water loss (up to 30 l/day) and extreme thirst.

In this disorder, the posterior pituitary may be diseased or have a tumor that interferes with the production of ADH. In this disease, the resorption of water by the renal tubules is not stimulated and the patient excretes a large volume of very dilute urine. Patients with diabetes insipidus can be successfully treated. Interestingly, their treatment consists of providing the hormone in an aerosol that allows the patient to inhale the hormone through the nose.

An even rarer disease of water balance is a form of diabetes insipidus that does not involve the production and release of ADH by the posterior pituitary but is primarily of renal origin. In this disorder, the kidney is unresponsive to the hormone. The reasons for this unresponsiveness are not known, nor has a suitable treatment been devised.

Edema

Of the conditions where a disordered water balance is secondary to the primary disease, edema is perhaps the most common. In this condition, water is accumulated in the tissues distal to the kidneys. Urine volume is very low and highly concentrated. As the fluids in the extracellular compartment increase, the functionality of the patient decreases. At first, the edema is noted in the extremities. Feet, ankles, legs, and hands become swollen, then, noticeably, there is an accumulation of fluid in the abdominal cavity and in the pericardial sac. This fluid accumulation makes it difficult for the patient to walk and, eventually, interferes with the vital functions of the internal organs such as the heart. Depending on the primary disorder, the edema can be treated. If due to inadequate protein or thiamin intakes, these nutrients can be supplied and the edema will subside as the patient's nutritional status improves. If, however, the edema is due to heart disease characterized by an impaired ability to pump the blood throughout the body, a loss in the pressure differential needed for peripheral fluid exchange and circulation through the renal tubules will occur. In this instance, the treatment is much more difficult, since it depends on the successful treatment of the diseased heart. Edema can also result from a loss of vascular elasticity, which characterizes high blood pressure (hypertension). Hypertension occurs when the vascular system is continually stimulated to constrict. In this disorder, the pressure of the blood is so high in the peripheral tissues that water cannot flow from the tissues to the blood in response to the usual pressure differential between the arteries, arterioles, capillaries, venules, and veins and the tissues they serve. However, if the blood pressure can be reduced through antivasoconstrictor medication, sodium intake restriction, and, if needed, weight reduction, then the edema will also be reduced.

While these disorders are all related to the excretion of water through the kidneys, disturbances in other routes of water loss can also result in an abnormal water balance. Excess environmental temperatures can result in excessive water losses (as well as electrolyte losses) through the skin as sweat. Unless compensated for by an increase in fluid and electrolyte intake and a decrease in urine output, dehydration results. The extracellular fluid becomes concentrated and hypertonic to the cells. Water then shifts from the intracellular compartment to the extracellular compartment. The obvious result of this shift is cell death and, unless water is provided, death of the patient is imminent.

Diarrhea

Excess water loss can also occur through the intestine. Large watery stools characterize diarrhea and can arise as a result of a variety of disorders. Perhaps the most common of these is that associated with food contamination. Various organisms such as those from the Salmonella family or the *Vibrio cholerae* can cause massive diarrhea and fluid loss. In the case of the latter, the cholera-causing organism produces a toxin that binds to specific receptors on the intestinal cell wall. The toxin activates adenylate cyclase by causing ADP-ribosylation of the GαS protein (Figure 2.9) involved in regulating the cyclase. This results in an elevation in cAMP levels, which affects electrolyte movement and inhibits the active transport processes necessary for the absorption of nutrients (and water) from the gut. While the water can pass freely from the intestine, other materials cannot and, thus, create an osmotic pull on the water. In turn, the water and unabsorbed nutrients fill the intestine, stimulating peristalsis and evacuation of the colon. If the massive fluid and electrolyte losses are not replaced, the cholera victim does not survive and recover. Cholera victims can be given an oral solution rich in glucose (~ 110 mM), sodium (99 mM), chloride (74 mM), bicarbonate (39 mM), and potassium (4 mM). This solution takes advantage of the fact that the cholera toxin does not "poison" the sodium-dependent, ATP-dependent, glucose uptake system. By giving excess glucose, sodium is "pushed" into the cell and electrolyte balance is restored. If the victim cannot swallow, an intravenous replenishment must be followed. If untreated, the victim becomes severely dehydrated and death ensues. In countries where fresh human excreta is used as fertilizer for the fields, epidemics of cholera occur frequently. Epidemics are particularly evident in very warm climates, since the cholera organisms multiply very rapidly under these conditions. Food contamination by organisms other than *Vibrio cholerae* is also common in areas where both animal and human excreta are used in the untreated state. If the waste is allowed to ferment, the heat generated by the fermentation process will kill most of the organisms likely to cause food-borne illness.

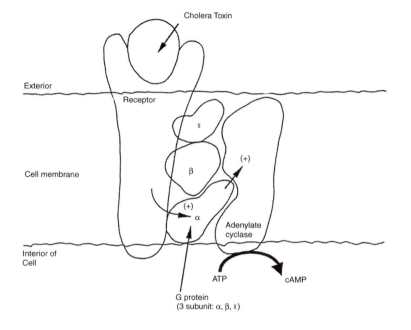

FIGURE 2.9   Mechanism of action of the cholera toxin showing its binding to a receptor that stimulates the α unit of the G protein and that, in turn, stimulates adenylate cyclase, which converts ATP to cAMP. Since many nutrients are absorbed through the epithelial gut cell via an energy-dependent active process, the toxin binding results in less ATP to support this process. The toxin also promotes K^+ secretion.

Diarrhea can also result if the individual develops an irritable colon. A hyperirritable intestine may be the result of a particular medication or it may be permanent due to a genetic error. Genetic errors resulting in the absence of a particular digestive enzyme will result in an accumulation of that substrate in the gut. This in turn will "pull" water into the intestine and diarrhea will result. Lactose intolerance due to the absence of the enzyme lactase is an example of a disorder characterized by diarrhea. Gluten-induced enteropathy is another example. In this instance, the patient is unable to digest the wheat protein gluten. Diarrhea is characteristic of this condition, and, if allowed to continue untreated, the intestinal villae will be abraded and the absorption of nutrients in addition to the gluten will be seriously impaired. Treatment for these types of diarrhea is fairly straightforward. If the offending nutrient is eliminated from the diet, the patient will gradually rebuild the absorptive surface of the intestine and will recover.

XI.   SUPPLEMENTAL READINGS

Adreoli, T.E. and Schafer, J.A. (1979) External solution driving forces for isotonic fluid absorption in proximal tubules. *Fed. Proc.* 38:154-160.

Andersson, B. (1978) Regulation of water intake. *Physiol. Rev.* 58:582-603.

Berlin, N.I., Watkin, D.M., and Gevirtz, N.R. (1962) Measurement of changes in gross body composition during controlled weight reduction in obesity and body density – body water technics. *Metabolism* 11:302-314.

Brozek, J. (Ed.). (1963) Body composition. *Annals of N.Y. Acad. Sci.* 110:1-1018.

Brozek, J. and Keys, A. (1955) Composition of tissues accounting for individual differences in body density. *Fed. Proc.* 14:22-27.

Christian, J.E., Combs, L.W., and Kessler, W.V. (1963) Body composition: Relative *in vivo* determinations from potassium-40 measurements. *Science* 140:480-490.

Clark, R.R., Kuta, J. M., and Sullivan, J.C. (1993) Prediction of percent body fat in adult males using dual energy x-ray absorptiometry, skinfolds and hydrostatic weighing. *Med. Sci. Sports Exerc.* 25:528-535.

Cote, K.D. and Adams, W.C. (1993) Effect of bone density on body composition estimates in young adult black and white women. *Med. Sci. Sports Exerc.* 25:290-296.

Dibona, D.R. and Mills, J.W. (1979) Distribution of Na^+-pump sites in transporting epithelia. *Fed. Proc.* 38:134-143.

Fesus, L. (1993) Biochemical events in naturally occurring forms of cell death. *FEBS* 328:1-5.

Fishman, P.A. and Atikkan, E.E. (1980) Mechanism of action of cholera toxin: Effect of receptor density and multivalent binding on activation of adenylate cyclase. *J. Membrane Biol.* 54:51-60.

Forbes, R.M., Cooper, A.R., and Mitchell, H.H. (1953) The composition of the adult human body as determined by chemical analysis. *J. Biol. Chem.* 203:359-366.

Forbes, R.M., Mitchel, H.H., and Cooper, A.R. (1956) Further studies on the gross composition and mineral elements of the adult human body. *J. Biol. Chem.* 223:969-975.

Fuller, M.F., Fowler, P.A., McNeille, G., and Foster, M.A. (1990) Body composition: The precision and accuracy of new methods and their suitability for longitudinal studies. *Proc. Nutr. Soc.* 49:423-426.

Ganong, W.F. (1994) Origin of the angiotensin II secreted by cells. *Proc. Soc. Exp. Biol. and Med.* 205:213-219.

Hacker, G., Vaux, D.L. (1997) A chronology of cell death. *Apoptosis* 2:247-256.

Kreitzman, S.N. (1992) Factors influencing body composition during very low calorie diets. *Am. J. Clin. Nutr.* 56:2175-2235.

Krolmer, G., Petit, P., Zamzame, N., Vayasiere, J-L., and Mignotte, B. (1995) The biochemistry of cell death. *FASEB* J 9:1277-1287.

Kumanyika, S.K., Landis, J.R., Mathews-Cook, Y.L., Almy, S.L., and Boehmer, S.J.S. (1998) Systolic blood pressure trends in U.S. adults between 1960 and 1980. *Am. J. Epidemiology* 148:528-538.

Lotem, J. and Sachs, L. (1998) Different mechanisms for suppression of apoptosis by cytokines and calcium mobilizing compounds. *Proc. Nat. Acad. Sci.* 95:4601-4606.

Malina, R.M. (1999) Progress in human body composition research. *Am. J. Human Biol.* 11:141-200.

Maurico, D. and Mandrys-Poulsen, T. (1998) Apoptosis and the pathogenesis of IDDM. *Diabetes* 47:1537-1543.

McCargar, L.J., Baracos, V.E., and Clandinin, M.T. (1989) Influence of dietary carbohydrate to fat ratio on whole body nitrogen retention and body composition in adult rats. *J. Nutr.* 119:1240-1245.

Meador, C.K., Kreisberg, R.A., Friday, J.P. Jr., Bowdoin, B., Coan, P., Armstrong, J., and Hazelrig, J.B. (1968) Muscle mass determination by isotopic dilution of creatinine[14]. *Metabolism* 17:1104-1108.

Mignotte, B. and Vayssiere, J-L. (1998) Mitochondria and apoptosis. *Eur. J. Biochem.* 252:1-15.

Nagy, L., Thomazy, V.A., Heyman, R.A., and Davies, P.J.A. (1998) Retinoid induced apoptosis in normal and neoplastic tissues. *Cell Death and Differentiation* 5:11-19.

Pace, N. and Rathbun, E.N. (1945) Studies on body composition; body water and chemically combined nitrogen content in relation to fat content. *J. Biol. Chem.* 158:685-691.

Reeds, P.J. and Fiorotto, M.L. (1990) Growth in perspective. *Proc. Nutr. Soc.* 49:411-420.

Schafer, J.A. (1979) Water transport in epithelia. *Fed. Proc.* 38:119-120.

Shimabukuro, M., Zhou, Y.T., Levi, M., and Unger, R.H. (1998) Fatty acid-induced ß cell apoptosis: A link between obesity and diabetes. *Proc. Nat. Acad. Sci.* 95:2498-2502.

Siri, W.E. (1956) The gross composition of the body. *Adv. Biol. M. Physics* 4:239-280.

Smalley, K.J., Kneer, A.N., Kendric, Z.V., Colliver, J.A., and Owen, O.E. (1990) Reassessment of body mass indices. *Am. J. Clin. Nutr.* 52:402-408.

Sohlström, A., Wahlund, L.-O., and Forsum, E. (1993) Adipose tissue distribution as assessed by magnetic resonance imaging and total body fat by magnetic resonance imaging, underwater weighing and body water dilution in healthy women. *Am. J. Clin. Nutr.* 58:830-838.

Szondy, Z., Reichert, U., and Fesus, L. (1998) Retinoic acids regulate apoptosis of T lymphocytes through an interplay between RAR and RXR receptors. *Cell Death and Differentiation* 5:4-10.

Tsai, M.-J. and O'Malley, B.W. (1994) Molecular mechanisms of action of steroid/thyroid receptor super family members. *Ann. Rev. Biochem.* 63:451-486.

Van der Kooy, K., Leenen, R., Serdell, J.C., Dourenberg, P., and Hautvast, J.G.A.J. (1993) Effect of weight cycling on visceral fat accumulation. *Am. J. Clin. Nutr.* 58:853-857.

Young, C.M., Martin, M.E.K., Chihan, M., McCarthy, M., Manniello, M.J., Harmuth, E.H., and Fryer, J.H. (1961) Body composition of young women. Some preliminary findings. *J. Am. Diet. Assoc.* 38:332-344.

Books

Hargrove, J.L. (1998) *Dynamic Modeling in the Health Sciences.* Springer-Verlag, New York.

Lee, R.D. and Nieman, D.C. (1993) Anthropometry, Chap. 6, pg. 121-163. In: *Nutritional Assessment*, Wm. C. Brown Publishers, Dubuque, IA.

Mitchell, H.H. (1962) *Comparative Nutrition of Man and Domestic Animals.* Academic Press, New York.

3 Energy

CONTENTS

After water, the most important requirement to sustain life is energy. It is expressed in heat units known as calories or joules. No other nutrient requirement can be met if the energy intake is insufficient to meet the body's needs.

DEFINITION

Classical nutritionists use the term Calorie or kilocalorie (kcal) to represent the amount of heat required to raise the temperature of 1 kilogram of water 1°C. The international unit of energy is the joule. One Calorie or kcalorie is equal to 4.184 kilojoules or 4.2 kjoules (KJ). There are cogent reasons to express energy in terms of kjoules. Nutritionists have realized that the energy provided by food is used for more than heat production. It is also used for mechanical work (muscle movement) and for electrical signaling (vision; neuronal messages) and is stored as chemical energy. The joule is 107 ergs, where 1 erg is the amount of energy expended in accelerating a mass of 1 g by 1 cm/s. The international joule is defined as the energy liberated by one international ampere flowing through a resistance of one international ohm in one second. Even though the use of joules or kilojoules is being urged by international scientists as a means to ease the confusion in discussions about energy, the student will still find the term Calorie or kcal in many texts and references. In some texts, the term calorie, spelled with a lower case "c," is used. This heat is actually 1/1000th of the heat unit spelled with an upper case "C." Physicists use the term calorie to represent the amount of heat required to raise the temperature of one gram of water 1°C. Note that this definition uses 1 g, not 1 kg, as stated above. Even though it is not correct, the term calorie is used in some nutrition literature when in fact Calorie or kcal is intended.

When foodstuffs are burned in the presence of oxygen, heat is produced. The quantity of heat produced can be measured in a bomb calorimeter and used as an estimate of the energy value of the food. The bomb calorimeter is an instrument used to measure heat production when a known amount of food is completely oxidized. It is a highly insulated, box-like container. All the heat produced during the oxidation of a dried sample of food is absorbed by a weighed amount of water surrounding the combustion chamber. A thermometer registers the change in the chamber temperature. The instrument's name is derived from the design of the combustion chamber, which is, indeed, a small bomb. The energy value of protein foods obtained in this manner is higher than the actual biologic value, for in biologic systems, the end products of oxidation must be excreted as urea, a process that costs energy. For instance, in a bomb calorimeter (Figure 3.1), the combustion or oxidation of protein yields 5.6 Calories (23.5 kJ)/g; the energy yield from the oxidation of protein after correction for urea formation and digestive loss by the body is about 4 Calories (16.8 kJ)/g. Corrections for digestive losses are also applied to the values obtained for the combustion of lipids and carbohydrates. The value of 4.1 Calories (17.22 kJ)/g is rounded off to 4 (16.8 kJ) for carbohydrates and the value of 9.4 (39.5 kJ) for lipids is rounded off to 9 (37.8 kJ). Listed in Table 3.1 are some common foods and their energy value.

The objectives of digestion, absorption, and metabolism in the animal system are to convert the chemicals in foods to the chemicals in the body. The conversion of food chemicals to body chemicals is stepwise and not 100% efficient. Energy exchange and conversion are an integral part of the process that converts the food chemicals to the body chemicals. Some of the chemical energy from food is trapped in high-energy storage compounds, but, at each step of the conversion process, some of the energy escapes as heat. This heat, generated by the body in the course of oxidizing various food components or converting them to body components, serves to maintain body temperature. However, because this heat is also lost from the body through radiation as well as through the various excretory processes, these losses must be replaced. Hence, the daily need for food and its associated energy value. Figure 3.2 illustrates the continuity of energy losses and gains by the living system. Energy is gained from oxidation of the fats, carbohydrates, and proteins consumed as food. This energy is transmitted via ATP (and other high-energy transfer compounds) to a variety of essential macro- and micromolecules in the body, which, in turn, are needed to sustain its optimal

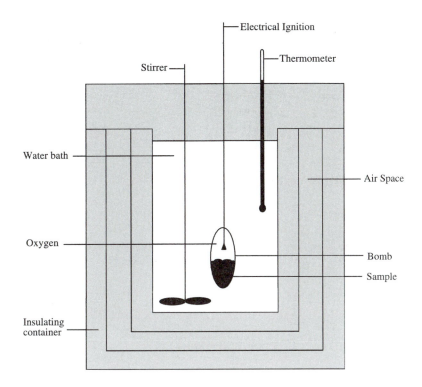

FIGURE 3.1 Cross section of a bomb calorimeter showing essential features.

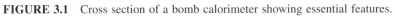

TABLE 3.1
Energy Content of Selected Human Foods

Item	Amount	Food kcal	Energy kJ
Milk (3.3% fat)	8 oz	150	628
Skim milk	8 oz	85	356
Butter	1 oz (~ 25 grams)	204	854
Egg	50 grams	80	335
Bacon	2 slices (15 grams)	85	356
Hamburger, lean	3 oz	185	774
Apple	138 grams	80	335
Avocado	216 grams	370	1548
Banana	119 grams	100	418
Grapefruit	241 grams	50	209
Orange	131 grams	65	272
Bread, white	25 grams (slice)	70	293
Brownie with nuts	20 grams	95	397
Peanut Butter	16 grams	95	397
Green Beans	1 cup, 125 grams	30	126
Corn	1/2 cup, 83 grams	65	272
Tomato, raw	135 grams	25	105

1 kcal = 4.184 kJ

function. As these functions also consume and release energy, more must be provided by the diet. Over and over this cycling occurs; this is the nature of the dynamic state of the living body. No reaction or process is ever completed and stops. The only time this happens is at death.

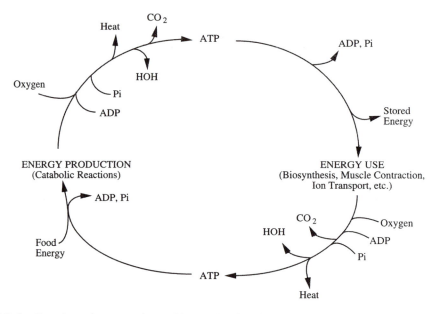

FIGURE 3. 2   Overview of energy gains and losses showing the high-energy compound ATP as the medium of exchange. Other high-energy compounds, e.g., GTP, UTP, and creatine phosphate are also involved in the cycle of energy intake and expenditure.

ENERGY NEED

Although the Food and Nutrition Board of the National Academy of Sciences has made recommendations for the energy intake (Table 3.2) for people of different ages, these Figures should not be considered immutable. The energy need is so variable that what would result in obesity in one person would be totally inadequate for another. Genetics and lifestyle choices have profound effects on energy balance and energy need.

Perhaps the best way of understanding the dimensions of the energy requirement is to examine what happens to the energy provided by food when it is consumed.

The energy provided by food (gross energy) can be determined using a bomb calorimeter as already mentioned. Not all of this energy is available to the consumer. Some is lost in preparation of the food and some is lost through digestion. The energy value of the feces subtracted from the gross energy of the food provides an estimate of the digestible energy available to the body. During digestion, energy is lost to the system through the breakdown of food to its appropriate absorbable components. Where energy is needed for absorption (active transport), this is also deducted from the gross energy of the food. It is difficult to accurately measure these losses, therefore, animal nutritionists typically correct the gross energy of food by deducting the energy of the feces. Altogether, these losses are about 10% of the gross energy of the diet if that diet is a mixture of fats, proteins, and carbohydrates. An additional deduction of the energy value of the urine accounts for energy lost as a result of metabolism of the food mixture. Again, this is an estimate, not an absolute value. When the deductions for these losses are made, the energy available to the body is the metabolizable energy (ME). Thus, ME is the gross energy minus the energy lost in feces and urine. Most tables of food composition giving the gross energy value of specific foods make the correction for these losses. The energy of the urine and feces is deducted from the gross energy

TABLE 3.2
Recommended Energy Intakes for Infants, Children, and
Adults Based on Weight and Height

Category	Age	Weight (lb)	Height (inches)	Daily Average Energy Allowance kcal	kJ
Infants	0–6 mo	13	24	650	2720
	6–12 mo	20	28	850	3556
Children	1–3 yrs	29	35	1300	5460
	4–6	44	44	1800	7560
	7–10	62	52	2000	8400
Males	11–14	99	62	2500	10500
	15–18	145	69	3000	12552
	19–24	160	70	2900	12180
	25–50	174	70	2900	12180
	51+	170	68	2300	9660
Female	11–14	101	62	2200	9240
	15–18	120	64	2200	9240
	19–24	128	65	2200	9240
	25–50	138	64	2200	9240
	51+	143	63	1900	7980
Pregnant	1st trimester:	No change			
	2nd trimester			+300	1260
	3rd trimester			+300	1260
Lactation	1–6 mo			+500	2100
	7–12 mo			+500	2100

1 kcal = 4.184 kJ

because this excreta represents or approximates the food energy lost via the digestive tract and the urinary tract. The energy of the feces consists of exfoliated intestinal cells, the residual of food not absorbed, and residual enzymes and lubricants used in the course of digestion and absorption. The energy of the urine represents the cost of excreting nitrogen as well as some small metabolites that are end products of degradative and one-way reactions. Metabolizable energy consists of the energy needed to keep the body warm (the heat increment) and to run the body processes. Each of these major divisions is subdivided as illustrated in Figure 3.3. The heat increment (HI) is composed of the heat released through work done by the body, for example, muscle contraction, and the heat released as food is oxidized and converted to usable body components. The latter is sometimes referred to as the specific dynamic action of food, or diet-induced thermogenesis (DIT). In animal nutrition, the heat increment is defined as the increase in heat production following the consumption of food by an animal in a thermoneutral environment. Utilizable energy (UE) is that which is used for body work. Net energy (NE) likewise has two components. One is basal energy (BE) or the absolute minimum amount of energy that is needed to keep the body alive, while the other is the energy that is either available for storage or is withdrawn from storage (EB).

DIGESTIVE ENERGY

The energy lost through digestion can be measured by collecting the feces and determining its energy content. Some of the fecal energy is due to the desquamated intestinal cells and intestinal flora (and their end products) and some from the nondigested portion of food. However, for the

$$GE - (FE + UE) = \text{apparent digestible energy (DE)}$$

$$DE\text{--}HI = \text{net energy} = \text{basal energy} + \text{utilizable energy} + \text{energy balance}$$

In the above, GE = gross energy of consumed food; FE = energy lost in the feces;

UE = energy lost in the urine; HI + diet-induced thermogenesis.

FIGURE 3.3 Energy equations representing the various losses of energy from the body.

purposes of determining the energy balance of the individual, all of these components of fecal energy can be grouped together because they represent energy lost from the body.

Basal Energy

By definition, basal energy reflects the energy used to sustain life. It is the sum of the energy lost as heat or used by anabolic and catabolic processes that are involved in body maintenance. It excludes energy used for growth, production/reproduction, lactation, movement, or work. The clinical definition for basal energy is the amount of energy used by the body at rest (not asleep), in the postabsorptive state (not starving), at sexual repose, and in a comfortable (thermoneutral) environment where neither shivering nor sweating occurs.

The measurement of energy need based on energy lost as heat or on the consumption of oxygen needed to oxidize fats, carbohydrates, and proteins to provide energy has been well studied and several methods are available. The energy need is additive. That is, energy is needed to maintain the body (basal energy) and sustain its various activities such as voluntary movement, work, or growth. Methods developed for estimating the basal energy requirement are listed in Table 3.3. The methods vary from very simplistic ones based on height and weight to those based on actual measures of heat production or estimates of heat production based on the heat needed to evaporate water lost by the body. Each method has its advantages and disadvantages. In those methods where actual measurements are made, the basal energy need must be measured in the postabsorptive state and the energy needed for growth and activity added to it. The postabsorptive state occurs after consumed food is digested and absorbed, but before the state of starvation ensues. Starvation involves a series of hormonal responses that can affect the fuel used by the different tissues. In the human, the postabsorptive state is about 12 to 14 hours after the last meal. In the mouse, it is 10 hours; the rat, 17 hours; guinea pig, 22 hours; rabbit, 60 hours; pig, 96 hours; and the ruminant, 5–6 days. The time needed to achieve the postabsorptive state depends on the length of the digestive tract and whether the animal is a ruminant or has a sizable "fermentation vat" within the gastrointestinal tract. In some species, the cecum serves this function, while in others, an enlarged intestinal tract has this function. At any rate, the postabsorptive state is characterized by a respiratory quotient (RQ) of 0.8, indicating that a mixture of fat and carbohydrate is being oxidized. If only fat were being oxidized, the RQ would be about 0.7. If only carbohydrate were being oxidized, the RQ would be 1.0. If energy need was being assessed by measuring heat production, the postabsorptive state would be that heat released at the point (in a continuous measurement) where the slope of the line changes, as shown in Figure 3.4.

TABLE 3.3
Methods and Equations Used for Calculating Basal Energy Need

Method	Equation
1. Heat production, direct calorimetry	kcal (kJ)/m² (surface area)
2. Oxygen consumption; indirect	O_2 cons./$W^{0.75}$
3. Heat production; indirect	Insensible Water Loss (IWL) = Insensible Weight Loss (IW) + (CO_2 exhaled – O_2 inhaled)
	Heat production = IWL $\times$ 0.58 $\times \left(\dfrac{100}{25}\right)$
4. Energy used; indirect	Basal energy = $\dfrac{\text{Creatinine N (mg/day)}}{0.00482\ (W)}$
5. Estimate (energy need not measured) (Harris Benedict equation)	BMR = 66.4730 + 13.751W + 5.0033L – 6.750A (men)
	BMR = 655.0955 + 9.563W + 1.8496L – 4.6756A (women)
6. Estimate (energy need not measured)	BMR = $71.2W^{0.75}\left[1 + 0.004(30 - A) + 0.010\left(\dfrac{L}{W^{0.33}} - 43.4\right)\right]$ (men)
	BMR = $65.8W^{0.75}\left[1 + 0.004(30 - A) + 0.018\left(\dfrac{L}{W^{0.33}} - 42.1\right)\right]$ (women)

Abbreviations are as follows: W = weight in kg; L = height in cm; A = age in years

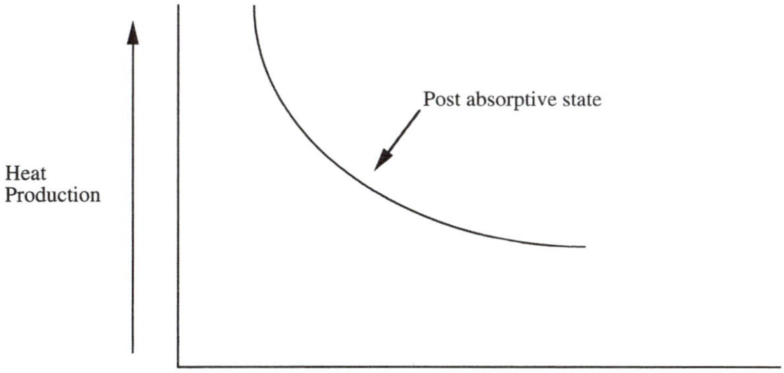

FIGURE 3.4 Changes in heat production mark the post absorptive state.

Energy released as heat can be determined directly by using a calorimeter. This instrument is nothing more than a large insulated box with sensors that can detect very small differences in temperature. Using a calorimeter is extremely tedious and the instrumentation is very expensive.

Subjects are placed in the box, kept at a comfortable temperature, and the heat transfer from the body to the chamber measured. The food energy available to the subject is carefully measured, as is the weight of the subject (before and after the period in the box) and the energy content of the feces and urine. Usually 24 hours must elapse to acquire good measurements of heat production. The basal energy is presumed to be that heat produced by the subject upon waking. Smaller time intervals can be used to assess heat production as a result of specific treatments such as the responses to hormone treatments or specific dietary ingredients or as a result of physical activity. The box is kept at a temperature that elicits neither sweating nor shivering. This temperature range is called the zone of thermic neutrality. Both sweating and shivering are energy-using processes. Sweating allows the individual to lose heat energy through water evaporation and loss. Shivering generates heat gain through surface muscle contraction and relaxation. Both processes are important to body heat regulation at environmental temperatures above and below the zone of thermic neutrality. If one were to measure energy loss above, at, and below this zone, increased energy loss would be observed at each extreme, as shown in Figure 3.5.

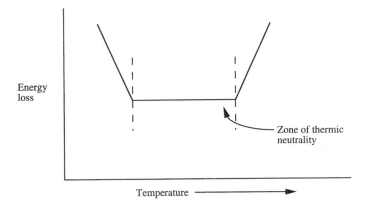

FIGURE 3.5 Energy is lost when the environmental temperature is below or above the zone of thermic neutrality.

The temperatures that mark the limits of the zone of thermic neutrality can vary between species as well as between individuals within a species. The zone of thermic neutrality is influenced by body covering. The winter coat of many species is longer and thicker than the summer coat. The winter coat can trap a layer of air around the body, which insulates it against the lowered environmental temperature. Humans do the same thing with their clothing choices. Heavier, more-insulating clothing is selected for winter wear, which affects the temperature at which shivering as a heat-generating mechanism begins. In the summer, the reverse occurs to allow heat dissipation without the need for sweating to facilitate body-heat loss. Heated houses and social behaviors such as huddling also work to decrease the need to generate heat via shivering. Air conditioning has the reverse effect. For humans, these environmental controls (heating/air conditioning) serve to decrease energy wasting and this, in turn, affects energy balance, adding to the amount of energy available for storage as fat and for use to maintain the body's metabolism.

Directly measuring the energy lost as heat from the body is not always convenient or possible. Few clinical settings can afford the time and expense to assess energy needs in this way. There is an alternative. Metabolic processes not only produce heat but also consume oxygen. The consumption of oxygen and heat production are direct correlates of each other. Oxygen consumption can thus be measured as an indirect method of assessing energy use and need. The oxidation of energy-providing nutrients (detailed in Units 4, 5, and 6) requires oxygen, which is used to make water and carbon dioxide. For every molecule of oxygen used to make water, there is an associated release of energy that is trapped in the high-energy bond of ATP and an associated release of energy as heat. The process whereby water and ATP are synthesized simultaneously is called oxidative phosphorylation. Actually, there are two processes — one, respiration, joins hydrogen and oxygen ions to make water, and the other, ATP synthesis, uses some of the energy so released to synthesize ATP. These coupled processes occur in the mitochondria of the cell.

Mitochondrial Structure and Function

The number, size, and shape of mitochondria within the cell are influenced by many factors: cell type, age, genotype, hormones, and nutritional state. However, within a given cell type and within the same animal, the number is relatively constant. For example, rat liver cells taken from a young, well nourished, nonstressed, normal animal contain between 800 and 1200 mitochondria per cell. These mitochondria are scattered throughout the cytosol and are in proximity to other organelles that have a high ATP requirement. Thus, electronmicrographs of cell cross sections often show mitochondria near the nucleus and ribosomes where protein synthesis is taking place. High rates of protein synthesis demand large amounts of ATP, since every amino acid incorporated into the protein macromolecule must first be activated by ATP. Thus, if the protein being synthesized contains 300 amino acid residues, 300 molecules of ATP will be required in addition to that used for RNA transcription and translation. Similarly, one will find large numbers of mitochondria in muscle located close by the contracting muscle fibrils. The ATP molecules produced by the mitochondria need diffuse only a very short distance to where they are used. Mitochondria are frequently located near fat droplets that serve as sources of metabolic fuel. Stored triacylglycerides are hydrolyzed in the cytosol to glycerol and fatty acids. The fatty acids are then transferred, via the acylcarnitine transferase mechanism, into the mitochondria and oxidized. Unit 6 gives the details of fatty acid oxidation. The ova contain many more mitochondria than the hepatocyte or the myocyte. Estimates vary from 2,000 to 20,000 depending on species. The sperm cell contains far fewer mitochondria and these are located in the tail of the cell. This tail facilitates the movement of the sperm through the vaginal canal and this movement requires ATP as its energy source. When fertilization takes place, only the head of the sperm penetrates the egg. Hence, very little of the sperm mitochondria enter the egg at this time. The estimate of the contribution of sperm mitochondria to the fertilized egg is about 1%.

Mitochondria are of many shapes. In the brown fat cell, they are spherical, in hepatocytes they are oval, in the kidney they are cylindrical, and in fibroblasts they are threadlike. The organelle consists of two membranes separated by a space called the intermembrane space. The membranes of the mitochondria differ not only in appearance but in function as well. The outer membrane is smooth and somewhat elastic, whereas the inner membrane is, as mentioned, convoluted. These convolutions serve to increase the surface area of the inner membrane, which is covered with regularly spaced spheres on stalks called inner membrane spheres. These spheres are not present on the outer membrane. The two membranes have been separated and their functional components studied. Within the inner membrane is the matrix, which can change in volume and organization as it changes its respiratory activity. The matrix contains, in addition to its enzymes, DNA and ribosomes with which it synthesizes 13 subunits of the respiratory chain and F_1F_0 ATPase.

The Mitochondrial Genome

In contrast to nuclear DNA (nDNA), which exists as a linear molecule, mtDNA is a closed circular molecule. The size of mtDNA ranges from approximately 16 kb in animals to more than 100 kb in plants. Mitochondrial DNA in animals is nearly identical in size and has the same organization and content of genes, which encode homologous products. In the rat, the size of the mitochondrial chromosome is 16,298 bp; in the human it is 16,569 bp. The mitochondrial genome has been sequenced and mapped in many organisms including the human and the rat. Figure 3.6 illustrates the location of each of the genes on the mitochondrial chromosome. This DNA encodes 22 tRNAs, 2 ribosomal RNAs, and 13 structural genes, which are all components of oxidative phosphorylation

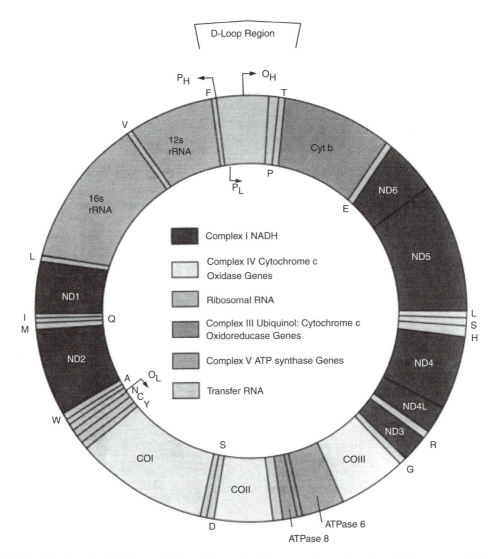

FIGURE 3.6 Transfer RNAs are indicated by a single-letter amino acid code with these encoded by the light strand on the inside and those encoded by the heavy strand on the outside of the circle. OL: origin of light strand; OH: origin of heavy strand; PH: heavy-strand promoter; PL: light strand promoter.

(OXPHOS). The structural genes include seven of the 39 units of Complex I (ND1, 2, 3, 4, 4L, 5, and 6), one of the 10 units of Complex III (Cyt b), three of the 13 units of Complex IV, Cytochrome C Oxidase (CO I-IV) of the respiratory chain and two units of the Fo portion of Complex V, the F_1F_0ATPase. Approximately 6% of the bases in the mitochondrial genome are noncoding. Ninety-seven percent of this noncoding DNA is located in the two controller regions, the 30 bp origin of replication for the light strand (O_L) and the 898 bp unit of the heavy strand (D_H) called the displacement loop or the D-loop.

The D-loop region is sandwiched between the genes for tRNA^{Phe}, which is downstream, and tRNAPro, which is upstream. This control unit contains the origin of replication for the heavy strand (O_H), the origins of both heavy- and light-strand transcription, major dedicated promoters for both heavy- and light-strand transcription, two transcription-factor binding sites, three conserved sequence blocks associated with the initiation of replication, and the D-loop strand termination associated sequences. The light-strand promoter region serves two purposes; it is not only the major promoter for light-strand transcription, but is also the site of priming for leading strand mtDNA replication.

The entire length of the genome contains genes situated on both strands. The heavy strand is the main coding strand, and codes for two rRNA species, 14 tRNA species, and 12 structural genes. The light-strand codes for eight tRNA species and one structural gene for a subunit of NADH dehydrogenase (ND6). The genome sequence shows extreme economy in that the genes have few noncoding bases between them. In fact, the largest space between two genes in mtDNA (excluding the controller regions) is the five-base pair sequence between the genes for tRNA^{Glu} and the cytochrome b gene. There is gene overlap as well. In six cases, there are genes that share coding nucleotides. In half of the cases, the shared nucleotides are not really shared in that they are on the heavy and light strands such that the shared bases are on the 3' ends of two genes. In the other three cases, the shared genes are actually shifts in the reading frame to allow the same nucleotides to code for two different proteins. The genes that share nucleotides include the ATPase 6 and 8 genes, which share 52 base pairs; ND4 and ND4L, which share seven; the tRNA$^{Ser}_{Agn}$ and tRNA^{Leu} share 1; ND 5 and ND6* share 31; the tRNA$^{Ser}_{unc}$ and the cytochrome oxidase 1 gene share four; and tRNA^{Ile} and tRNA^{Gln*} share three. Interestingly, only 56 base pairs are all that separate the different genes on the mt chromosome, and 98 base pairs are shared by neighboring genes.

The initiator codon of each reading frame, which can be AUG, AUA, AUU, or AUC, follows immediately or only a few bases after the 3' termination sequence of its upstream neighbor. Most reading frames lack termination codons and only code a T or a TA after the last sense codon. Completion of the termination codon occurs at the time of RNA processing by polyadenylation. Introns, common in nDNA, are not a feature of mtDNA. The tRNA genes are used as intervening sequences and come into play during RNA processing. Transfer RNA removal from primary transcripts causes the production of both the tRNA species themselves as well as mature mRNAs.

The mt genome of most mammals has a GC content between 36 and 44%. In the rat there is a bias toward the avoidance of using guanine in the third codon position that reflects the generally low amount of this base in the genome. Some G-ending codons are not used at all in this species, i.e., TAG, AGG. ATG is fairly abundant because of its function as an initiator codon. TAA is used as the stop codon in the mtDNA. One of the peculiar features of the mtDNA is the use of TGA as the codon for tryptophan. Considering the number of tRNAs present in this organelle, wobble rules have been determined. In the sets of four synonymous codons, an unmodified U exists in the first position of the anticodon and "wobble-pairs" with all four bases in the third position of the codon. Uridine is the only base that can form a "stable" pair with all four nucleotides in the third position of the codon in either a two out of three or a U:N wobble. In two-codon sets, post-transcriptional modifications restrict the pairing of U to A and G. For each of the eight "genetic code boxes" containing four synonymous codons, there is a single specific tRNA gene with a T in the first position of the anticodon. In the case of tRNA genes corresponding to the sets of two synonymous codons ending with a purine, a T is also found at the first position of the anticodon and it is thought that the corresponding U in the tRNAs is modified to restrict the codon recognition to two codons.

Nuclear-encoded enzymes and proteins play an important role in the transcription of mtDNA, the processing of mtRNAs, and in the translation of mitochondrial messages. These additional nuclear-encoded enzymes are needed for the synthesis of the entire complement of mitochondrially encoded proteins. Other nuclear genes also have functions that relate to the expression of individual mitochondrial gene products such as cytochrome *b* and the subunits 1 and 2 of cytochrome oxidase. The expression of these genes depends on nuclear genes that code for proteins involved in 5' end processing, base excision of the pre-mRNA, and translation of the mature message.

In addition to the above, the development of functional mitochondria requires structural and regulatory genes called PET genes located in the nucleus. The expression of these genes is required for the biogenesis of respiration-competent mitochondria. These genes code for products that have a direct function in mitochondrial respiration and ATP synthesis, yet they affect mitochondrial oxidative metabolism indirectly.

The fact that genetic information is distributed among two spatially separate compartments implies the existence of some mechanism for ensuring a coordinate expression of the proteins and/or RNAs encoded in the two genomes. Growth and division of eukaryotic cells is accompanied by a concomitant increase in mitochondrial mass. This is accomplished not only by the *de novo* formation of the organelle, but also by the addition of lipid and newly synthesized proteins to preexisting mitochondria. The latter condition depends on the balanced rates of synthesis of both the nuclear and mitochondrially encoded constituents of this organelle. In some single cell organisms such as yeast, mtDNA may be absent, yet the organism is able to function somewhat. There are some compensatory reactions that serve as respiratory components. In complex animals, compensation can occur in respiration-deficient cells; however, this compensation is quite limited.

Finally, the transcription of mtDNA is controlled not only by nuclear-encoded transcription factors but also by mitochondrial-specific factors that seem to target mtDNA. Thyroid hormone appears to act in this way, but the mechanism of its action has not been clearly described. Other mtDNA binding molecules have been suggested, but the details of such regulatory effects are lacking.

Respiration

Respiration is the process by which aerobic cells obtain energy from the oxidation of fuel. When coupled with ATP synthesis, the process is called oxidative phosphorylation or OXPHOS. Carbon dioxide, water, heat, and ATP are the products of this process.

Glycolysis, as well as fatty acid and amino acid oxidation, results in the production of an activated two-carbon residue, acetyl CoA. This common metabolic intermediate is joined to oxalacetate to form citrate and is then processed by the citric acid cycle. This cyclic sequence of reactions is found in every cell type that possesses mitochondria. The cycle is catalyzed by a series of enzymes and yields reducing equivalents (H^+) and carbon dioxide. It is illustrated in Figure 3.7. Reducing equivalents are produced when ketoglutarate is produced from isocitrate, when ketoglutarate is decarboxylated to produce succinyl CoA, when succinate is converted to fumarate, and when malate is converted to oxalacetate. These reducing equivalents, one pair for each step, are carried to the respiratory chain by way of either NAD or FAD. Reducing equivalents from succinate are carried by FAD, while those produced by the oxidation of the other substrates are carried by NAD. Once oxalacetate is formed, it can then pick up another acetate group from acetyl CoA and begin the cycle once again by forming citrate. Thus, for every turn of the cycle, two carbon dioxide molecules and eight pairs of reducing equivalents are produced. As long as there is sufficient oxalacetate to pick up the incoming acetate, the cycle will continue to turn and reducing equivalents will continue to be produced and these, in turn, will be joined with molecular oxygen to produce water, the end product (with carbon dioxide) of the catabolic process.

The above simplistic description of the citric acid cycle implies that it is free of controls, and, given adequate supplies of substrates, enzymes, and molecular oxygen, proceeds unhindered. This is not true. There are numerous controls in place that regulate the cycle. The citric acid cycle produces the reducing equivalents needed by the respiratory chain, and the respiratory chain must transfer these hydrogen ions and their associated electrons to the oxygen ion to produce water. In doing so, it generates the electrochemical gradient (the proton gradient) necessary for the formation of the high-energy bonds of ATP. Obviously, then, these processes, citric acid cycle, respiratory chain, and ATP synthesis, are regulated coordinately.

Respiratory Chain

The pairs of electrons produced at the four steps described above in the citric acid cycle, as well as electrons transferred into the mitochondria via other processes, are passed down the respiratory chain to the ultimate acceptor, molecular oxygen. The respiratory chain is shown in Figure 3.8.

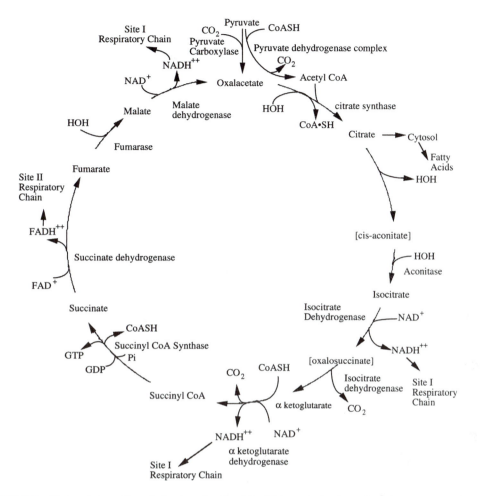

FIGURE 3.7 Krebs citric acid cycle in the mitochondria. This cycle is also called the tricarboxylate cycle (TCA).

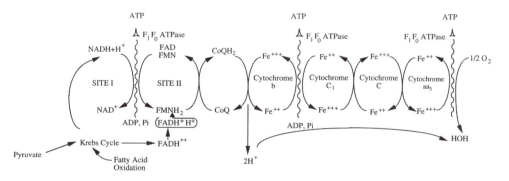

FIGURE 3.8 The respiratory chain showing the points where sufficient energy has been generated to support the synthesis of 1 molecule of ATP from ADP and Pi. Each of the segments generates a proton gradient. This energy is captured by the F_0 portion of the ATPase and transmitted to the F_1 portion of the ATPase. If uncouplers are present, the proton gradient is dissipated and all of the energy is released as heat.

The enzymes of the respiratory chain are particularly complex. They are embedded in the mitochondrial inner membrane and are difficult to extract and study. They catalyze the series of oxidation-reduction reactions that the respiratory chain comprises. Each reaction is characterized by a redox potential that can be calculated using the Nernst equation,

$$E_h = E_0^1 + \frac{2.303\ RT}{nP} \log n\left(\frac{[\text{electron acceptor}]}{[\text{electron donor}]}\right)$$

where E_h = observed potential, E_0^1 = standard redox potential (pH = 7.0, T = 25°, 1.0 M concentration), R = gas constant (8.31 J deg^{-1} mol^{-1}), T = Temperature (°K), n = number of electrons being transferred, P = Faraday (23,062 cal, V^{-1} = 96, 406 J V^{-1}).

The more positive the potential, the greater the affinity of the negatively charged acceptor for the positively charged electrons. It is this potential that drives the respiratory chain reactions forward toward the formation of water. Each succeeding acceptor donor pair has a higher affinity for the electrons than the preceding pair, until the point in the chain where the product, water, is formed. By comparison with the preceding pairs, water itself has little tendency to give up its electrons, and, unless this water is immediately removed, the chain reaction will stop. Of course, water does not accumulate in the mitochondria; it leaves as quickly as it is formed and thus does not feed back to inhibit the chain. If it did accumulate, it would dilute the concentration of the chain components. When water accumulates, the mitochondrion swells; if in excess, the mitochondrion would burst and die. This does not happen. Obviously, then, water must exit the organelle as soon as it is formed so as to maintain optimal osmotic conditions.

Although the respiratory chain usually proceeds in the forward direction (toward the formation of water) due to the exergonic nature of the reaction cascade, it should be realized that, except for the final reaction, all of these steps are fully reversible. In order to be reversed, sufficient energy must be provided to drive the reaction in this direction. For example, the reducing equivalents derived from succinate are usually carried by FAD (as FADH+H+). These can be transferred to NAD (as NADH++H+) with the concomitant hydrolysis of ATP. Electron transport across the other two phosphorylation sites can also be reversed, again, only if sufficient energy is provided.

Overall regulation of respiration or the activity of the intact respiratory chain is vested in the availability of the phosphate acceptor, ADP. A rapid influx of ADP into the mitochondrial compartment is what is needed to ensure a rapid respiratory rate. For example, the working muscle uses the energy provided by the hydrolysis of ATP and creatine phosphate. ATP is hydrolyzed to ADP and Pi and the ADP travels into the mitochondria and stimulates respiration and thence ATP synthesis.

ATP Synthesis

As electrons pass down the respiratory chain, ATP is synthesized. The sequential reactions of the respiratory chain generate an electrochemical gradient of H$^+$ ions across the inner mitochondrial membrane. This gradient serves as the means for coupling the energy flow from electron transport and water formation to the formation of ATP. This involves the mitochondrial membrane. The membrane, and the enzymes and transporters that are embedded in it, couple the energy gradient of the electron flow of the respiratory chain to the synthesis of ATP. To do this, the membrane must be intact and in the form of a continuous closed vesicle. If the membranes are disrupted, coupling will not occur. Respiration may occur, but ATP synthesis will not. The enzymes of the respiratory chain are arranged so as to transport hydrogen ions from the matrix across the inner membrane so that the gradients will develop in proximity to the F_1F_0 ATPase (ATP synthase) complex and provide a proton gradient sufficient to drive ATP synthesis by causing a dehydration of ADP and Pi. This energy capture in the ATP molecule is only a fraction of the energy generated by the respiratory chain. The rest of the energy is released as heat.

The components of oxidative phosphorylation are divided into five complexes. Complexes I through IV plus ubiquinone (Q) and cytochrome C comprise the respiratory chain. Complex V is the F_1F_0 ATPase. The electron carriers are the quinoid structures (FMN, FAD, Q) and the transition metabolic complexes. At three stages in the chain, oxidative energy is conserved (Figure 3.8) via coupled vectorial proton translocations and the creation of a membrane proton gradient ($\Delta\mu H^+$). This protonic energy is what drives the synthesis of ATP. Should this energy be dissipated, as happens when agents such as dinitrophenol or one of the uncoupling proteins are present, ATP synthesis does not occur, or occurs to a more limited extent. Uncoupling takes place because protons are transported through the membrane from the intramembrane space to the matrix. This "short circuits" the normal energy flow through complex V. In such a circumstance, electrons continue down the respiratory chain but the protonic energy thus generated is not captured in the high-energy phosphate bond. Instead, this energy is released as heat. There are variations or degrees of protonic energy capture *in vivo* that are related to the presence or graded absence of naturally occurring agents that serve to either inhibit the action of complex V or uncouple the respiratory chain energy-generation process from the energy-capture process of ATP synthesis.

Uncoupling Proteins

Uncoupling proteins (UCPs) are inner mitochondrial membrane transporters that dissipate the proton gradient, thus releasing heat. The uncoupling proteins are similar in size and homologous in both amino acid sequence and gene sequence for the majority of their structures. Three distinct UCPs have been identified so far. UCP_1 is uniquely expressed in brown adipose tissue. It uncouples OXPHOS in this tissue and this action can be stimulated by norepinephrine. Cold exposure and starvation, two events characterized by an initial rise then fall in norepinephrine, stimulate UCP_1 release and heat production by the brown fat. After the initial use in heat production, there is a fall as the animal attempts to conserve energy. UCP homologs have also been found in skeletal muscle and white adipose tissue. However, the control of their release and their function in the heat economy of the whole animal is somewhat different. UCP_2 is found in heart, liver, muscle, and white adipose tissue. It is subject to dietary manipulation and, as well, probably functions in body weight regulation. UCP_3 is found in skeletal muscle and is down regulated during energy restriction or starvation. Actually, this down regulation probably explains the increased metabolic efficiency that occurs in the food-restricted individual. Following refeeding, some of this increased efficiency is immediately lost, while the rest disappears over time. During the starvation period, the mRNA for these UCPs are up regulated, but the message is not translated. Translation does not occur immediately when food is restored but takes up to 10 days to appear, thus allowing for maximum food efficiency during the immediate recovery period. This up regulation of the UCP mRNA may also play a role in the rapid weight regain following food restriction.

Long-chain free fatty acids can act as partial uncoupling agents. A large influx of fatty acids increases the volume of the mitochondrion and this in turn serves to specially separate the respiratory chain and the ATPase. Other naturally occurring compounds can also reduce coupling efficiency. These agents increase body-heat production. This is an important defense reaction against invading pathogens. Increased body heat (fever) serves to reduce the viability of these pathogens. Some of these compounds are catabolic hormones and their effect on coupling is dose dependent. These include the thyroid hormones, glucocorticoids, sex hormones, catecholamines, insulin, glucagon, parathyroid hormone, and growth hormone. Some of these hormones have direct effects on mitochondrial respiration and coupling through affecting the synthesis and activation of the various protein constituents of the five complexes. These effects are listed in Table 3.4.

Other hormones have their effects on the exchange of divalent ions, notably calcium, and/or on the phospholipid fatty acid composition of the inner mitochondrial membrane. Some hormones,

TABLE 3.4
Effects of Hormones on the Coupling of Respiration to ATP Synthesis

Hormone	Effect
Thyroxine	Increase
Triodothyronine	Increase/decrease; dose dependent
Epinephrine	Decrease
Norepinephrine	Decrease
Insulin	Increase
Glucocorticoid	Increase/decrease; dose dependent
Glucagon	Increase
Parathyroid hormone	Increase; dose dependent
Growth hormone	Increase

thyroid hormones, for example, influence enzyme synthesis/activation, calcium flux, and membrane lipid composition. Clearly, Mother Nature created a very carefully regulated system with checks and balances to ensure the continuity of life. Without this careful control, survival during times of energy stress could not be assured.

The mitochondrial genome also affects mitochondrial function. It serves as a site for a number of genetically determined degenerative diseases in addition to diabetes mellitus. Some of these diseases (Table 3.5) are relatively rare while some, i.e., diabetes, "may" be quite common. The word may is in quotation marks because the prevalence of these mutations is only now being widely studied. As with any genetic disease, the severity and time course of development is determined by the location of the mutation within a specific gene. A mutation in a part of the gene that is translated into an active portion of the resultant protein would be far more devastating than a mutation in a more distal location. In turn, those mutations that result in devastating lethal diseases are rare and usually the result of a spontaneous mutation in that individual. Such a disease markedly shortens the life span of the individual who, in turn, would not likely contribute this gene mutation to the population's gene pool.

TABLE 3.5
Diseases Associated With Mutations in the Mitochondrial Genome

MELAS – Mitochondrial encephalomyopathy, lactic acidosis and stroke-like symptoms
LHON – Leber's hereditary optic neuropathy
MERRF – Myotonic epilepsy and ragged red fiber disease
NARP – Neurogenic muscle weakness, atoxia, retinitis pigmentosa
Diabetes mellitus
Parkinsons disease?
Alzheimers disease?

Errors in mt DNA can be inherent ones (point mutations) or caused by oxidative stress. Mitchondria are rich in lipids and consume ~ 90% of oxygen used by the cell. Free oxygen radicals and fatty acid radicals can form in these organelles attacking the mt DNA and these attacks can result in deletions of portions of the code. Intermittent anoxia followed by reperfusion of oxygen-rich blood can set the stage for such free radical attack. Because the mtDNA has little self repair, the code error (damage) would be sustained. Luckily, the cell has many mitochondria and not all would be affected. The cell can survive but may be somewhat compromised in function.

In contrast to diseases caused by mutations in nuclear DNA, mutations in mtDNA might not be fully expressed. This is because there are many mitochondria in each cell. The liver, for example, has between 500 and 2500 mitochondria per cell with the average value of about 1300. Each mitochondrion has about eight copies of the genome. Cells differ in the number of copies and thus the range is broad (1000–10,000 copies per cell). This is in contrast to nuclear DNA, of which there are only two copies per cell. If some of the mtDNA copies have a normal base sequence and others have a mutated sequence, the cell is heteroplasmic. Homoplasmic cells are those containing mtDNA with identical sequences. If the mutation is a point mutation, that is, a substitution of a base that in turn results in an amino acid substitution in the translation product, this mutated DNA will coexist with normal DNA in the same cell. Depending on where the base pair substitution occurs with respect to the active site of the translation product, the effect of the mutation could be minimal, modest, or profound with respect to the function of that particular mitochondrion. As mentioned, there are many mitochondria in any given cell, so if a small percentage is aberrant, the existence of the mutation might not be known. However, should a large percentage be aberrant, there could be measurable consequences.

Both heteroplasmic and homoplasmic mutations have been reported and these include both point mutations and deletion mutations. Large and small deletion mutations have been reported. Deletion mutations can occur due to slipped mispairing between repeated sequences during DNA replication or by erroneous RNA splicing. Domains containing tandemly repeated DNA sequences are often highly polymorphic in length due to the propensity of repeat units to undergo addition or deletion events. Slipped mispairing between adjacent or nearby repeat sequences during replication is one of several proposed mechanisms for mtDNA deletion mutation. Slipped mispairing between distant repeats can also occur and may be responsible for larger-scale deletions associated with a variety of neuromuscular diseases in humans. Deletions can also occur as a result of free radical attack on the genome. Age-dependent deletion has been reported in human liver and skin. These deletions were found to parallel an age-related decline in respiratory function and are illustrated in Figure 3.9. The age-related mutations are usually random deletions induced by the free radical attack on the genome. Altogether, these deletions plus those possible inherited base substitutions can explain the gradual change in function with age. Individuals may differ in their vulnerability to free radical attack of mtDNA. Some genomes may have more areas of direct repeats and because deletions are more likely to occur in or near these areas, these genomes might be more vulnerable to this type of mutation.

Just as cells can be heteroplasmic with respect to normal mtDNA and DNA with a point mutation, so too can cells be heteroplasmic with respect to mtDNA that has a deletion mutation. However, in the instance of the heteroplasmic cell with the deletion mutation there is the tendency to drift toward deletion mutation homoplasmy. The reason this drift occurs is that mitochondria reproduce themselves at a rate that is 5 to 10 times faster than the rate of cell replication and shorter strands of DNA are replicated at a faster rate than strands of normal length. Thus, a deletion mutation might become evident faster than a point mutation, all other factors being equal. In this scenario, age is a critical determinant of the percentage of the mtDNA with a deletion mutation. As the animal or human ages, there is a drift toward deletion mutation homoplasmy. Several investigators have reported that age, as well as dietary fat as a source of free radicals, are critical factors in the accumulation of mitochondrial DNA deletion mutation.

Point mutation in the codes for the 13 structural genes as well as in the codes for the tRNAs have been reported as well as mutations in the controller regions. Controller region sequence mutation has been reported to occur at rates faster than mutation rates elsewhere in the genome. Rates of base pair substitution in this region vary among the different sites of this region and these sites are distributed along the region rather than being clustered. Polymorphic variation occurs as well, with few or no effects on the activities of the gene products.

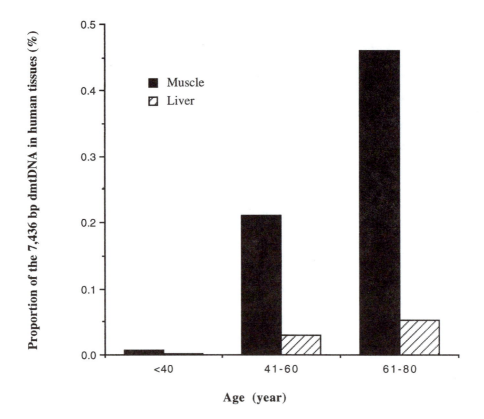

FIGURE 3.9   Age-dependent increase in the proportion of the 7436 bp-deleted mitochondrial DNA in human muscle and liver.

Metabolic Control: Oxidative Phosphorylation

Metabolic regulation is defined as the sum of all of those processes and reactions designed to provide a continuous supply of substrates for the maintenance of cell life. It includes both catabolic and anabolic processes as well as both energy-producing and energy-using pathways. In other words, it is the sum of all these reactions and their controls that defines the steady state. Living cells must interdigitate these pathways so that they are able to survive times of energy deficit and surfeit. They must be able to replace their functional parts as they are used up or worn out or damaged.

The regulation of metabolism can be viewed either as the controls exerted on a single reaction in the cell or as the control of an animal's response to a change in its environment. Neither view is wholly correct because regulation can and does occur at many levels in the body. The simplest level of control is that which is exerted over a single enzymatic reaction. This reaction is controlled by the amount of available substrate, the amount and activity of the enzyme that catalyzes the reaction, the presence of appropriate amounts of required cofactors or coenzymes, and the accumulated product.

One can calculate the strength of the control exerted by the enzyme that catalyzes a reaction or by factors that affect that enzyme using measurements of substrate, products, cofactor amounts, coenzyme amounts, and enzyme amounts using the equation for the calculation of the flux control coefficient. This is an expression of the rate at which a substrate passes to a product through one or more reactions in a series. The flux control coefficient for an individual enzyme E_i within a pathway is defined as $C \dfrac{J}{E_i} = (\partial J/J)/(\partial e_i/e_i)$, where J is the flux of the system and e_i is the activity of any enzyme. Control strength can vary among enzymes in a given reaction sequence and this can be estimated using metabolic control analysis. The elasticity and responsivity of a reaction or series of reactions to perturbations in reactants or environment can also be calculated. It is expressed as $\varepsilon_x^y = x\partial v/v\partial x$, where v is the rate of the reaction and x is a variable that modified v. Thus, the flux through a single reaction or a series of reactions can be estimated. Elasticity, response, and control coefficients determine how a steady-state response will be affected by changes in one or more constituents or conditions needed by this reaction or reaction sequence. This provides a quantitative approach to assessing metabolic control.

Oxidative Phosphorylation

Changes in the dietary or hormonal status of the individual result in large changes in the cytosolic pathways for glucose and fatty acid use as well as changes in protein turnover. All of these are orchestrated by changes in oxidative phosphorylation, which is governed by these changes in cytosolic activity. Starvation and diabetes, for example, result in decreased cytosolic glycolytic activity and lipogenesis while increasing fatty acid oxidation in the mitochondrion. These coordi- nated decreases and increases have in common a change in compartment redox state (ratio of oxidized to reduced metabolites) and phosphorylation (ratio of ATP to ADP) state. Reducing equivalents generated in the cytosol and carried by NAD^+ or $NADP^+$ must be transferred to the mitochondria for use by the respiratory chain. Through transhydrogenation (Figure 3.10), reducing equivalents generated in the cytosol through NADP-linked enzymatic reactions are transferred to NAD. In turn, since NAD cannot traverse the mitochondrial membrane, these reducing equivalents must be carried on suitable metabolites into the mitochondrial compartment. Several shuttle systems exist, with the malate–aspartate shuttle (Figure 3.11) thought to be the most important. The shuttle requires a stoichiometric influx of malate and glutamate and efflux of aspartate and α-ketoglutarate from the mitochondria. Alterations in the rate of efflux of α-ketoglutarate can significantly alter the shuttle activity in terms of the rate of cytosolic NADH utilization. α-Ketoglutarate efflux is dependent on mitochondrial ATP/ADP ratios and on the concentration of cytosolic malate. Shuttle activity is controlled by cytosolic ADP levels, malate levels, and availability of NADH.

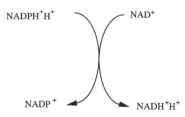

$NADPH^+H^+$ NAD^+

$NADP^+$ $NADH^+H^+$

FIGURE 3.10   Transfer of reducing equivalents from $NADPH^+H^+$ to NAD^+ via transhydrogenation.

Malate can also be exchanged for citrate (Figure 3.12) or for phosphate. The malate–citrate exchange involves transport of malate into the mitochondria, where it is converted to citrate via oxaloacetate. The citrate is then transported out of the mitochondria and the reactions reversed. This exchange is thought to be particularly active in lipogenic states, since it provides citrate to the cytosol for citrate cleavage. Because the cleavage of citrate provides the starting acetate for fatty acid synthesis, this exchange plays a key role in lipogenesis. As shown in Figure 3.12, other exchanges also take place to varying degrees. One can recognize the components of the malate shuttle among these exchange systems as well as identify the system for the exchange of adenine nucleotides. When the activity of the malate–aspartate shuttle is increased, the redox state of the cytosol is decreased, as is lipogenesis, whereas gluconeogenesis is increased. All of these exchanges

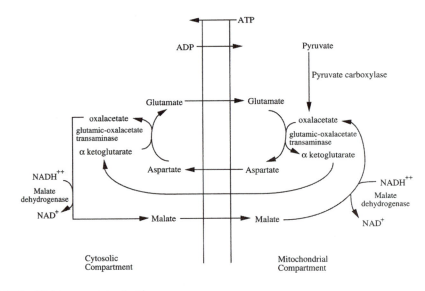

FIGURE 3.11   Malate aspartate shuttle.

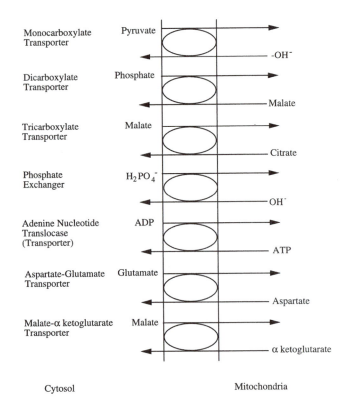

FIGURE 3.12   Metabolite exchanges across the mitochondrial membranes.

of metabolites are related to each other via a coordinated control exerted by the phosphorylation state, the latter, in turn, being controlled by ADP/ATP exchange.

Of importance to the control of glycolysis (see Unit 5) is the α-glycerophosphate shuttle (Figure 3.13). This shuttle is located at the outer side of the mitochondrial inner membrane. Transport of α-glycerophosphate and dihydroxyacetone phosphate across the mitochondrial inner membrane is not required. The activity of the shuttle is related to the availability of α-glycerophosphate and the activity of the mitochondrial α-glycerophosphate dehydrogenase. It is particularly responsive to thyroid hormone, which is thought to act by increasing the synthesis and activity of the mitochondrial α-glycerophosphate dehydrogenase.

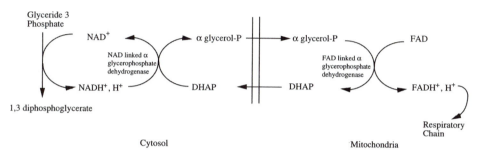

FIGURE 3.13   The α glycerophosphate shuttle.

Adenine nucleotide translocation, or the exchange of adenine nucleotides across the mitochondrial membrane (Figure 3.12), also plays a role in the regulation of oxidative phosphorylation. Although any one of the adenine nucleotides could theoretically exchange for any other, this does not happen. AMP movement is very slow (if it occurs at all). Under certain conditions, ADP influx into the mitochondria is many times faster than ATP efflux. This occurs when the need for ATP within the mitochondria exceeds that of the cytosol. An example of this occurs in starvation, where ATP is needed to initiate urea synthesis and fatty acid oxidation and to support gluconeogenesis. Under normal dietary conditions, however, the exchange of ADP for ATP is very nearly equal. For every 100 molecules of ADP that enters the mitochondrial compartment, about 87 molecules of ATP exit.

The number of molecules of ATP produced by the coupling of the respiratory chain to ATP synthesis depends on where the reducing equivalents enter the chain. If they enter carried by NAD, they are said to enter at site I. If they enter carried by FAD, they are said to enter at site II. Site I substrates are those that are oxidized via NAD-linked dehydrogenases. Pyruvate, for example, is a site I substrate, while succinate is a site II substrate. Reducing equivalents entering at site I will generate the energy for the synthesis of three molecules of ATP. Those entering at site II will generate enough energy to result in two molecules of ATP. Knowing how a substrate provides its reducing equivalents to the respiratory chain allows estimation of how many ATPs will be generated by a particular reaction sequence. Since each ATP has an energy value of about 30.5 kJ or 7.3 kcal/mol, the amount of energy each sequence will produce or use can also be estimated. Going one step further, the oxygen consumed can be measured and the amount of energy released estimated. This, then, is the basis for the indirect measure of energy expenditure through the measurement of oxygen consumed. The basal oxygen consumption can be measured, as can the increase in oxygen consumption with activity. The difference between growing and nongrowing animals can be obtained so that the energy cost of growth can be estimated. Similarly, if a person or animal is either gaining or losing weight, the energy cost of this weight gain (or loss) can be estimated.

The details of each of the major metabolic pathways are given in Units 4, 5, and 6. Each pathway is characterized by the number of ATPs it uses or produces. Not all of the ATPs are produced by the mitochondrial oxidative phosphorylation process. Some are produced as a product of substrate oxidation. Shown in Table 3.6 are the number of ATPs used or produced by these pathways. This number assumes that the reducing equivalents produced enter the OXPHOS system, which produces three ATPs if site 1 is used and two ATPs if site 2 is used.

As can be noted in Table 3.6, if the metabolic mixture consumed and oxidized is known, the energy change can be calculated. Rarely is this possible. Usually, the oxygen consumed and the carbon dioxide produced can be measured, and it can be determined whether the subject is gaining or losing weight and whether the subject is in nitrogen balance. Nitrogen balance means that the nitrogen from the protein in the food is replacing that of the proteins being degraded in the body. (The nitrogen balance concept is discussed in greater detail in Unit 4.) Energy balance has a similar meaning. The energy used by the body is replaced by the energy provided by the diet. A subject in energy and nitrogen balance is neither losing nor gaining weight. By measuring the respiratory gases, the respiratory quotient (RQ) can be calculated. RQ is the ratio of carbon dioxide produced to oxygen consumed.

TABLE 3.6
ATP Produced or Used by the Major Metabolic Pathways

			ATPs Produced
Glycolysis	a)	Gluco or hexokinase	−1
	b)	Phosphofructokinase	−1
	c)	Glyceraldehyde 3 phosphate dehydrogenase-2 NADH$^+$H$^+$ produced	+6
	d)	Phosphoglycerate kinase	+2
	e)	Pyruvate kinase	+2
Krebs Cycle	a)	Pyruvate dehydrogenase (2NADH$^+$H$^+$)	6
	b)	Isocitrate dehydrogenase (2NADH$^+$H$^+$)	6
	c)	α ketoglutarate (2NADH$^+$H$^+$)	6
	d)	Succinate thiokinase	2
	e)	Succinate dehydrogenase (2FADH$_2$)	4
	f)	Malate dehydrogenase (2NADH$^+$H$^+$)	6
Urea Synthesis	a)	Carbamyl synthetase	−4
Protein Synthesis	a)	Amino acid tRNA binding	2/amino acid
	b)	Amino acid tRNA bound to ribosome	−1/amino acid
	c)	Amino acid chain formation	0
	d)	RNA degradation	−2
Fatty Acid Synthesis	a)	Formation of methyl malonyl CoA	−1
Fatty Acid Oxidation	a)	Activation of fatty acid (thiokinase)	−1
	b)	Acyl CoA dehydrogenase (FADH)	2/acetyl unit
	c)	L(+), β hydroxyacyl CoA dehydrogenase (NAD$^+$H$^+$)	3
	d)	Krebs (citric acid or TCA)cycle	24/acetyl unit

When glucose is the sole substrate being oxidized, then the RQ is 1, since the oxidation of glucose uses and releases equal amounts of oxygen and carbon dioxide.

$$C_6H_{12}O_6 + 6\,O_2 \rightarrow 6\,CO_2 + 6\,HOH$$

$$RQ = 1.0 = \frac{6\,CO_2}{6\,O_2}$$

This complete oxidation to CO_2 and HOH will produce 36 molecules of ATP. When fatty acids are being oxidized, the RQ is close to 0.7. This is because fatty acids require far more oxygen for their oxidation than they produce as carbon dioxide.

$$\text{palmitic acid, } C_{16}H_{32}O_2 + 23\,O_2 \rightarrow 16\,CO_2 + 16\,\text{HOH}$$

$$RQ = \frac{16\,CO_2}{23\,O_2} = \sim 0.7$$

When it is considered that the fatty acids are mobilized from the stored triacylglycerols and the RQ is computed on this basis, a slightly higher RQ results. For example, using a theoretical triacylglycerol consisting of two molecules of stearic acid and one of palmitic acid attached to a glycerol backbone the equation is as follows:

$$C_{55}H_{106}O_6 + 76.5\,O_2 \rightarrow 55\,CO_2 + 53\,\text{HOH}$$

$$RQ = \frac{55\,CO_2}{76.5\,O_2} = 0.719$$

A molecule of glucose will, when oxidized to pyruvate, yield a net of 8 molecules of ATP (2 molecules of ATP are needed for glycolysis). When glucose is oxidized to CO_2 and HOH, 36 molecules of ATP are formed. A fatty acid such as palmitate will yield a net of 129 molecules of ATP (2 molecules of ATP are needed for activation). If each ATP has an energy value of 7.3 kcal (30.5 kJ)/high-energy bond, then, in theory, glucose oxidation to pyruvate should yield 7.3 kcal (30.5 kJ/mol) × 8 ATP or 58.4 kcal (244.3 kJ) per molecule. Complete glucose oxidation should yield 262.8 kcal (1099.6 kJ) and palmitate should yield 7.3 kcal × 129 ATP or 41.7 kcal (3940 kJ) trapped in the high-energy bond of ATP. However, these figures do not correct for the energy trapped in the ATP molecule through substrate phosphorylation, nor do they correct for energy lost as heat. The assumption is also made that the reducing equivalents produced by these catabolic reaction sequences will be sent to the OXPHOS system for ATP synthesis. This does not always occur. When palmitate is oxidized in a bomb calorimeter, 2609 kcal (10,958 kJ) of heat is released per molecule. In a living system, not all of the energy of nutrient oxidation is released as heat. Some is captured in the chemical bonds of high-energy compounds such as ATP, GTP, and UTP. The difference in the energy released as heat in the bomb calorimeter and that captured in these high-energy bonds is the energy lost as heat in the body plus that amount of energy captured in the bonds of CO_2 and water. If a ratio were to be made of the amount of energy captured in the ATP to that totally available (941.7:2609) the finding would be that about 36% of the total inherent energy of palmitate can be captured in the chemical bonds of ATP versus ~ 64% that is released as heat and used to make CO_2 and water. Note that palmitate oxidation produces more than three times the amount of ATP than does glucose. This is the reason that fats are more dense energetically than carbohydrates. Per gram, fat provides 9 kcal (37.6 kJ) and carbohydrate 4 (16.7 kJ).

The ratio of glucose to fatty acids being oxidized will be reflected in the measured RQ. Most humans consuming a mixed diet will have an average RQ of about 0.87. It will vary throughout the typical feeding-fasting day-night cycle followed by most people who work during the day and sleep at night. Just before breakfast, the RQ will be at its lowest, while after the evening meal it will likely be at its highest. This, of course, is dependent on the composition of the meals consumed as well as on their spacing. As mentioned in the beginning of this section, the basal heat production or oxygen consumption is usually measured in the postabsorptive state. This usually means a measurement made before breakfast and it also usually means that the metabolic fuel mix is that of glucose (from glycogen) plus fatty acids (from the fat depots).

ENERGY RETAINED

After the heat production associated with exercising muscles and the inefficiency of energy capture as described above are accounted for, two other components must be included. These are the energy that is either stored in the fat and glycogen depots or needed to sustain growth or production. This is quite straightforward. If weight is neither gained nor lost, then the energy balance (energy retained) is zero. If weight is gained as fat, the energy value of that fat must be accounted for. If the fat is deposited as preformed fat, that is, the fat in the diet is hydrolyzed at the gut, transported to the depot, and reesterified for storage, the energy cost of this storage is minimal. This is a very efficient way to accumulate body-fat stores. On the other hand, if glucose is used to make the stored triacylglycerols, the process is quite inefficient. To make one molecule of tripalmitin (palmitate is a 16 carbon fatty acid), 12 molecules of glucose would be needed and 45 molecules of ATP would be needed to make 3 molecules of palmitoyl CoA. Another half molecule of glucose and four ATPs would be needed to make the glycerol phosphate. Altogether, 12.5 moles of glucose plus 49 moles of ATP would be necessary to make 1 mole of tripalmitin. To generate the ATP for this synthesis, 1.3 moles of glucose would have to be completely oxidized since one mole would give only 36 ATPs, and 49 are needed. Thus, the efficiency of energy storage as fatty acids synthesized from glucose is much less than if the dietary fat were to be stored in the depot and dietary carbohydrate used to supply whatever ATP is needed. Humans consuming a mixed diet will have RQ closer to 1 than to 0.7 because they will oxidize glucose in preference to fatty acids. Table 3.7 illustrates these calculations.

TABLE 3.7
Efficiency of Storing Energy from Dietary Fat Versus that Using Glucose Triglyceride Synthesis (Tripalmitin) from Palmitate

Cost

$3\ \text{pal} + 3\text{ATP} + 3\text{CoASH} \rightarrow 3\ \text{palCoA} + 3\text{AMP}$ (2 ATP/palmitate $\rightarrow$ pal CoA)

$4\text{ATP} + 0.5\ \text{glucose} \rightarrow \alpha GP + 4\text{ADP}$

$3\ \text{pal CoA} + \alpha GP \rightarrow \text{Tripalmitin}$

10ATP/36ATP per mole glu = 0.27 moles glucose

$0.5 + 0.26 = 0.76$ moles glucose + 3 moles palmitate + 10 moles ATP $\rightarrow$ 1 mole tripalmitin.

Using protein for energy is even more costly and less efficient. Each amino acid that is incorporated into a polypeptide chain requires an ATP for its activation. In a protein containing many hundred amino acids, the requirement for ATP is enormous. ATP is also required for the synthesis of the RNA coded for the protein being synthesized. Because protein synthesis is so energy dependent, the energy requirement to support growth (protein synthesis) can be quite large. If, instead of using the amino acids from the dietary protein to synthesize body protein, they are used to provide energy, the cost of this energy must be corrected for the costs of synthesizing urea from the amino groups liberated prior to the oxidation of the amino acid carbon skeleton for energy. Approximately 20% of the gross energy of a typical protein is lost because of the need to synthesize urea.

The energy cost is therefore 10 ATP, each with a value of 7.3 kcal or 30.5 kJ. The total cost would be 73 kcal or 305 kJ. If the total energy value of tripalmitin was 7597 (31,907 kJ), then the efficiency of storing preformed fat would be $(7597–73) \div 7597$ or ~ 98%.

Tripalmitin synthesis from glucose is energetically more expensive because only four of the six glucose carbons are used to make the 16-carbon fatty acid, palmitate. It will take four glucoses to make one palmitate and 12 glucoses to make three palmitates.

$$12\ \text{glucose} + 45\ \text{ATP} + 0_2 \rightarrow 3\ \text{palmityl CoA} + 24\ CO_2$$

$$0.5\ \text{glucose}\ \frac{+\ 4\ \text{ATP}}{49\ \text{ATP}} \rightarrow \alpha\ \text{glycerophosphate} + \text{ADP}$$

3 palmityl CoA + α glycerophosphate → tripalmitin
1 mole of glucose completely oxidized yield 36 ATP
49 are needed
∴ 49/36 = 1.4 moles of glucose are needed to provide the ATP or 1.4 × 294.8 = 412.72
12 + 0.5 + 1.4 = 13.8 moles of glucose needed to produce 1 mole of tripalmitin; each glucose has a value of 294.8 kcal or 1238 KJ.

The cost of making tripalmitin would be 412.72 kcal (1726.82 kJ). The efficiency would therefore be (7597–412.72) ÷ 7597 = ~ 94%. However, if this cost was computed using the energy value of tripalmitin (7597 kcal or 31,907 kJ) corrected for the energy value of all the glucose needed to make the palmityl CoA and all the ATP used, the cost would be (7597–4068–412.72) ÷ 7597 or 41% of the total energy value of the tripalmitin.

Using dietary protein for body protein synthesis can be either very efficient or very inefficient, depending on the amino acid content of the diet and the body proteins being synthesized. This aspect of metabolism will be described in Unit 4. However, the energetics of protein deposition using dietary protein is quite straightforward.

Disregarding amino acid oxidation, urea formation, and the growth process, if the energetic efficiency of protein turnover is examined, an efficiency of about 82% is found. This figure is arrived at using the assumption that the dietary protein is used completely *and exclusively* to replace degraded body protein. For ease of description, the amount of protein degraded and replaced is 100 grams. This 100 grams would have a gross energy value of 570 kcal or ~2384 kJ. For every amino acid incorporated into this protein, 5 ATPs would be used plus 1.2 ATPs for rearrangements of the structure. This would mean an energy cost of about 694 kcal or ~2904 kJ. Dividing the energy value of the protein produced by the cost of its production $\left(\dfrac{570 \text{ or } 2383}{694 \text{ or } 2902} \right)$ gives an efficiency of about 82%. Practically speaking, for the average human adult in the United States, the energy efficiency of protein turnover is of little importance. The typical U.S. diet is not limiting with respect to protein or energy.

ENERGETIC EFFICIENCY

The food that provides the energy does so by providing fuel for oxidation to provide heat, ATP, CO_2, and water. The heat produced through this oxidation is needed to keep the body warm, but it is also a measure of the energy need. That is, the heat produced (and that can be measured) is the energy that is lost from the body and must be replaced. For example, if a molecule of palmitate is oxidized in a bomb calorimeter, the amount of heat released is 2,609 kcal (10,958 kJ). However, when oxidized in the body, it yields 130 ATPs, 146 molecules of water, and 1,384 kcal (5812 kJ) of heat. Of the inherent energy of palmitate, 36% is trapped by the body when this fuel is used and 64% is released as heat. This 40/60 (rounded figures) distribution of energy available to the body vs. that released as heat is an average distribution. More or less can occur in each category. The pattern of distribution is influenced by the composition of the diet and the genetics of the consumer. An example of the former occurs when an essential fatty acid-deficient diet is fed. This deficiency state is characterized by a decrease in the efficiency of use of food for body weight gain.

Feed efficiency is a term used to designate the efficiency with which an animal (or human) uses the food it consumes to build new tissue as it grows or rebuild body tissue that is lost through the normal conditions of life. Those animals that can gain more body weight on less food are more efficient than those animals that require more food for the same gain. Meat-animal production research has been devoted to increasing energetic efficiency using dietary and nondietary techniques. Selective breeding, for example, of beef animals has resulted in bovines that grow rapidly and consume less food per pound of weight gained than animals used for this purpose a century ago. Whereas it used to take 3 years to produce a bovine of a size suitable for use, it now takes 2 years or less to produce a meat animal ready for market. Furthermore, the meat produced today is of higher quality in terms of tenderness, flavor, and nutrient content than that produced 100 years ago. Other meat animals (sheep, pigs, chickens, goats) likewise have been selectively bred to produce a rapidly growing, energetically efficient animal. With the growing emphasis today on the production of meat with a lower fat content, animal scientists are continuing to use genetics and dietary maneuvers to produce an animal that meets the consumers' demands.

Just as the diet and genetics of the meat animal determine its energetic efficiency, so too can these same effects be expected in humans. Genetic and dietary factors interact and, in so doing, determine the rate and extent of longitudinal growth as well as the development of muscle mass and fat mass. At present, the segregation of humans by genotype is not possible. However, genes that appear to be important in the development of obesity (excess fat mass) are being identified. How diet, particularly the sources of energy, can affect the phenotypic expression of these obesity-related genes is not known.

UTILIZABLE ENERGY

The energy expended to do the body's work is referred to as utilizable energy. This is the energy used by muscles as they contract in the course of voluntary activity or work. This energy is sometimes referred to as the activity increment. That is, it is the energy cost associated with body movement, which is added to the basal energy need when the energy requirement is calculated. For sedentary persons, only a small increment is needed but for very active persons, a large increment will be needed to sustain activity. As much as a 200% increment above basal energy need may be required to sustain a high level of activity and maintain body weight. Shown in Table 3.8 are some representative activities and their associated energy cost given as heat units per kilogram body weight per hour.

In the course of muscle contraction, oxygen is used for the oxidation of metabolic fuels by the working muscle. Heat is released and water and carbon dioxide are produced. The more active a person is, the more oxygen is needed for the oxidation of metabolic fuel by the muscle. Trained athletes are more efficient in their use of metabolic fuels than are nontrained, sedentary individuals. Training involves an increase in use of specific muscle groups as well as an increase in lung and heart action. Muscle contraction, which is usually supported by the oxidation of glucose (from blood glucose or glycogen breakdown) in the sedentary person, can use fatty acids as fuel after training. During exercise, the respiratory quotient (RQ) in the trained individual decreases. This means that fat is being oxidized, since the oxidation of fatty acids results in a lower RQ than the oxidation of glucose. Fatty acid oxidation by working muscle will spare glucose and will decrease the rate of lactate production. The muscle does not store large amounts of lipid for use during work, but it can use fatty acids liberated from fat depots through the action of the catabolic hormones. Part of training is to increase muscle fatty acid oxidation while also increasing the glycogen–glucose reserve in the muscle. The so-called glycogen-loading technique dictates the exhaustion of the muscle glycogen store followed by rest and glycogen repletion just prior to the competitive event. During the rest/repletion period a high carbohydrate diet is consumed. This exhaustion/repletion routine results in an increased supply of glucose from glycogen within the muscle. Since the first phase of glycolysis is anaerobic, an enlarged supply of glucose from glycogen can be oxidized in the absence of oxygen, and thus exhaustion, which is characterized by an oxygen debt, is delayed. Training or adaptation to exercise or work is thus characterized by decrease in RQ due to both an increase in the oxidation of fatty acids and an increase in the anaerobic use of glucose from glycogen. Table 3.9 summarizes the effects of exercise on metabolism, while Table 3.10 gives some typical results of a comparison of trained and untrained subjects with respect to their oxygen and glucose use during a bout of exercise. Note that the untrained and trained subjects consumed the same amount of oxygen, but the trained subjects had a lower RQ. This means that the trained subjects were oxidizing some fatty acids.

TABLE 3.8
Energy Cost of Activities Exclusive of Basal Metabolism and Influence of Food

Activity	kcal/ kg/hr	(kJ)	Activity	kcal/ kg/hr	kJ
Bedmaking	3.0	12.6	Playing cards	0.5	2.1
Bicycling (century run)	7.6	31.9	Playing Ping Pong	4.4	18.4
Bicycling (moderate speed)	2.5	10.5	Piano playing (Mendelssohn's Song Without Words)	0.8	3.3
Boxing	11.4	47.9	Piano playing (Beethoven's Appassionata)	1.4	5.9
Carpentry (heavy)	2.3	9.7	Piano playing (Liszt's Tarantella)	2.0	8.4
Cello playing	1.3	5.5	Reading aloud	0.4	1.7
Cleaning windows	2.6	10.9	Rowing	9.8	41.0
Crocheting	0.4	1.7	Rowing in race	16.0	66.9
Dancing, moderately active	3.8	16	Running	7.0	29.3
Dancing, rhumba	5.0	21	Sawing wood	5.7	23.8
Dancing, waltz	3.0	12.6	Sewing, hand	0.4	1.7
Dishwashing	1.0	4.2	Sewing, foot-driven machine	0.6	2.5
Dressing and undressing	0.7	2.9	Sewing, electric machine	0.4	1.7
Driving car	0.9	3.8	Singing in loud voice	0.8	3.3
Eating	0.4	1.7	Sitting quietly	0.4	1.7
Exercise, Very light	0.9	3.8	Skating	3.5	14.6
Light	1.4	5.6	Skiing (moderate speed)	10.3	43.1
Moderate	3.1	13	Standing at attention	0.6	2.5
Severe	5.4	22.7	Standing relaxed	0.5	2.1
Very severe	7.6	31.9	Sweeping with broom, bare floor	1.4	5.9
Fencing	7.3	30.7	Sweeping with carpet sweeper	1.6	6.7
Football	6.8	28.6	Sweeping with vacuum sweeper	2.7	11.3
Gardening, weeding	3.9	16.4	Swimming (2 mi/hr)	7.9	33.1
Golf	1.5	6.3	Tailoring	0.9	3.8
Horseback riding, walk	1.4	5.9	Tennis	5.0	20.9
Horseback riding, trot	4.3	18.0	Typing, rapidly	1.0	4.2
Horseback riding, gallop	6.7	28.0	Typing, electric typewriter	0.5	2.1
Ironing (5-lb iron)	1.0	4.2	Violin playing	0.6	2.5
Knitting sweater	0.7	2.9	Walking (3 mi per hr)	2.0	8.4
Laboratory work	2.1	8.8	Walking rapidly (4 mi per hr)	3.4	14.2
Laundry, light	1.3	5.4	Walking at high speed (5.3 mi per hr)	8.3	34.7
Lying still, awake	0.1	0.4	Washing floors	1.2	5.0
Office work, standing	0.6	2.5	Writing	0.4	1.7
Organ playing (1/3 handwork)	1.5	6.3			
Painting furniture	1.5	6.3			
Paring potatoes	0.6	2.5			

That fatty acids were used is seen in the last column, showing that the trained subjects consumed less glucose per minute than did the untrained subjects.

THERMOGENESIS

Another way energy is lost from the body as heat is the heat lost as one or more of the uncoupling proteins are activated. In early years, it was thought that this heat was associated with the degradation of the food components in preparation for its use by the body for its maintenance. Hence, it was called diet-induced thermogenesis. Now, however, there seems to be another explanation having to do with the production and release of proteins called uncoupling proteins. The first of these, UCP_1, was identified in the brown fat depots. These brown fat depots are located at the base of the neck,

TABLE 3.9
Summary of the Effects of Training on Metabolism and Body Composition

Decreased RQ during exercise
Decreased fat mass
Increased muscle mass[1]
Increased fatty acid mobilization during exercise
Increased glucose synthesis by the liver
Increased aerobic capacity of muscle
Improved glucose tolerance
Decreased need for insulin to facilitate glucose use
Decreased heat production via activation of uncoupling proteins in muscle[1]

[1] May be localized; depends on the types of muscles used for the activity

TABLE 3.10
Effect of Training on Oxygen Uptake and Fuel Use

Subject	O_2 L	RQ $\frac{[CO_2]}{[O_2]}$	Glucose Used mmol/min
Trained	3.0	0.90	10.6
Untrained	3.0	0.95	13.3

along the backbone and, in males, across the shoulders. The brown fat cell differs from the white fat cell in that it contains many more mitochondria in the cytosol than does the white cell. Both cell types have stored lipid droplets that, if sufficiently large, can push all of the other organelles off to the side of the cell. In contrast to the white cell depots, the brown fat depots are highly innervated and vascularized as shown in Figure 3.14. This increase in vascularization gives the depot its brownish color and name, brown fat.

As described above, much of the structure of the white cell is similar to that of the brown fat cell. Whereas white depots are distributed throughout the body, brown depots are found in just a few locations. Brown fat cells, if allowed to accumulate lipid, may change in appearance and look like white fat as the lipid droplets enlarge. Histochemical studies have failed to reveal any qualitative differences between the fat depots of the two cell types. More brown fat can be observed in newborns than in adults and it is thought that thermoregulation in the immature animal is dependent on the activity of the brown fat depot with respect to its ability to generate heat. Both cell types can store lipid and this lipid can be readily mobilized. However, when it mobilizes its stored lipid, the brown fat oxidizes its lipid *in situ* rather than releasing it for utilization by other tissues. When stimulated, the brown fat can produce more heat during metabolism than can the white fat cell.

In the newborn, brown adipose tissue has the function of generating heat as part of the body's thermoregulatory process. However, it is not the only tissue that contributes to thermoregulation. Heat production due to uncoupling protein also occurs in muscle and white adipose tissue. The heat produced in this way is especially important to newborns because they lack the insulation provided by the subcutaneous fat store. This fat layer helps conserve body heat. Additional heat production is provided by the newborn's metabolic processes, which are relatively immature with respect to energy conservation. Heat loss from these processes can be quite large. As the newborn

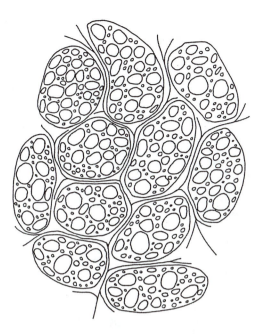

FIGURE 3.14   Anatomy of the brown fat deposit. This depot is more highly vascularized that is the white depot. It also has many more sympathetic nerve endings than does the white fat depot.

matures biochemically as well as physiologically, the importance of these uncoupling proteins in energy balance subsides. The baby begins to accumulate a subcutaneous fat layer and no longer has to endure the penalty of an inadequate energy store. Glycogen accumulation and utilization patterns mature as well, so that the infant and young child can be fed less frequently.

ABNORMAL ENERGY STATES

Starvation and Undernutrition

The basic metabolic response to starvation of an otherwise healthy individual is conservation. As the gut receives less food, it slowly empties. First, the stomach, then the duodenum, the jejunum, the ileum, and the large intestine lose their contents and shrink in size. Simple mono- and disaccharides are the first to disappear, followed by the products of the progressively more complex nutrients: polysaccharides, proteins, and lipids. As the sugars disappear, there is less stimulus for insulin release and basal insulin levels are approached. As glucose is less available from the gut, the body begins to mobilize its glycogen stores and when they are close to being depleted, the body will begin to mobilize its stores of triacylglycerol and, to a lesser extent, its body protein. It can use certain of the amino acids and glycerol from the triacylglycerols to synthesize glucose via gluconeogenesis and utilize the carbon skeletons of deaminated amino acids plus the fatty acids liberated from the triacylglycerols for fuel. In 1915, Benedict, in an extensive monograph on the metabolic responses to starvation, reported that the body carbohydrate (glycogen and glucose) provided only a small fraction of the total fuel needed for maintenance. Cahill later estimated that a 70-kg man had approximately 75 grams of glycogen stored in the muscle and liver, which provides approximately 300 kcal (1255 kJ) during the initial 24 hours of starvation. The glycogen and the glucose synthesized via gluconeogenesis thus provide only a small percentage of the 2000–2500 kcal (8368–8577 kJ) needed per day for maintenance. Benedict estimated that mobilizable body protein could provide about 15% of the body's fuel needs and that the fat stores of the adipose tissue provided the rest. Although Benedict did not have today's sophisticated technology at his disposal, his estimates were remarkably close to those of Cahill. Cahill estimated that a "normal" 70-kg man required about 2000 kcal (8368 kJ) per day to maintain his body and that he had sufficient fuel stores to sustain life for about 80 days. As shown in Figure 3.15, adapted from Cahill's paper, most of the energy comes from the lipid stored in the adipose tissue. While Cahill and others evaluated the energy losses from the whole animal, interorgan fuel fluxes have been studied as well. Figure 3.16 illustrates these fluxes during the first 24 hours of starvation.

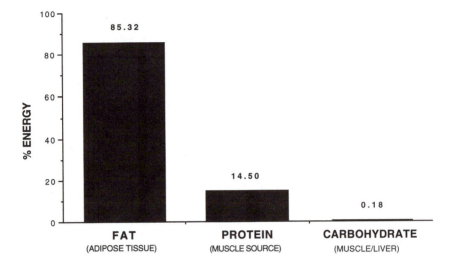

FIGURE 3.15 Sources of metabolic fuel for starving man. The lipid utilized is primarily the fatty acids released from triacylblycerol by the adipose tissue depots, the protein is mainly that raided from the muscle and the carbohydrate utilized is that released by the liver and muscle glycogen and that synthesized by the kidney and liver via gluconeogenesis from selected amin acids and from the glycerol moiety of triacylglycerol released by the adipose tissue. (Adapted from Cahill et al., and Sandek and Felig.)

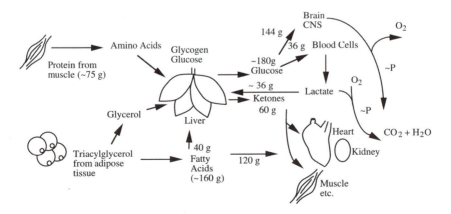

FIGURE 3.16 Inter-tissue fuels fluxes after 24 hours of starvation. Note the central position of the liver. This organ uses glycerol, lactate, fatty acids, and amino acids to produce ketones and glucose, which serve as fuel sources for blood cells, the brain and central nervous system, heart, kidney, and muscle. These fuels are oxidized to carbon dioxide and water, requiring only the presence of molecular oxygen and energy from the high-energy phosphate bonds as provided by the adenine and guanine nucleotides.

Lipids, primarily triacylglycerols, are hydrolyzed to fatty acids and glycerol through the action of hormone-sensitive lipase. This enzyme, located on the interior aspect of the fat cell membrane, is activated by the catabolic hormones, epinephrine, and glucocorticoid, and its activity is increased when glucagon is high and insulin is low. The glycerol is converted to glucose via gluconeogenesis in the liver and kidney. The fatty acids are oxidized to ketones and then to carbon dioxide and water. Whereas the liver can oxidize the fatty acids completely to carbon dioxide and water, the muscle is unable to do so and thus ketones, the end products of muscle fatty acid oxidation, rise. These ketones can be used by the brain as a fuel when the supply of glucose becomes more limited. After about 40 days of starvation, the brain has been shown to obtain nearly 65% of its energy from the ketones. These fuel fluxes are diagrammed in Figure 3.16. Under normal (i.e., fed) conditions, the central nervous system uses 115 g of glucose/day while erythrocytes, bone marrow, renal medulla, and peripheral nerves use about 36 g of glucose/day. Most of this glucose can be synthesized through gluconeogenesis from glycerol, lactate, and selected amino acids during the early phase of starvation. However, as the starvation continues, the body attempts to protect its protein component and the amino acid substrates for gluconeogenesis become less available. This, coupled with the rising ketone level (ketones can cross the blood–brain barrier), serves to induce the utilization of the ketones by the brain as a metabolic fuel.

Proteolysis, initially increased, after 48 hours of starvation is suppressed by rising levels of growth hormone as the body attempts to conserve its body proteins. The initial proteolysis, however, serves to provide the needed amino acids for the synthesis of enzymes needed for survival (enzymes needed for energy mobilization and conservation). Once these mechanisms are established, body protein is conserved. The temporal relationship of fuels and the hormones that control their availability is diagrammed in Figure 3.17.

Protein–Energy Malnutrition

Starvation is the extreme state of malnutrition that occurs when the individual is provided little or no food to nourish the body. Between starvation and the state of adequate nourishment to meet nutrient needs, there are graded levels of inadequate nutrient intake. Although infants and children of third-world nations come to mind when malnutrition is pictured, people of all ages in all countries are vulnerable. Where the intake of macronutrients is inadequate, the syndrome is called protein-calorie malnutrition (PCM) or, more correctly, protein energy malnutrition.

Chronic malnutrition is characterized not only by energy deficit (energy need exceeding energy intake) but also by a deficit in the protein intake and the intake of micronutrients. The needs for these nutrients and energy are determined by the age and health status of the individual. Rapid growth, infection, injury, and chronic debilitating disease can drive up the need for food and the nutrients it contains. Infants and young children have been described as having PCM. The characteristics of PCM are described in Unit 4.

Just as infection or trauma potentiates the needs for protein, energy, and micronutrients in third-world children, so these conditions also increase the need for nutrients in developed nations. Injury and sepsis both increase energy needs. Both adults and children may have increased nutrient needs under these circumstances and if these needs are not met, varying degrees of malnutrition or PCM will be observed. Malnutrition has been documented in hospitalized patients in the U.S. and this malnutrition may have a negative effect on the time course of recovery as well as on mortality.

Trauma And Energy Needs

Since Cuthbertson first described the body's disproportionate catabolic response to trauma, physicians, nutritionists, and physiologists alike have accepted this as an obligatory and necessary response to illness or injury. With the advent of parenteral and enteral feeding techniques, it has been possible to show that this loss, formerly thought to be obligatory, is not. Indeed, losses due

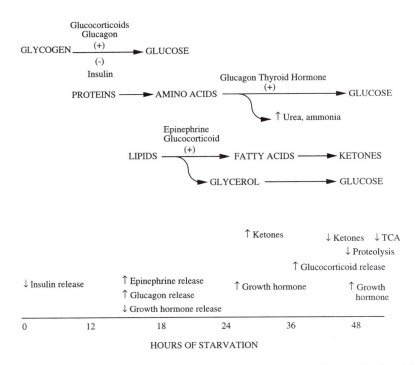

FIGURE 3.17 Temporal relations of fuels and hormones during starvation. During the first 24 hours, there is a decrease in blood glucose levels and an increase in proteolysis. After 18 hours, measurable increases in gluconeogenesis due to glucose production from glycerol can be observed. There is a rise in lipolysis, initially stimulated by epinephrine but then maintained by rising glucocorticoid, glucagon, and growth-hormone levels. As these hormones rise, they serve to decrease peripheral tissue sensitivity to insulin and decreased glucose tolerance can be observed. With rising growth-hormone levels, proteolysis is decreased and the body attempts to conserve body protein. By 48 hours, ketosis, having been high, now begins to decline as the body adapts to using ketones and fatty acids as metabolic fuels.

to surgery, infection, or burn have been shown to be minimized and even reversed (in some cases) with the provision of adequate nutritional support. This implies then, that the catabolic response to trauma or illness is more a response to inadequate nutrition in the face of a greatly increased set of nutrient requirements than to the trauma or illness itself.

The endocrine and metabolic responses to injury are closely related (Figure 3.18). Increased production of some hormones and the inhibited release of others are integral parts of the body's basic defense mechanism. The primary function of this mechanism is to provide a continuous fuel supply to the central nervous system and the required substrates for the repair of body tissue. While the body may respond to trauma with an increased release of the hormones that regulate metabolism through cAMP or through the phosphatidylinositol cycle, this response, in comparison with the overall metabolic response to injury or illness, is relatively short lived. It appears, therefore, that the hormonal responses to injury serve as initiators or inducers of metabolic events that must occur if recovery is to proceed. As relief from the trauma occurs, these hormonal responses recede and other metabolic control mechanisms assume command. These, in turn, give way to the normal metabolic control mechanisms as recovery proceeds. Aging patients and children likely will have a more exaggerated metabolic response to trauma than young, otherwise healthy adults. Although the sequence of hormonal and metabolic response may be similar, the time frame and intensity of response will differ. Sometimes these differences can be life threatening if close monitoring is not practiced. The elderly may already have peripheral tissue insulin resistance, which is made worse by the trauma. The child may be more likely to quickly exhaust energy stores and have little reserve. In each instance, the difference between death and survival may rest with the provision of adequate

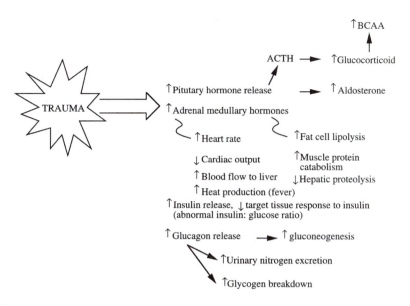

FIGURE 3.18 Trauma elicits both hormonal and metabolic responses that result in increased energy need.

nutrition support in terms of amounts of energy, glucose, and amino acids plus appropriate amounts of insulin to facilitate the return to normal fuel homeostasis.

The temporal changes in the choice of metabolic fuels are characterized by subtle transitions from one fuel source to another. These are orchestrated by the hormonal response to the trauma or infection, which in turn may be influenced by the pre-injury nutritional status of the patient and the nutrients provided during the recovery period.

Basal energy requirements can increase by as much as 200% in traumatized patients. Part of this increase can be attributed to the thermogenic effects of the catecholamines released in response to the injury. In addition, increases in energy requirement may be due to the increased energy needed to support protein synthesis. Protein synthesis is highly dependent on energy intake. New proteins are needed for tissue repair and for the inflammatory and immunologic responses of the body to infection or injury or both. If the diet is inadequate, the synthesis of these proteins occurs at the expense of muscle protein. Amino acids not used for protein synthesis are deaminated and the resulting ammonia converted to urea. Urea production likewise is energetically expensive. Thus, large increases in both protein synthesis and ureagenesis represent an increase in the basal energy requirement and an increase in the protein requirement in the traumatized or severely ill individual. Unless this additional energy and protein are provided, weight loss will occur.

OBESITY

Although excess body-fat stores, or obesity, is considered a risk factor in a number of diseases, we have no permanent cure for the disorder. Listed in Table 3.11 are some of the reasons that excess body fatness develops. Obesity is probably the result of an interaction between genetics and environment. An individual may have inherited one or more mutated genes that influence the efficiency with which that individual uses the intake energy and converts it to stored energy. When provided with an ample food supply, these individuals may become fat. However, if the food supply is limited, the excess fat store might not develop. In addition, there may be cultural overrides that influence the phenotypic expression of an individual genotype. Individuals may consciously limit food intake and increase physical activity so as not to phenotypically express their genotype. Obesity, therefore, may be considered a multifactorial phenotype.

TABLE 3.11
Suggested Causes of Obesity

Mutations in Genes for	Hormonal Imbalance	Other Causes
a) Leptin, Leptin Receptor	a) Excess glucocorticoids	a) Injury to hypothalamus and brain stem
b) Cholecystokinin, Cholecystokinin Receptor	b) Hypothyroidism	b) Sociocultural feeding behaviors
c) Glucagon-like peptide, Glucagon-like peptide receptor	c) Hyperinsulinism	c) Inactivity
d) Tumor Necrosis Factor (TNFα)		
e) Neuropeptide Y (NPY), NPY Receptor		
f) Corticotropin-Releasing Hormone (CRH), CRH Receptor		
g) Adipocyte Specific Transcription Factor C/EBPα		
h) Agouti protein		
i) Carboxypeptidase E		
j) Phosphodiesterase		
k) β adrenergic receptor		
l) Growth Hormone Receptor		
m) Glucocorticoid Receptor		
n) Insulin Receptor		
o) UCPs		

Genetics

Research on the genetic basis for excess body fatness is very active. More than 20 candidate genes have been identified as being associated with excessive body fat. Several investigators have shown that the familial trait for body fatness has a much stronger influence on body composition than environmental influences such as culture, socioeconomic status, or food-intake patterns. Stunkard and associates as well as Bouchard and Despres have published extensively on the responses of twins to dietary manipulation and exercise. They found that identical (monozygotic) twins are more nearly alike in these responses than are siblings or nonidentical (dizygotic) twins. These and other workers have also examined the home environment with respect to body fatness. This work attempts to answer the question of whether people become overly fat because of environmental influences such as the daily coaching by the parents to eat or not eat. Most revealing in this respect are the studies of monozygotic and dizygotic twins reared by their biological parents or by adoptive parents. In one study, adopted children and their biological and adoptive parents were compared with respect to body weight and body fatness, while in other studies twins reared together or apart were compared. Allison and colleagues have calculated that the heritability of the body mass index is between 0.50 and 0.70, depending on the definition of obesity and body mass index used. Overfeeding studies of twins have been conducted by Bouchard and associates that showed that identical twins will gain a similar amount of weight, whereas siblings or unrelated subjects will be highly variable. After the overfeeding period, there were also genetic differences in weight-loss patterns. This is also true for those attempting to lose weight via energy restriction. Some people can lose weight far more easily than others. These differences are probably of genetic origin. All these studies showed that the genetic influence on body fatness far outweighed the environmental influence.

    A number of genetic diseases are characterized by obesity. The Prader–Willi, the Bardet–Biedl, the Laurence–Moon, the Cohen, the Boyeson, and the Wilson–Turner syndromes are all characterized by obesity as well as by other abnormalities. All of these syndromes are rare and none seem to correlate with any of the mutations listed in Table 3.11. The Prader–Willi syndrome occurs as a result of a partial deletion of the long arm of chromosome 15. It occurs in 1/5000 to

1/10,000 live births. Individuals with this syndrome are developmentally delayed, have poor muscle tone and are growth retarded. Once the child with Prader–Willi syndrome reaches the age of 2 or 3, other behavioral features develop. The child has a persistent food-seeking behavior that can be self destructive. Patients with Bardet–Biedl syndrome, although obese, have a different set of characteristics. Most are mentally retarded with polydactyly (extra fingers/toes) and hypogonadism. The prevalence of this condition is about 1/17,500 live births. These patients do not have the aggressive, persistent food-seeking characteristic of the patient with Prader–Willi syndrome. Patients with the Laurence–Moon syndrome are similar to those with the Bardet–Biedl syndrome except that they are frequently diabetic and paraplegic. They do not have the polydactyly feature. The prevalence of this disorder as well as the others listed above is of the order of 1/20,000. As might be anticipated, all of these disorders are characterized by a shortened life span.

A number of spontaneous genetic errors in the animal kingdom have obesity as one of their characteristics. Genetically obese rats, mice, dogs, and desert animals have been described. In the rodent species, the mode of inheritance and, in some instances, the chromosomal location of genes for obesity have been found. Obesity can be inherited via an autosomal recessive or dominant or sex-linked mode. In each of these mutations, an error occurs that affects energy balance. Errors in the perception of hunger and/or satiety by the brain can explain the excess food intake (hyperphagia) that characterizes several of these mutants. Inappropriate hunger signals, satiety signals, and their receptors have all been implicated. The central integrator of this seemingly unrelated set of characteristics may reside in that group of compounds called the cytokines. This group of small peptides has intercellular, interorgan signaling functions that in turn define them as hormones. These compounds have receptors in specific cells or target cells, and current evidence suggests that mutations in either the genes for the target cell receptors or for the cytokine itself or for its production and release could explain a number of clinical conditions. The cytokines, their receptors and their signaling mechanisms are listed in Table 3.12. The interleukins (IL-1-8) are mainly concerned with the immune system, although one or two may also play a role in adipocyte apoptosis. The cytokines of interest to researchers in energy balance are TNF (α and β) and leptin. TNF is found in many cell types but of interest is the TNF α. This cytokine induces adipocyte apoptosis. Thus, this cytokine has a two-pronged attack on energy balance. First, through suppressing hunger it reduces energy intake and second, because it stimulates adipocyte apoptosis, it has the effect of reducing fat stores.

Another cytokine that has a similar mode of action is leptin. Leptin is produced by the adipocyte and transported to the hypothalamus, where it serves to signal satiety. Mutations in the gene for leptin have been found in genetically obese rodents as well as in humans. Leptin gene mutation is uncommon. However, mutations in the leptin receptor in the brain have been found in several obese rat and mouse strains and they are presumed to be more common than mutations in the leptin gene. Mutations in either gene result in obesity due to a lack of this satiety-inducing cytokine.

Leptin also can stimulate adipocyte apoptosis so, like TNF α, it affects both food intake and energy store through an effect on the number of fat cells available for fat storage. Leptin also upregulates the muscle UCP_3 and thus increases heat production via an effect on OXPHOS. In addition, leptin regulates fatty acid homeostasis. It suppresses fatty acid deposition in nonadipocytes. Counteracting TNFα and leptin is neuropeptide Y (NPY), which stimulates appetite. While present in most neural tissues, the NPY that is closely associated with feeding is synthesized by cells of the arcuate nucleus. It is released primarily in the paraventricular nucleus, whereupon it stimulates feeding. NPY has the opposite effect of corticotropin-releasing hormone (CRH) within the hypothalamus with respect to signaling feeding. Leptin regulates both of these compounds. It downregulates NPY and upregulates CRH.

Greater than normal food intake may also characterize the genetically obese human. Yet, there are many overfat people who are not hyperphagic. There are those who cannot dissipate their surplus intake energy as heat, i.e., thermogenesis. (See text on the UCPs) and who do not tolerate cold well. The common thread to these two conditions is the apparent inability of tissues to uncouple

TABLE 3.12
Cytokines, Their Receptors and Their Signaling Mechanism

Cytokine	Receptor Distribution	Signaling Mechanism
IL-2	T cells, B cells, Monocytes, Myeloid precursors, NK cells	High affinity binding induces phosphorylation of tyrosine kinase
IL-1	T cells, B cells, Fibroblasts, Endothelial cells, Keratinocytes	(a) A GTP binding motif suggests G protein activity (b) May involve cAMP and PLC activation
IL-5	B cells, Eosinophils, Basophils	Cellular tyrosine kinase induces phosphorylation of several proteins and this proline rich receptor protein may be one of them
IL-4	T cells, B cells, Monocytes, Macrophages, Granulocytes, Megakaryocytes, Erythroid products, NK cells, Fibroblasts, Endothelial cells	Cellular tyrosine kinase induces phosphorylation of this serine and proline rich receptor protein
IL-6	T cells, B cells, Monocytes, Fibroblasts, Megakaryocytes, Hepatocytes, Keratinocytes, Mesangial cells	Tyrosine kinase mediated signaling system
IL-8	Neutrophils, basophils, monocytes, T cells (3 Types of receptors)	Tyrosine kinase mediated signaling system
IL-3	Myeloid precursors, basophils, mast cells, macrophages, megakaryocytes	Involves tyrosine kinase protein kinase C
IL-7	Two types: high and low affinity, B cell progenetors, Thymocytes	Tyrosine kinase
IL-3	Basophils, myeloid precursors, mast cells, macrophages, megakeryocytes	Tyrosine kinase
SCF	Pluripotent stem cells, lymphoid precursors, myeloid precursors, megakaryocyte precursors, erythroid precursors	SCF binding initials dimerization of receptors. Also involves the tyrosine kinase, phosphorylation of PLC γ, c-raf, and PI-3 kinase. Ca^{++} is also involved as a second messenger
LIF	Hematopoitic stem cells, megakaryocyte progenitors, osteoblasts, neurons, myoblasts, adipocytes, embryonic stem cells, hepatocytes, kidney epithelial cells, placental cells	Involves the tyrosine kinase system
G-CSF	Granulocytes, pluripotent stem cells, myeloid progenitors, T cells, fibroblasts, endothelial cells	Involves G proteins and the tyrosine kinase
EPO	Erythoid precursors, megakaryocytes	?
GM-CSF	Myeloid precursors, monocytes, macrophages, eosinophils, neutrophils, megakaryocytes, endothelial cells, osteoblasts, Langerhans cells	Involves the tyrosine kinase system
M-CSF	Monocytes, macrophages	Involves the tyrosine kinase system
TGF α, β	Several related cytokines and receptors. Found in most cells	Involves the tyrosine kinase system
NPY	Found in most neural cells	Involves the tyrosine kinase system
TGF α, β	Found in many cell types	?
Leptin	Found in brain cells as well as other cell types	?

oxidative phosphorylation so as to release heat to keep the body warm. Thus, ATP is continuously synthesized, in turn transferring its energy to the synthesis of fat. Obesity has also been attributed to a failure of these cells to respond to the stimulatory effects of norepinephrine and is associated with an anomalous central regulation of the sympathetic input to this tissue.

It has been suggested that genetically obese individuals become obese because they are unable to increase their heat production when overfed or when suddenly thrust into a cold environment. It has been hypothesized further that genetically obese animals develop subcutaneous fat pads as insulation against heat loss or gain, thereby circumventing their relative inability to thermoregulate. To increase their insulation layer, they must overeat to provide the requisite substrates for lipogenesis. Such a hypothesis has some elements of validity. The ob/ob mouse, for example, is unusually sensitive to cold and is incapable of increasing its heat production when suddenly exposed to cold or injected with norepinephrine. If gradually exposed to cold, these mice can slowly adapt to the gradual change in temperature. These features of the ob/ob mouse precede the development of both hyperphagia and obesity and have been attributed to a mutation in the gene for leptin. These mice do not produce normal leptin and this deficiency means that there is no leptin to travel to the brain to suppress feeding. Hence, these mice are hyperphagic. These mice also do not turn on thermogenesis very well when exposed to cold. This is because leptin has another role — that of stimulating the production of UCPs. Since the mobilization of body fuel (induction of lipolysis and glycogenolysis) is not abnormal in the obese ob/ob mouse, it would appear that only the release of heat when these fuels are oxidized is defective. In other words, more energy is trapped in the chemical bonds of high-energy compounds than is released as heat. This, of course, is related to the increased energetic efficiency of these animals as well, since they also gain more fat per unit food consumed (and release less heat) than lean animals.

Impaired thermoregulation has also been reported in genetically obese Zucker rats. These rats produce ample amounts of leptin but they have a mutation in the gene that encodes the leptin receptor. Thus, although they produce the cytokine it is without effect because its receptor is abberant. It cannot bind the leptin and signal the cell accordingly. Zucker rats, like ob/ob mice, are hyperphagic and obese. Similarly, they do not respond well to sudden cold exposure. Again, the missing link is not leptin but its intracellular effects on satiety signaling and UCP production. Zucker obese rats and ob/ob mice are not the only animals affected. Lower body temperatures in neonates and an impaired ability to increase thermogenesis in response to overeating, cold exposure, or to norepinephrine, have been reported in a variety of genetically obese animals models. Perhaps obese humans may also have this defect. A few humans have been described with leptin defects, but whether leptin or its receptor can explain all the cases of obesity is doubtful. When stimulated by cold or infusions of norepinephrine, normal-weight subjects increased their heat production while obese subjects did not.

Normal-weight humans appear to regulate their body-fat mass by increasing their heat production when overfed or exposed to cold. Several investigators developed an animal model that showed that when overfed, thermogenesis was stimulated. They showed that when offered a variety of energy-rich snack foods, normal animals increased their heat production to maintain a normal weight. However, this mechanism is far from perfect in that, over time, these overfed animals did become fatter than their control-fed littermates. Nonetheless, the observation that heat production will increase in response to fluctuations in energy intake is a very interesting facet of energy balance. The mechanism whereby heat production is increased above basal involves the synthesis and release of UCPs. These proteins are not always present and active. In the starved animal, for example, they cannot be found. This means that extra heat production induced by UCPs can be switched on and off. The synthesis of UCPs is rapid. Exposure to cold or hyperthyroidism or birth or starvation-refeeding triggers a rapid and marked increase of messenger RNA for this protein as well as a marked increase in the level of protein. In most animals, the increase in the level of UCPs parallels an increase in nonshivering thermogenesis. In lean animals, surplus food intake seems to signal UCP synthesis. The regulation of this synthesis occurs at the level of messenger RNA transcription. The genes that encode these proteins have been isolated and sequenced. The protein completely traverses the inner mitochondrial membrane and has a C-terminal region that projects from the outer surface of the membrane. It works by dissipating the proton gradient that is developed when pairs of reducing equivalents are passed down the respiratory chain to make water. The energy that is developed by the respiratory chain is not captured in the high-energy bond of ATP but is, instead, released as heat. The control of its uncoupling function is through the external C terminal region that contains the nucleotide (ADP)-binding site. If UCP binds the nucleotide, it is not available to the F_oF_1 ATP synthase for ATP synthesis. Fatty acids interact with the nucleotide binding site so that ADP binding is increased. These fatty acids are released from the stored triacylglycerols via a hormone-stimulated cyclic AMP mechanism. This explains how norepinephrine can stimulate brown fat thermogenesis (BAT). Norepinephrine works by increasing the cAMP levels in the cytosol. This, in turn, stimulates the activity of the cytosolic lipoprotein lipase, which serves to release the fatty acids from the stored lipid. Norepinephrine is particularly effective with respect to intracellular fatty acid release in the brown fat. Other lipolytic hormones that work through increasing adenylate cyclase activity and cAMP levels also work to increase heat production. Diets rich in polyunsaturated fatty acids potentiate these hormone effects on this process.

While insulin is not thought of as a lipolytic hormone, it too has a role in regulating the synthesis and activity of the UCPs and heat production. Both the synthesis of the uncoupling protein and the ability of various tissues to assist in the regulation of body temperature via the UCPs that help to dissipate the energy provided by excess food intake is impaired in the insulin-deficient animal. Once insulin is restored, the impairment is corrected. Of interest is the observation that many genetically obese rats and mice are hyperinsulinemic.

As mentioned in the sections on starvation and anorexia, hormonal balance is important to the regulation of energy balance and normal body weight. Hypercortisolism and hyperinsulinism are associated with obesity. Cortisol and its related compounds, corticosterone and cortisone, play an important role in the regulation of lipogenesis as well as in the signaling of apoptosis. While these hormones are usually catabolic hormones, there are circumstances when they stimulate anabolic processes, such as fat synthesis.

Finally, there are social and cultural influences that can ensure or potentiate genetic tendencies to develop obesity. Anthropologists and medical historians have identified examples of cultural groups that consider excess body fat a mark of beauty as well as an indication of economic status within their society. Examples of this are the various statuary of different ages all the way from the upper Paleolithic period through the Renaissance to the 18th and 19th centuries. Women have been represented with large bellies and breasts that, to the eye of the contemporary observer, are overfat. Men, too, are of ample proportions. In fact, there is an old German expression that indicates the desire of men to have overweight women as wives: "A fat wife and a full barn never did a man harm." Even today there are cultures, notably in Africa, that have customs that include preparing girls for marriage by fattening them. Malcom, for example, described this practice for elite Efik girls in traditional Nigeria, as well as the custom in Kenya of demanding high bride prices for fat brides. In these cultures, female fatness may not only be a testament to the families' wealth, it may also be a symbol of maternity and nurturance. This is important to the woman if the only way she gains status is through motherhood. A fat woman is thus assumed to be very maternal and nurturing.

With respect to societally determined fatness and the values of fatness, it can be assumed that the fatter a person is in a society that values fatness, the more likely that person will be to marry and produce children carrying genetic tendencies to be fat and who will be similarly taught to eat enough to be fat also. Lean people will be less likely to contribute to the gene pool because they will be considered less-desirable mates. While people in the U.S., as well as other developed nations, may not have these values, there is no doubt that eating behaviors can be taught. If young children are constantly reminded and coached to overeat, there may be a continuing stimulus to overconsume food. Added to this may be cultural and social dictates with respect to physical activity. A decrease in energy expenditure ensures a positive energy balance that may well result in excess body fatness.

Frequently, those who are overfat are told that they could become lean if they would reduce their food intake. However, simply restricting one's food intake does not cure the problem; it merely treats the result of the positive energy balance — excess body fat. Once this fat is lost, the formerly obese person frequently abandons the restricted diet, returns to previous eating habits and, as a result, returns to the prior weight. In some, there may also be an increase in body fatness, not just a return to the prior body weight.

Set Point Theory in Body Weight Regulation

The idea that each body has its own unique size and weight has been discussed, denied, and supported by a wide variety of researchers. The hypothesis that adult body weight is closely regulated at its own unique level was developed from observations of both humans and animals. The mechanism(s) that serve to regulate this steady state body weight are not fully known.

Healthy adult humans vary very little over the years in their body weight. They may be overweight and/or overfat but, for most humans, that weight is maintained for years until some event occurs that results in a body weight change. In women, pregnancy or menopause, two normal physiological events, may perturb the system sufficiently to establish a new steady-state body weight (or new set point) which, again, will be defended tenaciously. A change in the endocrine system, an insult to the body, or a conscious decision to eat more (or less) over a prolonged period (months to years) are other examples of events that might perturb the system sufficiently to result in a new set point — a new body weight that is maintained from that time on.

Similarly, animals appear to regulate their body weight within fairly tight limits. Much of the research on the set-point hypothesis has used rats and mice. Studies using rats that were either over- or underfed revealed that they had a body weight that was related to their food intake. That is, if they were forced to consume more energy than they would voluntarily consume, they would become overfat. If they were underfed, they would be leaner than normal. After these feeding treatments were discontinued, the rats that were overfed significantly reduced their food intake and used their fat stores to provide their energy needs while those rats that were underfed dramatically increased their voluntary food intake until they gained the weight they would have gained had they not been food restricted. When both these groups of rats attained the weight of their untreated controls, they resumed normal feeding behavior.

Although the body weight returned to normal in these over- or underfed rats after the treatment was terminated, the composition of the body was not the same as their untreated counterparts. The percent of the body that was fat was affected. Those rats that were underfed recovered by significantly increasing the synthesis and deposition of body fat. This recovery was faster than the recovery of body protein. In the overfed rats, the body protein normalized within days of cessation of the overfeeding, yet the body fat content remained elevated weeks after overfeeding ended.

Other studies have used parabiotic rats or mice to study the consequences of overfeeding or underfeeding on body weight and composition. Parabiosis is a technique where two weanling animals are joined together surgically at the skin so that they have a common circulation. Hervey, Harris, and others have used this technique to answer the question of whether there are blood-borne factors that are involved in the regulation of feeding and body weight. Genetically obese animals have been joined to genetically lean ones, as have normal weight partners in which one was either over- or underfed, or was lesioned in either the feeding center of the hypothalamus or the satiety center. In each of these instances, the feeding behavior of both as well as their body weight and composition were monitored. In each instance where the one partner overate and became obese, the other underate or starved and subsequently lost its body fat as well as its lean body tissue. These results were interpreted as indications that there are blood-borne factors generated by the fat store that signal the feeding behavior. Indeed, some of these blood-borne factors have been identified (leptin, NPY, TNFα, etc.). In the preceeding section, a number of rodents (as well as other species) were described that carry mutations that result in obesity. Some are characterized by hyper-phagia (abnormally increased food intake) and some are diabetic as well as obese. Still others are hypertensive and obese. Some develop renal disease, while others do not. The range of phenotypes is large, suggesting that more than one mutation can exist having obesity as part of its phenotype. The results of studies using hyperphagic genetically obese animals suggested that these obese animals neither sent nor received appropriate satiety signals or were not able to respond to them by decreasing their food intake. Likely the nonresponsivity (that is, an error in the signaling system) is the explanation, since parabiotic pairs using genetically lean and obese rats behaved like the force fed and voluntary feeding pairs. While the genetically obese partner was hyperphagic and obese, the lean partner ceased eating and eventually starved to death.

It is apparent that although there may be controls that influence feeding and body weight, these controls may not fully regulate body fatness. That is, body weight may be set but body fat may change depending on food intake and physical activity. This may explain why aging humans may gain body fat while decreasing food intake to maintain their body weight. As humans age, they decrease their physical activity and their body composition changes; they lose muscle mass and gain body fat. Their body shape changes as well. They may observe an increase in the size of their fat mass in the abdomen and on the thighs and buttocks. Again, epidemiologists have noted the differences in health risks associated with the location of the excess fat stores; the so-called apple and pear shapes. Those persons whose fat stores are distributed equally between storage sites on shoulders, arms, abdomen, hips and thighs are said to be "apples." Their risk of developing obesity-associated disorders is greater than that in people who have accumulated fat stores at sites below the waist, the "pears." The depots differ in the degree of fatty acid turnover. That is, they differ in how readily they can release their stored fat for use by other tissues. In humans, studies of cells isolated from the femoral, gluteal, and omental (thigh, buttocks, abdomen) depots revealed significant differences in free fatty acid release. On the basis of the rate of free fatty acid release and the size of the depots, the half life of the fat depot in the femoral area was calculated to be 305 days. For the gluteal depot it was 326 days and for the omental depot it was 134 days. Estimates of the half life of the fat in the other depot sites have not been made. An estimate of half life is the estimate of time needed to exhaust one-half of the fat store. As the human uses the stored lipid, more lipid is synthesized to replace that which was used. Hence, the term fatty acid turnover means that fatty acids are both used and replaced. If they are used at a greater rate than they are replaced, a net fat loss will occur. As can be seen, however, different depots will shrink at different rates depending on their location. In addition to the aforementioned differences in depot fat use, there are also genetic and sex differences in the extent and location of the fat depots. Women, for example, have larger subcutaneous fat stores than men. Men have larger omental fat depots than women of the same age and weight.

Morbidity of Severely Obese People

Health care professionals have observed countless instances of the codevelopment of excess body fat with diabetes mellitus, hypertension, and cardiovascular disease. Epidemiologists have reported that obesity and overweight are risk factors in the development of these diseases. However, there are some inconsistencies with respect to the relationship of obesity to cardiovascular disease and total mortality. Studies by the CDC and those by Sjostrom suggest that weight loss by the obese does not positively affect life span. Long-term studies of mortality by formerly obese people conducted by the CDC suggest the reverse. Their preliminary report indicates an increase in mortality in people who have consciously reduced their body fat and remained lean. This report has raised serious questions about the efficacy of weight loss with respect to life-span extension.

Treatment of Obesity

In almost no other area of medicine have there been so many failures as have occurred in the treatment of obesity. Fully 90% of all those who lose weight regain it within 5 years. Data from the Chicago Gas and Electric Study suggest that one cycle of loss and regain is a risk factor for death from coronary heart disease independent of body fatness. The gain–loss group, when compared with subjects who neither gained nor lost weight, had 1.8 times the risk of death from heart disease. This suggests that weight cycling is not a healthy behavior. If weight is to be lost, it must stay lost if health benefits are to be gained. Often this does not occur. Weight cycling consists of intermittent periods of food restriction followed by periods of "normal" eating patterns. These patterns may include periods of gorging or binge eating. One of the major effects of calorie restriction on metabolism is a reduction in resting metabolic rate (RMR). This lowers the overall energy requirement and increases energy efficiency, thus allowing a greater percentage of dietary energy to be partitioned into fat synthesis upon refeeding.

The effects of weight cycling on energy efficiency may be due to the composition of the weight loss during calorie restriction. One of the consequences of rapid weight loss, especially when induced by very low-calorie, low-carbohydrate diets, is the loss of body protein or lean body mass. This is especially true when the individuals are physically inactive. Maintenance of lean body mass is an energy-expensive process. Lean body mass is the most metabolically active tissue in the body with respect to energy demands, accounting for the majority of calories to support the basal energy requirement (i.e., 60–70% of daily basal energy requirements for adults). Therefore, the less body protein, the lower the energy requirement. If weight loss consists of significant amounts of body protein, then the formerly overfat person will have a lower basal energetic requirement and an increased energy efficiency in terms of the weight regain as fat.

One of the responses of cycled humans is the tendency to overeat during the initial few days of the refeeding period. This suggests that the regulation of food intake is affected by the weight loss. The regulation of food intake is discussed in the next section. Signals sent to the brain by the starved body seem to set the stage for hyperphagia (increased food intake above normal) once food is no longer restricted. These signals must be fairly enduring because this hyperphagia is of about the same duration as the duration of the restriction period. The origin of these signals is not known, but no doubt they exist because food intake is an event regulated by the central nervous system. Studies of starved and refed rats showed that these rats had a preference for dietary fat if given a choice of several energy sources. As a result of this selection, cycled rats regained more body fat than if the food offered was rich in carbohydrate and/or protein. Again, this suggests the involvement of signals from the brain directing the individual to select energetically rich food. This signal, coupled with the increased efficiency of the body in retaining the ingested energy, helps to explain why the fat regain occurs in people who have restricted their energy intake to lose weight. Food restriction puts into place a metabolic machinery geared to save as much energy as possible and to stimulate the brain to signal the body to consume energy-rich foods. Thus, even though the patient tries to control eating and food intake, the body seeks to return to its prior overfat state. Constant vigilance is required of the patient to override these biological signals that direct the body to be fat. However, even when the patient carefully monitors food-energy intake and consciously decides to regulate it, weight regain may occur due to the body's increased energetic efficiency and its tendency to synthesize and store fat in preference to protein. Here is where a good exercise program might be useful. Exercise, on a regular basis, stimulates muscle protein development and increases energy expenditure. Exercise can be a useful adjunct to energy-intake restriction because it redirects energy loss from the lean body mass. In the sedentary individual, weight loss occurs at the expense of both fat and protein components of the body. In the exercising food-restricted individual, the weight loss is primarily fat loss. Further, mild to moderate exercise seems to suppress food intake. Thus, food restriction together with exercise is additive in a beneficial way with respect to the loss and regain of body fat.

Drugs

Pharmacologic approaches to the treatment of obesity have captured the interest of numerous pharmaceutical companies worldwide. Table 3.13 lists some of these drugs. Drugs that target those mechanisms involved in hunger and satiety as well as drugs that target feed efficiency have been developed. The latter category includes compounds that interfere with normal digestion and absorption. Unfortunately, none of these compounds has a significant anti-obesity effect. Glucosidase inhibitors as well as lipase inhibitors have been developed. The glucosidase inhibitors, acarbose and miglitol, for example, inhibit the action of amylase and thus reduces its activity. This means that the long chain (straight and branched) starches found in many plant products are not digested as quickly as usual. In theory, this retardation of digestion should result in a retardation of absorption

TABLE 3.13
Drugs that May Have Anti-Obesity Properties

	Example	Effect
a) Anti nutrition drugs		
1. Gastric emptying inhibitors	(--) threochlorocitric acid	Delays gastric emptying, induces satiety
2. Glucosidase inhibitors	Acarbose, miglitol	Inhibits carbohydrate digestion
3. Inhibitors of lipid uptake	Cholestyramine	Binds bile acids, disrupts micelle formation
4. Pseudonutrients	Olestra	Fat substitute with less energy
	Artificial sweeteners	Sugar substitute, no energy
	Bulking agents, fibers	Induce satiety at lower energy intake
5. Lipase inhibitor	Xenecal	Inhibits hydrolysis of triacylglycides
b) Drugs that affect nutrient partitioning		
1. Growth hormone		Stimulates protein synthesis
2. Testosterone		Stimulates protein synthesis in males only
3. α_2 adrenergic antagonists		Enhances lipolysis
4. Thermogenic drugs		
β_2 and β_3 adrenergic	BRL-26830A, terbutaline	Stimulates protein synthesis and lipolysis; can have serious side effects
Dinitrophenol		Metabolic poison; not recommended
c) Appetite suppressors		
1. β phenethylamine derivatives	Fastin, Dexatrim	Interferes with hunger signaling via norepinephrine
2. Serotonergic agents	Fenfluramine, fluoxetine	Increases serotonin release and signals satiety
3. Amine reuptake inhibitor	Sibutramine	Blocks reuptake of norepinephrine and 5-HT and suppresses appetite

of the end products of starch hydrolysis. Unfortunately, this may not result in a reduction in intake energy. If starch digestion is not completed by the enzymes of the small intestine, flora of the large intestine take over and produce fatty acids that are then absorbed and used for energy.

Lipase inhibitors (Xenecal) or fat absorption inhibitors (cholestyramine, neomycin, perfluorooctyl bromide) also serve to reduce energy intake. Cholestyramine binds bile acids and disrupts micelle formation. This results in an inhibition of fat absorption and increased fecal fat loss. Despite this loss of food fat in the feces, clinical trials have not demonstrated a significant weight loss by obese subjects. Neomycin, an antibiotic, reduces fat absorption as well. However, it has the side effect of reducing the intestinal mucosa. This can result in diarrhea. Perfluorooctyl bromide, a product used as a contrast medium for gastrointestinal X-ray studies, also blocks fat absorption as well as amino acid and glucose absorption. While useful in studying the functional state of the gastrointestinal tract, because it interferes with the absorption of all the macronutrients, its usefulness as an anti-obesity drug is very limited.

Food companies have expanded into the "anti-obesity business" by developing noncaloric sweeteners, reduced-caloric sweeteners, fat substitutes, and bulking agents. All of these products are designed to reduce the energy value of food products. Aspartame, cyclamate, saccharin, and acesulfame K are sweeteners without energy value. They are used in soft drinks as well as a number of snack foods. Canned fruit and frozen desserts are also prepared with these noncaloric sweeteners. Some of the sugar alcohols, i.e., manitol, are also in use in prepared foods to reduce their energy content. Likewise, fat substitutes such as the sucrose polyester, olestra, are used to reduce the energy value of some foods. Bulking agents such as guar, pectin, and fiber are used as energy diluents in processed foods. All of these pseudonutrients can effectively reduce the energy intake when incorporated into a well-balanced diet that is energy restricted. This will help the overweight individual lose excess fat.

Listed in Table 3.13 are some hormones that affect protein synthesis as well as fat storage. None of these should be used therapeutically to stimulate weight loss. However, they are included in the table because fat weight loss may be a secondary effect when these hormones are used for other reasons. For example, growth-hormone supplements may be given to the growth-deficient child who may be very short and fat. The supplemented child will then grow and as this growth occurs, the fat depots shrink. In males, the percent body fat is inversely related to circulating testosterone levels. In females, increased upper abdominal and visceral fatness is associated with rising levels of testosterone. Glucocorticoid excess (Cushing's disease) usually results in an accumulation of abdominal fat whereas glucocorticoid deficiency (Addison's disease) is characterized by a depletion of fat stores. Thyroid hormone excess likewise is characterized by a reduction in fat stores, while thryoid hormone deficiency has the reverse feature. Hypothyroid individuals have enlarged fat depots. Among the pharmaceutical products we have drugs that are thermogenic. In other words, these are drugs that stimulate energy wastage as heat. None of the known thermogenic drugs are without risk. β adrenergic compounds frequently have serious side effects such as tremors. One of these, Terbutaline, is useful in asthma treatment. When used for this purpose, weight loss has been reported.

One group of drugs acts through the central nervous system in the regulation of hunger and satiety. The first of these is the β phenethylamine derivatives, which work through affecting either the release or reuptake of norepinephrine. These drugs suppress appetite. Some, however, have undesirable side effects on the cardiopulmonary system and may induce insomnia. In addition, with long-term use they lose effectiveness. The second group of drugs is the serotonergic drugs. These suppress appetite by increasing serotonin levels in that part of the brain (the hypothalamus) that controls food intake. Dry mouth and insomnia are side effects and, in some instances, pulmonary hypertension has been reported as a result of the use of fenfluramine. Fluoxetine, another of the serotonergic drugs, blocks serotonin reuptake. It too is an appetite suppressant. This drug is mainly used as an antidepressant, not as an anti-obesity drug. Subutramine, an amine uptake inhibitor, blocks the reuptake of norepinephrine, thereby suppressing food itnake. All of the drugs described above have some measure of risk associated with their use. Some are not available at all because they are too risky to use. Others are available by prescription only and should be used only under the supervision of a physician. Even when used appropriately, they may not result in significant and lasting weight loss.

REGULATION OF FOOD INTAKE

In the preceding section, the health concerns of obesity were discussed as well as a notation that it is sometimes characterized by hyperphagia (overeating). In this section, food intake and its regulation will be discussed not only from the physiological point of view but also from the sociocultural angle. It is important for those who study the processes by which man consumes and utilizes food to realize how complex the subject is. An individual does not ingest thiamine, vitamin A, protein, and selenium, those nutrients necessary for his well-being; he ingests food, be it sirloin steak, fresh juicy peaches, or chocolate-covered ants. He does not choose to eat a green salad because it is nutritionally sound to do so, but because of complex conscious and subconscious motivation peculiar to himself. This section is designed to explain the origin of his motivation — its psychological and physiological roots.

Psychological Aspects of Food Intake

Man consumes food, not nutrients. Although specific nutrients are necessary for the growth and maintenance of the human organism, it would be shortsighted to attempt to study man's basic nutritional needs without an appreciation of those factors that influence his intake of a sufficient variety of foods to obtain them. Most animals other than man eat primarily to satisfy this nutritional need; man's motivation for eating (or not eating) is frequently to satisfy nonnutritional requirements. His food selection is based on a combination of forces arising from his culture, his family, his educational level, his economic circumstances, and his individual needs and idiosyncrasies.

Culture is the integrated pattern of human behavior that is transmitted to succeeding generations. It dictates the role each person plays in society, as well as his responsibilities to himself, his peer group, and his family. Food habits are largely determined by one's culture. Many habits have existed for centuries and have been maintained as an integral part of a cultural heritage. The Judaic dietary law, based on passages in Leviticus and Deuteronomy in the Old Testament, have very specific regulations about meat consumption. The prohibitions include the flesh of birds and animals of prey, reptiles, creeping insects, animal blood, any animal that does not chew its cud and have a cloven hoof, and any species from the water than does not have fins and scales. This eliminates eagles, ostriches, snakes, lizards, grasshoppers, camels, pigs, rabbits, sharks, oysters, clams, shrimp, and mussels. A large portion of the world's population has its dietary habits controlled by the teachings found in Buddhism, Hinduism, and Jainism (a sect of dissenters from Hinduism). These philosophies support the belief that all life is sacred. This precludes killing animals for food. Such a prohibition does vary from religion to religion, and even within a religion, varies from cultural group to group. For example, the Hindu reveres the cow and will not kill it for food. However, when a cow or oxen dies, the Untouchables (the lowest class in Hindu society) take the animal, skin it for leather and eat the meat. Since this population ordinarily is the poorest in India, this distribution of energy and protein serves to ensure their survival.

Not only do cultural laws prohibit the eating of certain foods, cultural practices also influence the foods that are eaten. The Jamaican enjoys plantain, ackee (a native food, poisonous when ripe, that looks and tastes like scrambled eggs), eggplant, papaya, mangoes, fish, lobster, naseberries, and otaheite apples. The Otomi Indians of the Mezquital Valley in Mexico make their meals from tortillas and from local plants such as malva, hediondilla, nopal, maguey, garambullo, yucca, purslane, pigweed, sorrel, wild mustard flowers, lengua de vaca, sow-thistle, and cactus fruit. They drink an intoxicating beverage, pulque, made from the century plant. A North American raised in a different culture would look askance at this diet and view it as nutritionally deficient. However, nutritional analyses of the Otomi Indians' diet showed it to be better balanced than that of an urban group from the U.S. Persons from large sections of east and south Asia and tropical Africa refuse to drink milk; other African groups, on the contrary, prize milk as a precious food and serve it only to adult men. The Masai, an African tribal group, not only drink the milk from their cattle but draw blood from the jugular vein and drink that also. Entomophagy, the eating of insects, is accepted in many cultures; the Australian bushmen consume sugar ants and witchetty grubs; local inhabitants from Central Africa eat fresh and fried termites; some Japanese groups eat dytiscid beetles (fried and made into a sauce with sugar), grasshoppers, maggots, pupae of the wasp, and the larvae of silkworms.

Within a given culture, the family has a significant influence on food acceptance. This happens not because there is an active effort by elders to teach the children but because the children see the same daily ritual of food preparation. Unconsciously they assimilate it. In primitive societies, meals are important daily social events; females prepare the food and it is distributed on the basis of sex and age. In these societies as well as in our own, important family social events (christenings, weddings, funerals, etc.) are celebrated with food. These family practices become part of the cultural heritage and influence food choice.

Similarly, in progressive industrial societies, food customs are assimilated by children through the practices of their parents. As technological advances increase the complexity of a society, food as an element in its culture becomes less important. Sociologists who study contemporary society have observed that mealtimes have become less relevant as a time for family social interaction. In the U.S., a large part of the eating is done outside the family environment; convenience foods, sandwiches, fast foods, soft drinks, and many such items are picked up by individuals on a regular basis throughout the day. Forces outside the family influence food choices. Advertising, peer pressure, lifestyle, and age may well be more-important determinants of food choices than family food practices. There has also been a change in the roles of food in festive occasions. Whereas 100 years ago a large meal might have been served to celebrate an important life event, such as a wedding or a christening, today these events are more often celebrated with a cocktail party. As in less-industrialized societies, children observe these practices and apply them.

The impact that the family has on food choices is often a reflection of the educational level of the one who selects and prepares the food. If this person is limited in education, the diet frequently shows a poor supply of nutrients.

In more recent times in the U.S., a definite correlation has been shown between the education of a homemaker and the nutritional intake of her family. The data for this correlation come from two surveys conducted to examine the extent of malnutrition in the U.S.: (1) the Ten State Survey from 1968–70 mandated by the federal government; and (2) the Health and Nutrition Examination Survey (HANES) conducted by the Centers for Disease Control, U.S. Public Health Service. Food intake, clinical tests, physical examinations, anthropometric examinations, medical histories, and educational and financial status were evaluated. The surveys showed that the fewer the years of education the homemaker had, the greater the number of nutritional deficiencies in the diet of the family.

Economic circumstances also exert considerable influence on food choices. The aborigine, living in an arid barren land, is very poor. He hunts for the food he consumes. To increase his food supply, his culture has evolved to include a host of insects as part of his daily diet. At the other extreme, in a more-affluent society considerable amounts of money are spent on foods of no outstanding nutritional value. Caviar is a prime example. In 1979, Beluga caviar cost just over $300 per pound. Caviar is considered a prestigious food by many Americans and Europeans, and they delight in both serving it to guests and eating it themselves. It has no greater nutritional value than cheese, eggs, or hamburger but does impart a certain status to the consumer.

Additionally, there are a host of other interrelated factors that influence food choices: geography, climate, methods of distribution, and storage facilities. Although the New Zealanders and the Danes live many miles apart, both their diets include an abundance of dairy products. This is a function of, in part, the similarities in their geography and climate. Citrus fruits are easily grown in Egypt. However, the food distribution methods are antiquated. As a result, many people in the country do not enjoy these fruits because they spoil in the process of being shipped. In contrast, in the U.S., because of rapid transportation systems, imported foods such as papaya and plantain are frequently enjoyed and foods produced in one segment of the country are available throughout the nation and in all seasons.

Final among the factors that influence food choices are an individual's physiological and psychological idiosyncrasies. An example of the former is the situation in which individuals lack the intestinal enzyme, lactase, which is necessary to digest the milk sugar, lactose. When they drink milk, they experience abdominal bloating, cramps, and diarrhea. Needless to say, they elect to exclude milk from their diet. Countless food allergies have been observed: allergies to wheat, corn, peanuts, chocolate, eggs, strawberries, tomatoes, soy products, to name a few. If an allergy can be identified, frequently a very difficult task, the item is eliminated from one's diet. Sometimes a food item is eliminated instinctively without medical documentation simply because an individual senses a relationship between his food intake and his sense of well being.

Throughout history, there have been individuals who possessed bizarre appetites. During the 19th century, one Jeremiah Johnson, a mountain man, wandered the unexplored West, living off the land and the livers of Crow Indians. Presumably, during the course of his travels, he devoured the livers of 247 Indians. In Hungary in the early 1600s the Countess Elisabeth de Bathory had a penchant for the blood of young, buxomy virgins, for through their blood she hoped to regain her youth. In her efforts to do so, she is reported to have killed 650 girls, drinking their blood and using it as a fluid in which to bathe.

All in all, man's reasons for selecting the foods he eats is a very complex issue with apparently little consideration given to his nutritional requirements. The foods one person might consider an elegant repast, another would not deign to touch. Human behavior added to the study of nutrition makes a difficult subject even more complex.

PHYSIOLOGICAL ASPECTS OF FOOD INTAKE

Sensory Perception of Food

In addition to the social, cultural, and economic influences on food intake, the selection of foods involves a complex interaction among the special senses: reactions of the eye, ear, nose, mouth, and the sensations of pain and touch are all involved. The sensation of hunger, coupled with the appearance, texture, smell, and taste of food, which, in many ways, are inextricably bound to one's cultural heritage, determine whether the hand will reach out and grasp the food, transport it to the mouth, and consume it. The appearance of the food, its color, its consistency, and its temperature are perceived by the sensory system, which includes the eye, the sense of touch, the sense of temperature, and the sense of smell. Temperature, taste, texture, and smell are perceived via sensory receptor systems located in the nose and mouth. Recall that a receptor is a defined organization of molecules within a membrane or cellular organelle that recognizes and binds compounds or elements needed by the cell. A receptor may also serve to translate or transmit or initiate the sending of a message to other parts of the cell or to other parts of the body. For example, the sensory receptors in the oral cavity perceive food attributes such as texture and taste. The taste/smell/texture translates the stimulus into an electrochemical message that is relayed to the brain. Currently, far more is known about the anatomy of the area in which these events take place than about the physiology of the events themselves.

Appearance

Part of the social/cultural force that influences one's acceptance of food is the defined expectation of an acceptable food. In part, this expectation is based on the appearance of that food. Does it have the desired size and shape, and most important, is it the expected color?

Work done on the relationship between food acceptance and color has shown a striking dependence of one on the other. One study showed that when jellies were colored in an atypical manner, the fruit flavors were incorrectly identified. In another study, the flavoring of colorless syrups was incorrectly identified by most of a group of 200 pharmacy students; they were even less able to identify the correct flavor if the solutions were given unusual colors. In a third study, a trained panel of wine tasters showed a dependence on color in their evaluation of wine. Food coloring was added to dry white table wine to simulate the appearance of reisling, sauterne, sherry, rosé, claret, and Burgundy. The panel judged the rosé-colored wine to be the sweetest and the claret-colored wine to be the least sweet. Interestingly, subjects who seldom drank wine and participated in the same experiment did not relate color to sweetness.

So important are these visual aspects of food that the USDA food quality grading standards are based on the appearance of food. For example, color is an important characteristic for the grading standards of beef and of fruits. Other visual characteristics, such as the presence or absence of blemishes and bruises, are also important.

Food scientists have spent considerable time trying to relate visual characteristics to measurable physical parameters that determine the acceptance or rejection of a given food. Appearance may provide a clue about the juiciness of an apple or the tenderness of a steak; these properties, of course, are also determined in the mouth and perceived there as differences in texture.

Texture

The texture of food plays an important role in food acceptance because the sense of touch is highly developed in the mouth. Texture, traditionally defined in terms of how a food "feels" in the mouth, is perceived by four different sets of receptors: the pain, tactile, pressor, and sound receptors. The pain receptors may be activated if foods are extremely hot or cold or rich in such seasonings as cayenne pepper, for these items chemically burn the surfaces of the mouth and/or tongue. The tactile receptor receives messages about the geometrical characteristics of the food. The size, shape, and frequency of food particles will be ascertained and, if these characteristics are expected, the food will be accepted. If, however, the mashed potatoes are lumpy or the ice cream gritty, the tactile receptors will perceive this, and the food may be rejected. These tactile receptors are located in the skin of the tongue, oral cavity, and throat. Not only do they perceive characteristics such as "grittiness" or "lumpiness," they also detect differences in moisture and fat content. These latter characteristics may describe the richness, moistness, or slipperiness of a given food.

Texture is also perceived by pressor receptors located in the muscles, tendons, and joints of the mouth, jaws, and throat. These receptors are elements of the kinesthetic sense. The characteristic resistance to chewing, as in a tough piece of meat, is an example of the perception of texture by the kinesthetic sense. "Hard or tough to chew" means extreme physical resistance to the actions of the teeth and jaws. Strenuous exertion by the voluntary muscles is required; this, in turn, is perceived as changes in the position, movement, and tension of the teeth and jaws. The kinesthetic sense is difficult to study because it is not easily located and identifiable. However, through the use of such drugs as cocaine, which blocks the muscle receptors, it has been learned that the oral kinesthetic sense originates as much from the joints as from the muscles. Four sets of receptors are involved: two in the muscles, one in the tendon, and one in the fascia associated with the muscle. There are free nerve endings (also called pressor receptors) in the muscles that are activated by the chewing of such hard items as nuts, crackers, or bones, and that stimulate a sense of motion.

Some textural characteristics are sensed by sound receptors. The sounds a food makes when chewed contributes to the acceptability of the item. The crunch of crisp celery or the snap of a fresh potato chip contribute to the enjoyment of that food. The stimulation of tactile and kinesthetic receptors and auditory receptors play important roles in the evaluation of textural characteristics of the food. Individuals will vary in their preferences for smooth, chewy, crisp, hot, cold, or crunchy textures; all of these attributes, however, are based not on taste, smell, or appearance but on mouth "feel" and "food sounds." In addition, cultural influences will contribute to the textural expectations of individuals. For example, a soft, smooth, bland-textured food may be associated with the food needs of infants or invalids and may not be accepted by the young male with a strong "macho" self-image. Juicy, chewy textures requiring exertion of the jaw muscles may be very acceptable to the young adult but are much less acceptable to the school-age child.

Smell (Olfaction)

Olfaction and gustation are intimately related. Persons who have lost their sense of smell, as frequently happens with a cold, complain that food is not as tasty as when they are well. This is because part of their appreciation of food has decreased through a temporary impairment of their ability to smell.

Among the special senses, the sense of smell is the most sensitive. The average person can detect one part in a trillion parts of air for some high-potency odorants. For example, ethyl mercaptain (ethanethiol) can be detected at 4.0×10^{-11} mg/ml air. However, the perception of a particular aroma quickly diminishes if the aroma persists. This process is called olfactory adaptation and begins the first second after an aroma is perceived.

The perception of smell is a subjective phenomenon. Depending upon a person's expectations, an item can have an intrinsically pleasant or unpleasant aroma. One example of such subjectivity is the scent of a gardenia: many people enjoy it but some find the aroma too strong or overpowering. Another is that when Westerners first came to Japan, the Japanese found the body odor of these people offensive. This was due to the presence of small amounts of butyric acid in the sweat of their visitors. This butyric acid aroma arose because these people were heavy meat eaters. Only people who do not eat meat, as the Japanese did not do in any significant quantity during the late 19th century, notice the odor. However, as the Japanese have been exposed to greater numbers of

Westerners and as the consumption of meat by the Japanese has increased, the difference in body odor has lessened.

Because the perception of smell is so highly subjective, it is difficult to study it either qualitatively or quantitatively. Some physiologists contend that whereas taste perception involves the differentiation of four primary tastes, smell involves many primary odors. However, little progress has been made toward identifying and classifying these odors. Although it is difficult to study the phenomenon of smell, the anatomy of the area in which the event occurs has received considerable attention and is fairly well known.

The perception of smell is performed in a specialized area (Figure 3.19) located in the respiratory tract, which consists of the nose, nasal cavity, pharynx, larynx, trachea, bronchi, and lungs. Within this area, the nasal cavity is divided into two approximately equal and separate chambers known as the nasal fossae or nasal passages. Ambient air enters these chambers, proceeds to the nasopharynx, and exits through rear passageways known as the choanae. In man, olfaction occurs in an area that occupies 2–4 cm^2 in the superior portion of both nasal passages.

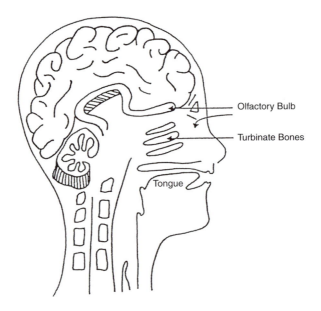

FIGURE 3.19   Anatomy of the major components of the olfactory system.

Although the entire nasal cavity is lined by a mucous membrane, that from the olfactory region is distinguished by its yellow to brown color and is known as the olfactory mucosa or olfactory membrane. Many small glands of Bowman secrete mucus onto the surface of the olfactory mucosa. The receptor cells for the sense of smell, known as the olfactory receptor cells or simply olfactory cells, are also found in the olfactory mucosa. The olfactory sensory unit is shown in Figure 3.20. The olfactory cells are long, slender, bipolar, modified nerve cells; they are interspersed and supported by columnar epithelial cells. Both cells have an underlying layer of basal cells. The dendritic end of the olfactory cell has numerous small (approximately 0.1 microns in diameter and 10–200 microns in length) olfactory hairs or cilia that project into the mucus that coats the olfactory mucosa. The cilia of the olfactory mucosa are distinguishable from the others of the respiratory tract by their motion. Whereas the respiratory tract cilia wave back and forth rhythmically and by their motion assist in removing impurities from the respiratory tract, the cilia of the olfactory mucosa do not. Their movements appear to be random and uncoordinated. The presence and action of the cilia have been confirmed by electron microscopic examination of mucosal tissue.

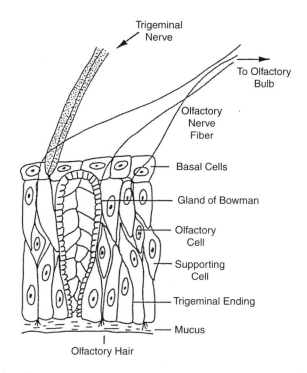

Olfactory Hair

FIGURE 3.20 Details of the olfactory sensory unit. The olfactory cells are supplied with both sensory and motor fibers. The sensory fibers proceed in three separate branches to the olfactory bulb.

From the other end of the olfactory cell extends an axon directly into the central nervous system. Axons from different olfactory cells converge and form the olfactory nerve. The olfactory nerve extends through the sievelike openings of the ethmoid bone located behind the bridge of the nose, to one of the two olfactory bulbs of the forebrain. The two bulbs lie on top of the ethmoid bone beneath the frontal lobes of the brain. Information about different odorants passes directly from the olfactory bulb to the cerebral cortex.

The trigeminal nerve in the cheek is involved in certain responses to odorants. The trigeminal receptors are bare nerve endings found in the nasal passages, mouth, throat, and mucosa around the eyes. They communicate with the brain through the trigeminal nerve. A trigeminally mediated component is part of the odor of such substances as chlorine, peppermint, and menthol. The extent of its involvement is a function of the nature of the odorant and its concentration in the air.

Even though the anatomy involved in olfactory reception is well described, the process by which smells are detected and discriminated is poorly understood. It has been established that the perception of smell involves both a preneural and neural phase. Several features are involved in the preneural phase. A volatile chemical will release molecules into the air. These molecules are inhaled, entering the nasal passages. Under normal conditions, about 2% of the inhaled air will reach the olfactory region and participate in the olfactory event. Sniffing enhances olfaction because inhaled air is forcefully drawn into the upper nostrils, thus increasing the number of odorant molecules to which the olfactory region is exposed. These molecules must then dissolve in the layer of mucus that covers the olfactory region. Once they have dissolved in the mucus, they can interact with the receptor site. At one time, it was thought that the receptor sites were located only on the cilia. However, although it is currently believed that the cilia are not the only possible place, the exact position of other sites has not been established. The nature of the interaction between the odorant molecule and the receptor site is the subject of considerable debate.

This interaction triggers the neural phase; an action potential is initiated in the axon of the receptor cell and transmitted via the olfactory nerve to the olfactory bulb and on to the cerebral cortex. Through this sequence of events, 2,000 to 4,000 smells can be discriminated.

In attempting to unravel the mystery of the mechanism of smell, the relationship between molecular structure and odor discrimination has been an active area of investigation. Regrettably, an odor cannot be predicted from knowledge of the structure of a molecule because often, but not always, minor alterations in the structure produce marked changes in the smell. The odor of vanillin is a familiar one, drawing to mind visions of fresh-baked cookies. A simple substituent change produces isovanillin, a compound that is practically odorless. Replacing the methoxy group with an ethoxy one makes ethylvanillin, a compound four times more aromatic than vanillin. In contrast, there is no marked change in odor quality if the aldehyde group is replaced with a nitro or cyano group. These structures are shown in Figure 3.21.

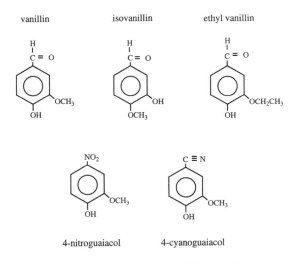

FIGURE 3.21 Structures of related compounds that vary little but that are perceived differently by the olfactory system.

More than 20 theories have been proposed to explain why a specific molecular structure will arouse a certain smell sensation. Most of them deal with the nature of the interaction between the odorant molecule and the receptor site. The "penetrate and puncture" theory of Davies and the stereochemical site theory of Amoore are two such theories.

Davies contends that the odorant molecule is adsorbed by the lipid layer of the membrane wall of the olfactory receptor cell (see Figure 3.20). This molecule can either desorb from the surface of the cell membrane or penetrate it. If it penetrates, it punctures the membrane and leaves a hole that closes slowly. The outer fluid of the receptor cell has a high sodium ion concentration; the inner fluid has a high concentration of potassium ions. Before the hole closes, ions enter the cell. This stimulates the initiation of an action potential and a signal is sent to the brain.

Amoore proposes an alternative explanation. His stereochemical site theory postulates that the size and shape of a molecule govern the type of odor perceived. An odorous molecule will find a complementary molecular structure in the receptor cells. Compounds with similar sizes and shapes will fit into the same site on the receptor cell and, thus, elicit the same smell perception. A necessary part of his theory is that primary odors exist, just as do primary tastes, except that there are far more primary odors than primary tastes.

These theories are highly speculative. The study of people with specific anosmias (no smell perception) are providing further insights into the process of olfaction. In albinism, a genetic mutation that results in absence of pigmentation, anosmia is frequently observed. This suggests that there may be a relationship between olfaction and pigment formation analogous to the relationship of visual acuity and visual pigments. However, the presence of a relationship does not imply that olfactory response is dependent on the presence of pigments in the olfactory region. It may mean, instead, that pigmentation and olfaction are dependent variables of a common genetic error in metabolism. If such as this were the case, pigmentation and olfaction would have no relationship to one another; they are manifestations of the same problem. Other kinds of specific anosmia have also been observed. Some persons are unable to detect the sulfur-containing compound, n-butyl mercaptan. Others are insensitive to the "sweet" smell of hydrogen cyanide or to the scent of freesia (a sweet-smelling flower). This suggests that specific chemical structures in both odorants and receptors are needed for odors to be detected. Parosmia (inappropriate odor perception) is probably due to anosmia of a particular substituent in an odorant grouping. Frequently a loss in olfactory sensitivity is the result of a severe bout of influenza or damage to the trigeminal or fifth cranial nerve. In this latter instance, the error in olfaction resides in the neural phase rather than the preneural phase, as has been the case in the other examples cited. In contrast to all these forms of anosmia, very high sensitivity to odors has been noted in persons with cystic fibrosis (a genetic error in electrolyte exchange characterized by an accumulation of mucous in lungs) or with Addison's disease (deficient adrenal cortical hormone release). In both these diseases, sodium ion loss is excessive; this indicates a need for the movement of sodium in odor perception and acuity. New data are constantly being added to that already accumulated. They may show, in time, that the present theories are inaccurate or incomplete.

Taste (Gustation)

The perception of taste is, as is the perception of smell, highly subjective. Despite this, physiologists have established that man perceives four primary tastes: sour, salty, sweet, and bitter. Chemicals that can elicit any one of these tastes are called tastants. The tastants must be in solution in order to be perceived. Both water-soluble and lipid-soluble compounds can serve as tastants.

Different substances evoke each of the primary tastes. The chemicals that elicit a sour taste are acidic compounds; the hydrogen ion, rather than the associated anion, actually stimulates the receptor. Generally, the sourness is proportional to the concentration of the hydrogen ion. A more acidic compound will trigger a stronger response than a neutral compound. An anion of an inorganic salt produces a salty taste. The halides, chloride, fluoride, bromide, and iodide are usually associated with a salty taste.

A variety of chemicals, mostly organic, trigger the sensation of a sweet taste; sugars, glycols, alcohols, aldehydes, ketones, amides, esters, amino acids, sulfonic acids, halogenated acids, and the inorganic salts of lead and berryllium. The sweetest compound known is the n-propyl derivative of 4-alkoxy-e-aminonitrobenzene. Such organic compounds as the glycosides amygdalin (found in almond kernels) and naringin (found in citrus fruit), and the alkaloids caffeine, quinine, strychnine, and nicotine taste bitter. These structures are shown in Figure 3.22. Inorganic salts of magnesium, ammonium, and calcium also taste bitter.

The average person is more receptive to a bitter taste than to a sour, salty, or sweet taste. For example, a 0.000008 M quinine solution tastes bitter, but a much higher concentration (0.0009 M) of hydrochloric acid is required to taste sour, and an even higher concentration (0.01 M) of sodium chloride to taste salty, or of sucrose to taste sweet.

Additionally, the pleasantness of a given taste relates to the concentration of the tastant. For example, as the concentration of sucrose in a solution is increased, its taste changes from unpleasant to pleasant; the pleasant sensation of sweet arises only at higher concentrations. In contrast, a bitter

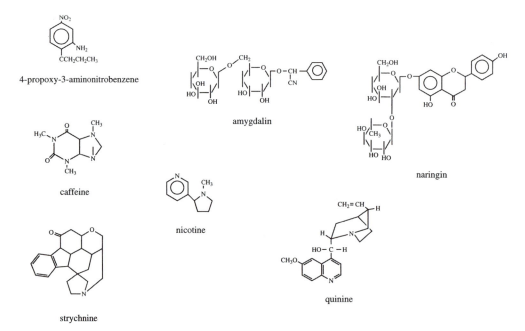

FIGURE 3.22 Chemical structures of compounds that elicit the bitter taste.

taste can be pleasant at low concentrations but become unpleasant at high ones. In small quantities, the white membrane of orange or grapefruit sections enhances the flavors of these fruits; however, they are seldom eaten alone because of their bitter taste.

Within a given taste modality, some chemicals can be tasted at a lower concentration than others. This can be expressed quantitatively by measuring the detection threshold and, from this, calculating the relative taste indices. Table 3.14 gives the relative taste indices of several substances with the intensities of each of the four primary sensations referred to a reference compound: the acidic substances to hydrochloric acid; the sweet substances to sucrose; the bitter ones to quinine; and the salty ones to sodium chloride. Each of these reference compounds is assigned an index value of 1.

Each of these primary tastes is perceived through the organ of taste, the taste bud. The taste bud is about 1/30 millimeter in diameter and 1/16 millimeter in length. It contains two kinds of cells; the receptor cell and the supporting cell. The gustatory receptor cells, also called the taste cells, are barrel-shaped, modified epithelial cells. From one end of each taste cell protrudes several microvilli or taste hairs. These microvilli extend through a taste pore within the tongue's surface to contact the fluids of the mouth. For a tastant to be perceived, it must be in solution. The other end of each taste cell is innervated with gustatory nerve fibers. One cell may be innervated with several fibers or several fibers may innervate one cell; there is no one-on-one line of communication between the individual taste cell and the central nervous system (CNS).

The traditional view of taste held that its perception was mediated only by taste buds (Figure 3.23a) found in the papillae on the surface of the tongue, and that there were specific areas where each modality, and only that modality, was perceived (Figure 3.23b). This is not wholly true. Taste buds are actually found several places within the oral cavity — on the surface of the tongue, palate, pharynx, and larynx, and sometimes on the cheeks.

The surface of the tongue is covered by small structures called papillae. Four distinct kinds of papillae have been described (Figure 3.23c). Filliform papillae, which contain no taste buds, are very small and are scattered over most of the surface of the tongue. Fungiform papillae are raised, pigmented papillae and are intermixed with the filliform papillae on the anterior two-thirds of the

TABLE 3.14
Relative Taste Indices of Different Substances

Sour Substances	Index	Bitter Substances	Index	Sweet Substances	Index	Salty Substances	Index
Hydrochloric acid	1	Quinine	1	Sucrose	1	NaCl	1
Formic acid	1.1	Strychnine	3.1	4-propoxy-3-amino nitrobenzene	5000	NaF	2
Chloracetic acid	0.9	Nicotine	1.3	Saccharin	675	$CaCl_2$	1
Lactic acid	0.85	Phenylthiourea	0.9	Chloroform	40	NaBr	0.5
Tartaric acid	0.7	Caffeine	0.4	Fructose	1.7	NaI	0.35
Malic acid	0.6	Pilocarpine	0.16	Alanine	1.3	LiCl	0.4
Potassium H tartrate	0.58	Atropine	0.13	Glucose	0.8	NH_4Cl	2.5
Acetic acid	0.55	Cocaine	0.02	Maltose	0.45	KCl	0.6
Citric acid	0.46	Morphine	0.02	Galactose	0.32		
Carbonic acid	0.06			Lactose	0.3		

(Adapted from A. C. Guyton, *Textbook of Medical Physiology*, 7 ed. (Philadelphia: W. B. Saunders, 1971) p. 639)

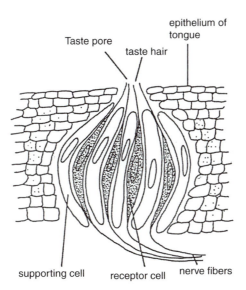
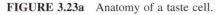

FIGURE 3.23a Anatomy of a taste cell.

surface. They are not found beyond the sulcus terminalis, a V-shaped groove near the back of the tongue. Circumvallate papillae are larger and taller and are prevalent on the posterior surface of the tongue. Foliate papillae are located along the sides near the back of the tongue. Moderate numbers of taste buds are found in the fungiform and foliate papillae, but most of the taste buds are found in the circumvallate papillae. The tongue, although it perceives all four of the taste modalities, is the most sensitive to salty and sweet (see Figure 3.23b). The palate, on the other hand, is more sensitive to the sour and bitter tastes than to the salty and sweet tastes. The pharynx also detects all four tastes but not to the same extent as the tongue and palate (see Figure 3.24). Scattered over the entire oral cavity of an adult are approximately 10,000 taste buds. The taste cells within the taste buds are epithelial cells, which are short-lived cells with a rapid turnover rate. A human taste cell has an approximate lifetime of 250 hours. The ability to quickly regenerate is in

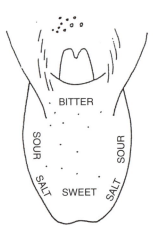

FIGURE 3.23b Taste areas of the tongue.

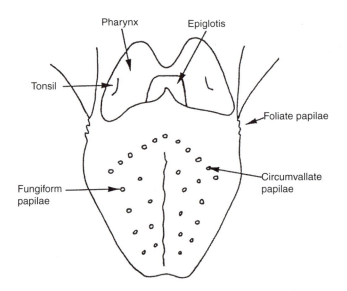

FIGURE 3.23c Upper surface of the human tongue.

marked contrast to most other elements of the nervous system. As one grows older, the rate at which taste cells are regenerated is decreased and, as a consequence, there is a concomitant decrease in quantity. With a decrease in number of taste cells, taste acuity declines.

The anatomical features involved with gustation have been well studied, as have the tastants that elicit the sensation. Organic chemists have long known that small structural changes can alter tastes. For instance, the sugars listed in Table 3.10 are structurally similar. The taste response they elicit, however, varies from very sweet (β-D-fructose) to bitter (β-D-mannose). The most remarkable feature of these compounds is that mutarotation about the anomeric carbon of α-D-mannose to make β-D-mannose changes the taste perceived from sweet to bitter. These structures are shown in Figure 3.25.

Saccharin is sweet, but its N-alkylated derivatives are tasteless. The alkali metal salts of cyclamate (cyclohexyl amine sulfate) are sweet, and the amine salt is nearly tasteless. It has been found that the dipeptide L-aspartyl-L-phenylalanine methyl ester (aspartame) and certain related compounds are nearly 200 times sweeter than sucrose. Since this compound is composed of natural

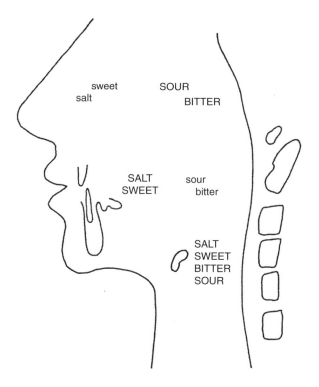

FIGURE 3.24 A schematic representation of taste localization on the tongue, palate, and pharynx of mormal man. The taste modalities in capital letters indicate more sensitive taste acuity, while those in small letters indicate less-sensitive tase acuity. Each of the taste modalities is represented in each anatomical area. However, salt and sweet are perceivd most acutely on the tongue, bitter and sour most acutely on the palate. (From R.I. Henkin, The role of taste in disease and nutrition. *Borden's Review of Nutrition Research*, 28 (1967):73.)

amino acids and is quite low in calories, it offers intriguing possibilities as a synthetic sweetener. If any other amino acids are substituted for the L-aspartate (even the closely related compound L-glutamate), the resulting product is tasteless. However, sweetness is maintained if phenylalanine is replaced by methionine or tyrosine. The dipeptide free acid of the methyl ester is not sweet, nor is the ethyl ester as sweet as the methyl ester.

Although much is known about the anatomy of the oral cavity and about the chemistry of the tastants, a thorough understanding of the mechanism of taste has not been assembled. As with smell, the process includes both a preneural and neural phase. The preneural event involves an interaction between the tastant and the receptor cell. It is generally believed that this is a steric interaction between these two sites, possibly involving conformational changes. Then, in some incompletely understood manner, this triggers the neural phase, which is the depolarization of specific taste nerves and the passage of impulses to the brain. Electrical signals generated when various tastants have been applied to the tongue have been measured.

For the auditory and visual senses, medical specialties have evolved to diagnose and treat, where possible, deviations from normal. Similar specialties have not been developed to solve problems of taste and smell, nor have great strides been made in the diagnosis and treatment of disorders of these senses. However, abnormalities in taste perception have provided a means for verifying and enlarging the understanding of the mechanism of the taste sensation.

Anatomic abnormalities of both the palate and the tongue have been associated with a decrease in taste sensitivity. Patients with abnormal palate structures have significantly elevated thresholds for sour and bitter tastes but not for sweet and salty ones. An increase in threshold means that a greater concentration of the tastant is required for detection and recognition of that tastant by a

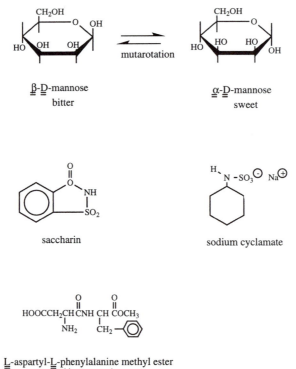

FIGURE 3.25   Compounds having a sweet taste.

subject. However, not all patients with anatomic abnormalities of the hard or soft palate exhibit taste disturbances. For example, those with gross clefts of the back part of the hard palate detect and recognize all four modalities of taste.

People who wear dentures report an increase in the detection and recognition thresholds for sour and bitter tastes, but no change in their response to sweet and salty tastes. Dentures fit close to the palate and cover part of the mouth area containing taste receptors. As a result, there may be an artificial masking of taste receptor sites in these parts of the mouth and taste perception may be affected.

Abnormalities on the surface of the tongue, such as lichen planus and tumors, cause a decrease in taste acuity. Diseases that affect the nerve supply to the tongue (such as postdiptheritic neuritis, sarcoidosis, and Bell's palsy), severe trauma, and irradiation of the oral cavity as part of treatment for a malignancy will result in a decrease in taste sensitivity. In all of these abnormal states, there is a reduction or omission in the number of taste receptor cells, which has been given as the reason for the decrease in taste acuity. Interestingly, however, congenital underdevelopment or absence of the tongue is not accompanied by a decrease in taste acuity.

Speculation about the specific functions of the taste bud in taste perception have resulted from studies of patients with Type I familial dysautonomia (Riley–Day Syndrome). In this syndrome, the tongue's surface is smooth; the sulcus terminalis, taste buds, and fungiform and circumvallate papillae are missing, and the number of unmyelinated free nerve endings is greatly diminished. Patients demonstrate significantly raised detection and recognition thresholds; some cannot consistently distinguish between water and saturated solutions of sodium chloride, sugar, urea, and 0.03 M hydrochloric acid. However, when treated with methacholine (an α-adrenergic drug), these patients have normal taste perception while the drug remains in their system. This has led to the suggestion that the taste buds function as a chemical sieve. It is proposed that taste buds have pores of a small, controlled size through which chemical stimuli may reach the nerves. Numerous factors, not yet identified, may control this pore size. In patients with familial dysautonomia, treatment with methacholine causes an increase in membrane permeability, including that of the lingual surface, which, in turn, allows a tastant to reach the unmyelinated, free nerve endings in the tongue. Thus, the taste threshold is lowered and the patient is more responsive to the tastant.

The divalent cations, particularly copper, zinc, and nickel, have been reported to affect taste sensitivity. When given to patients with hypoguesia, some improvement occurs. Observations of serum and tissue levels of copper in patients with rheumatoid arthritis and Wilson's disease have led to conjectures about copper's role in the regulation of taste acuity. Patients with either of these diseases are often treated with D-penicillamine. With this therapy, patients having Wilson's disease experience no change in their taste acuity; however, patients with rheumatoid arthritis frequently report a decrease. D-penicillamine therapy is associated with a decrease in serum and tissue copper levels. For arthritic patients, this does indeed happen. Not so in patients with Wilson's disease, which is characterized by abnormally high levels of serum copper. Penicillamine simply reduces this high level to a normal level. The taste acuity of arthritic patients, if given oral copper sulfate, returns to normal. Thus, copper appears to be directly involved with taste acuity and its depletion leads to hypoguesia.

Recent reports indicate that taste dysfunction may be associated with impaired zinc absorption and decreased levels of zinc in the saliva. Oral therapy of zinc or nickel returns the taste acuity to normal.

Steroid hormones have also been implicated in the taste mechanism through studies of diseases of the endocrine system. Patients with Addison's disease, decreased adrenal cortical function, or panhypopituitarism have lowered detection thresholds. Patients with Addison's disease are sometimes able to detect concentrations of tastants as low as 0.01 of that perceived by normal subjects. In both cases, the heightened taste sensitivity returns to normal when the missing steroids are given. The mechanism by which the steroids influence taste perception is not known.

A comprehensive, unified theory of taste perception has not yet been realized. But the taste of food, as well as its appearance, texture, and smell, is intimately involved in man's desire to eat.

NEURONAL SIGNALS FOR HUNGER AND SATIETY

Internal cues regulate food intake through a number of signals and responses that ultimately result in the initiation or cessation of feeding. These cues are in addition to those described above, which involve the cerebrum. Both short-term and long-term controls are exerted that, over time, serve to regulate the food intake of normal individuals so that they neither gain nor lose weight. Food-intake control rests, in part, with the integration of a variety of hormonal and nonhormonal signals that are generated both peripherally and centrally. The hypothalamus is thought to be the main integrator of these signals. Other discrete areas are also involved. The hypothalamus is located beneath the thalamus, a part of the forebrain, close to the pituitary (Figure 3.26). The hypothalamus is involved in both the initiation and cessation of food and water intake. It serves as an endocrine organ that produces the hormones that, in turn, modulate the release of hormones from the posterior pituitary. It also releases other hormones, called releasing factors or tropins, which control the activity of the anterior pituitary. The area of the brain that includes the thalamus, hypothalamus, and pituitary has been called the center of existence, because it controls much of what is known as instinctive behavior. In addition to its regulatory effect on appetite, satiety, and thirst, the hypothalamus serves, through its effect on the pituitary, as the main subcortical control center for the regulation of the parasympathetic and sympathetic systems; for the regulation of heart rate; and for the regulation of vasodilation and vasoconstriction, two important processes for the maintenance of body temperature. If the body temperature rises, vasodilation (increased blood flow through skin capillaries) along with increased respiration and increased sweat loss, occurs, thus increasing body heat loss. Conversely, if body temperature is below normal, vasoconstriction (decreased blood flow) occurs

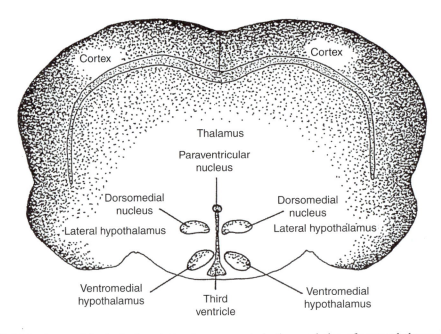

FIGURE 3.26 Areas of the brain thought to play some role in the regulation of energy balance are shown in a vertical cross section of the center of the rat brain. In the 1950s, it was thought that the ventromedial hypothalamus contained a "satiety center," which, when activated, inhibited a "hunger center" in the lateral hypothalamus. The paraventricular nucleus (located in a plane that is slightly in front of the other labeled areas of the hypothalamus, shown in white) appears to be involved in maintaining glucostasis, or the balance of blood gluscose. The dorsomedial nucleus is currently thought to be involved in determining body size rather than body-fat content.

and body heat is conserved. Vasoconstriction, vasodilation, and heart rate are also important to the regulation of blood pressure. Indirectly, the hypothalamus regulates the activity of the gastrointestinal system, the emotions, and spontaneous behavior.

The role of the hypothalamus in the control of eating behavior has been well studied. As early as 1840, extreme obesity in man was reported to occur in patients with hypothalamic tumors. Recognition of the involvement of the ventromedial hypothalamus in the regulation of food intake did not come until it was shown that if the ventromedial hypothalamic area was destroyed or lesioned, the animals overate, with a resulting increase in body fat. If the lateral hypothalamus was lesioned, animals became both adipsic (had no thirst response) and aphagic (did not eat). This relationship of feeding behavior to drinking behavior can be understood when the consequences of dehydration due to absence of fluid intake are realized. In adipsic animals, saliva production is significantly reduced; thus, laterally lesioned animals have difficulty, initially, in swallowing dry food. As the lesioned animal recovers or adapts to the lesion, he drinks when he eats dry food but does not eat when water deprived. In addition, the lesioned rat does not drink in response to serum hyperosmolarity (increased levels of solutes in the blood), hyperthermia (increased body temperature) or hypovolemia (decreased blood volume). Animals with lesions in the lateral hypothalamus do not respond to reductions in blood sugar levels (via insulin injections) and will die in severe hypoglycemia rather than eat readily available food. This observation suggests that both the lateral and ventromedial nuclei in the hypothalamus interact via chemical signals to control eating and drinking. Since eating and the cessation of eating are under hypothalamic control, it is reasonable to assume that this behavior is initiated or stopped by a series of signals emitted from and/or received by this tissue. The nature of this signal system is rather complex. As research continued in this area, it was learned that other areas of the brain are involved. The paraventricular nucleus located slightly in front of the dorsomedial nucleus (Figure

3.26) appears to be involved in the regulation of glucose intake as it relates to the maintenance of glucose homeostasis. The dorsomedial nucleus, found on either side of the third ventricle, seems to be involved in the control of body size but not body fat and, because of this involvement, is likely to play a role in food intake. In addition, the area postrema of the brain stem and the caudal medial nucleus have been implicated in food-intake regulation. The details of this involvement are not yet in hand, but we do know that the cytokines, bound to their cognate receptors, are intimately involved in determining eating behavior.

One school of thought is that eating is a response to variations in the level of circulating glucose. This theory, called the glucostatic theory, proposes that cellular energy requirements determine feeding behavior. In particular, it suggests that brain cells, which use glucose almost exclusively as their metabolic fuel, are exquisitely sensitive to fluctuations in blood glucose levels, and, as such, will activate the "feeding center" to initiate feeding when blood glucose levels dip below normal, or activate the "satiety center" to stop feeding when blood glucose levels are high. Support for this theory comes from the observation that feeding is initiated by animals injected with insulin and from the observation that gold thioglucose (which destroys the satiety center of the hypothalamus) is ineffective in diabetic animals. In the latter case, eating continues because gold thioglucose does not get into the hypothalamic cells of diabetic animals to destroy the satiety center. This occurs because the penetration of gold thioglucose into the hypothalamic cells is insulin dependent. This is a very simplistic approach to food-intake regulation, but it has provided a framework for the building of a more cohesive explanation of the systems that operate to ensure energy balance.

Another school of thought is that eating behavior is controlled by the fat-cell size and number. This is called the lipostatic theory. It speculates that there is a set point for each animal for the number of fat cells and their fat content and that when this set point is reached, the animal ceases to eat. In the absence of eating, these fat stores are mobilized and used until a lower set point is reached and feeding again commences. This theory is supported by observations of animals that had been starved. These animals ate large amounts of food when realimented after starvation until they regained their prestarvation weight; then, they resumed their prestarvation eating behavior. In other words, they overate to fill their fat depots, then ate only enough to maintain these depots. Modulation of food intake by signals arising in adipose tissue has been an important component of many theories of energy balance.

It is possible that the theories described above (as well as some others) may be integrated into one to more readily allow for the understanding of the signals needed to initiate, maintain, and stop feeding. In addition to the cytokines already described, both the brain and the gastrointestinal tract release a variety of hormones that regulate quite specific components of the food-intake and utilization system. Most of these hormonal signals have short-term effects on feeding, but do not affect overall long-term food consumption. These signals may truly be hunger or satiety signals, but one must not confuse a satiety signal with a food-intake-inhibition signal or confuse a hunger signal with a food-intake-initiation signal. The initiation may occur but not be sustained sufficiently to result in significant food consumption. Similarly, inhibition may occur but may not significantly alter overall food intake. Therefore, not only the stop and start signals need to be examined, but also the overall control of food intake that has a long-term effect on energy balance. Sustaining feeding or food abstinence may involve not only the factors listed in Table 3.12 but other factors as well. Initiation may be hormonally induced feeding but sustained because the food is found to be pleasing as per the discussion on the hedonistic qualities of food — its taste, smell, texture, etc. Similarly, cessation of feeding even though hormones have signalled initiation may occur if the food is not palatable or acceptable.

A number of hormones, diet ingredients, metabolites, and drugs have been shown to influence food intake and feeding behavior. Some of the more important ones are shown in Table 3.15. Hormones that can enhance food intake at one level can suppress it at another. Insulin is a prime example. Thyroxine is another. Normal individuals given a low dose of insulin will experience hunger. However, large doses of insulin can provoke a serious hypoglycemia that will have the

TABLE 3.15
Factors That Affect Food Intake

Enhances		Suppresses
Insulin	Leptin	Anorectin
Testosterone	Estrogen	Corticotropin-releasing hormone (CRH)
Glucocorticoids	Phenylethylamines[1]	
Thyroxine	Mazindol	Neurotensin
Low serotonin levels	Substance P	Bombesin
Dynorphin	Glucagon	Cyclo-his-pro
β endorphin	"Satietin" (a blood borne factor)	High protein diets
Neuropeptide Y	High fat diet	High blood glucose
Galanin	Serotonin	Enterostatin
Opioid peptides	Fluoxetine	Calcitonin
Growth hormone-releasing hormone	Pain	Thyrotropin releasing factor
	Histidine (precursor of histamine)	
Desacetyl-melanocyte stimulating hormone	Amino acid imbalance in diet	TNFα
	Tryptophane (precursor of serotonin)	
Antidepressants[2]	Cholecystokinin (CCK)	
	Somatostatin	
	Thyrotropin releasing hormone	

[1] These are drugs and except for the drug phenylpropanolamine are controlled substances. Many have serious side effects. They are structurally related to the catecholamines. Most are active as short term appetite suppressants and act through their effects on the central nervous system, particularly through the b adrenergic and/or dopaminergic receptors. This group includes amphetamine, methamphetamine, phenmetrazine, phentermine, diethylpropion, fenfluramine, phenylpropanolamine. Phenyl-propanolamine induced anorexia is not reversed by the dopamine antagonist haloperidol.
[2] All of these drugs are controlled substances and their use must be carefully monitored. This groups includes amitriptyline, buspirone, chlordiazepoxide, chlorpromazine, cisplatin, clozapine, ergotamine, fluphenazine, impramine, iprindole and others that block 5-HT receptors.

opposite effect. Campfield and Smith have studied the signals for feeding that occur in the rat. They have shown that feeding is initiated when the brain perceives a small fall in blood glucose. Transient declines within the normal range of blood glucose levels were found to precede meal initiation. This feeding response could be attenuated if blood glucose levels were elevated via an intravenous infusion of glucose. Preceding the transient fall in blood glucose was a transient insulin spike that probably was responsible for the transient fall in glucose. Individuals soon after a high-glucose meal will feel satiated; their blood and brain glucose levels have risen, as has blood insulin, and their appetite is suppressed. Other hormones are involved as well. In hypothyroidism, hunger signals are poorly perceived. The patient, although not anorexic, does not have a strong drive to eat. In contrast, hyperthyroidism is characterized by strong, almost unremitting hunger.

Within this framework are a number of afferent and efferent systems that influence food intake by providing information to the brain and relaying instructions via neuronal signals from the brain to the rest of the body. Bray has recently reviewed the actions of peptides that affect the intake of specific nutrients and the sympathetic nervous system. Food intake can be increased or decreased with reciprocal effects on the central nervous system when these peptides are administered. Galanin, neuropeptide Y, opioid peptides, growth-hormone-releasing hormone, and desacetyl-melanocyte-stimulating hormone increase food intake, whereas insulin excess, glucagon, leptin, cholecystokinen, anorectin, corticotropin-releasing hormone, neurotensin, bombesin, cyclo-his-pro, and thyrotropin-releasing hormone reduce food intake. Several of these hormones or peptides have specific actions with respect to the intake of specific food components. For example, increases in neuropeptide Y result in increased carbohydrate intake, while increases in the level of galanin and opioid peptides increase fat intake. Fat intake is suppressed when the blood level of enterostatin rises. Rising blood levels of glucagon suppress protein intake. All of the above are short-term signals that appear to regulate food selection as well as the amount of food consumed. Although most of these studies have been done in carefully prepared experimental animals (usually rats), there is sufficient indirect evidence to suggest that short-term food intake is similarly regulated in man. In humans, serotoninergic agents are being developed for use as treatments for obesity and eating disorders. These agents are successful because they either block the binding of serotonin (5-hydroxytryptamine, 5-HT) to its receptor, or upregulate the receptors' binding affinity. 5-HT receptors are widespread throughout the cerebral cortex, the limbic system, the striatum, the brain stem, the choroid plexus, and almost every other region of the central nervous system. Because serotonin suppresses feeding if the receptor is blocked, feeding is enhanced. Thus, drugs that block these receptors are useful in treating anorexia (decreased desire to eat) especially the anorexia that accompanies anxiety, depression, obsessive-compulsive disorders, panic disorders, migraine, and chemotherapy emesis. In contrast, drugs that potentiate the binding of 5HT to its receptor will result in a suppression of appetite and may be useful in treating the hyperphagia of Prader–Willi syndrome and that associated with genetic obesity. As the database on leptin and its receptor expands, doubtless there will be drugs that either interfere with this system or potentiate it. The latter might be useful in the treatment of obesity, while the former might be helpful in treating anorexia.

Drugs, particularly those used in cancer chemotherapy, frequently have appetite suppression as a side effect. In part, this reduction in food intake may be due to disease- or drug-induced changes in taste and aroma perception and, in part, due to the effects of the disease or drugs on the central nervous system, particularly the adrenergic and serotonergic receptors. Several of the drugs listed in Table 3.15 are appetite suppressants and are chemically related to the catecholamines. As indicated, some of these drugs can be addictive and are therefore controlled substances. It appears that none of the drugs listed in Table 3.15 are free of side effects.

Some steroids affect food intake. Adrenalectomized animals or humans with Addison's disease, both glucocorticoid deficient states, do not perceive normal hunger signals. If without food for extended periods of time, these individuals are difficult to realiment. However, once eating commences, a normal feeding pattern will be maintained. In excess, glucocorticoid stimulates feeding, and patients with Cushing's disease (excess glucocorticoid production) or patients who are receiving long-term glucocorticoid treatment will report increased hunger and food intake. Patients with Cushing's disease are often characterized by large fat depots across the shoulders and in the abdomen. In addition, obese patients are frequently characterized by excess blood levels of both glucocorticoids and insulin. As noted above, these hormones stimulate appetite and feeding.

Within the normal range, doses of testosterone and estrogen, although also steroids, have opposite effects with respect to food intake. In experimental animals, day-to-day variations in food intake by females will follow the same pattern as their day-to-day variation in estrogen level. When estrogen is high, food intake is suppressed and vice versa. Women who are anestrus due to ovariectomy or who are postmenopausal frequently lose their day-to-day estrogen-mediated food-intake pattern. With this loss is a more even (and somewhat increased) food intake and subsequent body fat gain. This has been found as well in castrated female rats.

The gain in body weight as fat is explained by the loss in food-intake control exerted by the estrogens rather than by an estrogen-inhibiting effect on lipogenesis. Testosterone increases food intake marginally, but also stimulates protein synthesis and spontaneous physical activity. As a result, body fat does not increase. As testosterone levels decline in males with age, protein synthesis declines and the body tends to sustain its fat synthetic activity. This results in a change in body composition with an increase in body-fat stores. The age-related decline in testosterone production may not be accompanied by a decline in food intake.

Although food intake can vary from day to day in response to minor day-to-day variations in food supply, activity, and hormonal status, body weight is relatively constant. The mechanisms that control body weight are very complex and the fine details of this regulation are far from clear. However, suffice it to say, major long-term deviations in either food intake or physiological state can affect body weight or energy balance. If food intake (energy intake) is curtailed for days to months, body weight will fall; similarly, if food intake is dramatically increased, body weight will increase. This relationship assumes no change in body energy demand. As described in the section on trauma, the energy requirement can be increased up to tenfold by major illness despite the fact that the patient may be recumbent and perhaps sedated. Similarly, individuals who have markedly changed their activity levels will affect their energy balance.

If strenuous exercise is added without an increase in food intake, this will increase energy expenditure and negative energy balance, or weight loss will occur. In most individuals, therefore, long-term changes in energy balance, either through changes in intake or expenditure, will result in a body-weight change.

Anorexia Nervosa

That food intake can be consciously controlled is evident in the condition known as *anorexia nervosa*. This condition is frequently observed in adolescent females and is related to their inaccurate perception of their body fatness. They become obsessed with the desire to be thin and either refuse to eat and adequately nourish their bodies or they eat, then force themselves to regurgitate the food. Self-induced vomiting is called *bulimia*. Additional behavior related to an obsession with body image includes the excessive use of laxatives and diuretics and the extensive participation in exercise designed to increase energy expenditure. Although the patients may be eating some food, they are not consuming enough food to meet their macro- and micronutrient requirements. Because of this, they are in negative energy and protein balance. These patients are characterized by little body fat. Because ovulation requires a minimal amount of fat in the body, ovulation ceases. Amenorrhea, hypothermia, hypotension also develop and, if unrecognized and untreated, anorexics may starve to death. Some people, for whatever reason, self recognize and resume eating. In many respects, anorexic people have physiological/biochemical features that are similar to those patients described in the section on starvation. Their catabolic hormone levels are high and their body-energy stores are being raided as a result. Insulin resistance due to the catabolic hormones is observed. Liver and muscle glycogen levels are low. Fat stores are minimal. As the weight loss proceeds further, these individuals have reduced bone mass, decreased metabolic rate, decreased heart rate, hypoglycemia, hypothyroidism, electrolyte imbalance, elevated free fatty acid and cholesterol levels, peripheral edema, and finally, cardiac and renal failure. When their fat stores fall below 2% of total body weight, they will die. This 2% represents the lipids essential to the structure and function of membranes as well as those complex lipids that compose the central nervous system. With this scenario in mind, the clinician faces the challenge of reversing the condition. Just as it is difficult to reverse starvation-induced changes in the metabolism of unintentionally starving humans (see sections on starvation, protein-calorie malnutrition, and trauma), reversing the weight loss of anorexic patients presents some special challenges. The energy requirements for weight regain in anorexic patients are highly variable and depend largely on the physiological status of the patient at the time of treatment initiation and on the pre-anorexia body weight. Those patients who had been obese prior to their self-induced anorexia regained their lost weight faster than patients who had been of normal body weight. Pharmaceutical agents to stimulate appetite and reverse depression (if present) can be used. If the person is clinically depressed, treatment of the depression will frequently have a positive effect on food intake. This is not always true, however. In contrast, treatment of the anorexia with appetite-stimulating drugs, nutritional support, and counseling can reverse the condition of weight loss and secondarily, positively affect the depression. Again, this is not always true. The outcome of the treatment depends on the time at which it is instituted. If anorexia nervosa is recognized early in the sequence of hormonal and metabolic change, then the chances of success are much greater than if treatment is initiated after irreversible tissue changes have occurred. While controversy exists as to the success of treatment as well as the accuracy of diagnosis, it is generally agreed that aggressive treatment can achieve reversal in 50% of the cases. Mortality is estimated in 6% of cases. This leaves an estimate of approximately 44% who recover spontaneously without medical intervention. Treatment success also depends on the degree of self-prescribed food-intake restriction. Total food abstinence is far more threatening than mild abstinence. Included in the mortality figure of 6% are those who commit suicide. This implies a relationship between the development of depression and anorexia — two self-destructive behaviors that represent abnormalities in the central nervous system (CNS).

Restoring the weight loss of the anorexic patient follows a slightly different pattern from the weight regain by traumatized individuals and formerly obese individuals. In the latter groups, the fat regain precedes the protein regain. In fact, in the genetically obese individual, fat regain takes precedence over protein regain. In the recovering anorexic who was not genetically obese prior to anorexia, protein regain keeps pace with fat regain. As both synthetic processes utilize micronutrients, these must be provided at levels similar to those prescribed for growing children. Recovering anorexics are "growing" new tissue to replace that which was raided during the energy deficit period. They must consume sufficient nutrients to support this regrowth.

Bulimic and nonbulimic anorexics differ in their weight recovery. Those who were bulimic recover their lost weight more rapidly than those who were anorexic only. This is probably due to the difference in rate of weight loss. Those anorexics who were also bulimic were more severely starved and lost weight faster than nonbulimic anorexics. Because of this, bulimics are more likely to be diagnosed and treated sooner than nonbulimic anorexics. In anorexics, as with prolonged starvation, gut absorptive capacity is compromised due to a loss of cells lining the gastrointestinal tract. In the early phase of treatment, malabsorption is likely to occur. For this reason, the diet offered during recovery must be gradually increased with respect to its energy content. A gradual 300 kcal (1255 kJ) thrice weekly increase from an initial 1200 kcal (5,040 kJ) diet which includes about 3g sodium is recommended. The recovery diet should also be a lactose-free diet and should be offered in six or more small meals over 24 hours. A low-fat diet is sometimes recommended, but this depends on the genetic background and pre-anorexia health status of the patient. Those with diabetic tendencies might not fare as well if faced with a low-fat–high-carbohydrate diet. The medical history of the patient and family will provide clues as to the most appropriate diet design. The recovering anorexic requires more food than the recovering bulimic anorexic. The recovering anorexic has lost more absorptive cells than the bulimic anorexic. Of interest is the report that even after weight regain, the recovered anorexic has a higher than normal energy requirement and, if this is not met, will begin to lose weight once again. This suggests that not all anorexia nervosa is self inflicted. It may begin with a conscious effort to consume less food but then may continue because of a change in the signals for food-intake initiation and cessation and a change in the efficiency with which the body uses the food consumed.

ABNORMAL APPETITE

Man, as well as some lower animals, will sometimes or habitually consume items of no nutritional value. In some cases, the item in question will have a deleterious effect on the person's health. The habit is called pica, after the Latin word for magpie, a bird that will consume all manner of food and nonfood items. Pica has been observed for centuries and was described by Aetius of Amida in 1542. Many different items are consumed; however, the most common are clay (geophagia), laundry starch (amylophagia), or ice (pagophagia). A number of studies on the prevalence of pica have shown that up to 70% of some population groups may have this habit. Pregnant women as well as children are the most frequently affected, and black women are three to four times more affected than white women of the same socioeconomic group. The most common cravings were for laundry starch (as much as

8 oz. a day) and clay. When both men and women were studied, few men exhibited the practice and it has been suggested that men use liquor or tobacco to meet their nonfood oral needs.

The question of why pica exists has not been satisfactorily answered. From the various epidemiological studies, age, sex, social status, and race appear to be important factors in the development of the habit. Several studies have noted that pica was associated with anemia. Reynolds et al. reported that frequent nosebleeds and other spontaneous losses of blood accompanied or preceded an increased craving for certain food and nonfood items. Clay, rice, French fries, ice, green vegetables, bread, hot tea, and grapefruit were mentioned as being consumed in large quantities by these patients. The patients were treated for their anemias with iron supplements and were tested for their iron-binding capacity. Some of the patients had low uptakes of iron while others were normal. Those with poor iron-binding capacities were usually the clay eaters; those with normal iron-binding capacities were ice cream eaters. Clay, even the small amount residing in the gastrointestinal tract of patients having no access to clay while hospitalized, could have adsorbed the oral iron supplements. Thus, it seems unlikely that an innate lowered iron-binding capacity was responsible for either the anemia or the pica. However, pica does appear to follow the development of anemia rather than precede it.

In addition to anemia, other conditions have been observed in pica patients. Muscular weakness and low serum potassium levels have been reported in geophagic patients. Both these conditions could be attributed to the binding of potassium in the intestine by the clay. This may also be true in patients consuming large quantities of laundry starch.

A more serious aspect of pica is the consumption of paint chips (plumbism) by young children. If the paint contains lead oxide as the pigment, lead intoxication can develop. This is characterized by anemia, low serum iron and copper values, growth depression, ataxia, kidney damage, coma, convulsions, and death. The ataxia, stupor, coma, and convulsions reflect the effect of lead on the central nervous system. This can be understood as the effect of lead on hemoglobin synthesis. Both copper and iron utilization are impaired and the anemia typical of lead intoxication is microcytic and hypochromic in character. In addition, lead may replace either copper, iron, or calcium in a number of tissues and, because it is metabolically inert, inhibit the functionality of that tissue. In the case of hemoglobin synthesis, it becomes obvious that the oxygen-carrying capacity of the red blood cells is decreased. Those tissues with a high oxygen requirement, i.e., the neural tissue, will be the most affected. Thus, one can understand the neuromuscular response to chronic lead ingestion. If neuronal tissue suffers from prolonged oxygen deprivation, it will die and this damage is irreversible. Subjects with lead poisoning can be treated with compounds such as EDTA that will bind the circulating lead and allow the body to excrete the EDTA–lead complex. It is not possible, however, to rid the body of all of its accumulated lead nor to protect the patients from future ill effects of their lead-induced pathology. Lead will remain in its storage sites, such as bone, and, when mobilized, will have untoward effects.

In the U.S. today, the majority of lead-intoxication cases are young children, ages 1 to 6, with pica. Adults who work in lead-related industries or consume lead-contaminated illicit beverages are also affected. Increasing the levels of lead exposure generally increases the blood and tissue lead levels, yet, individual variations due to age, sex, and nutritional status occur. The factors that determine the fractions of the body where lead is deposited have not been determined. It is known that well-nourished individuals are more resistant to the deleterious effects of lead than are poorly nourished individuals.

SUPPLEMENTAL READINGS

Articles

Allison, D.B., Kaprio,.J., Korkeila.,M., Koskenvuo, M., Neale, M.C., and Hayakawa, K. (1996). The heritability of body mass index among an international sample of monozygotic twins reared apart. *Int. J. Obesity* 20:501-506.

Alpert, S. (1990). Growth, thermogenesis and hyperphagia. *Am. J. Clin. Nutr.* 52:782-792.

Aw, T.Y. and Jones, D.P. (1989). Nutrient supply and mitochondrial function. *Ann. Rev. Nutr.* 9:229-251.

Benedict, F.G. (1915). A study of prolonged fasting. Carnegie Institute pub #203.

Booth, D.A. (1992). Integration of internal and external signals in intake control. *Proc. Nutr. Soc.* 51:21-28.

Bouchard, C. (1989). Genetic factors in obesity. *Med. Clin. North America* 73:67-81.

Bouchard, C., Savard, R., and Despres, J.P. (1985). Body composition in adopted and biological siblings. *Human Biol.* 57:61-75.

Bray, G. (1992). Drug treatment of obesity. *Am. J. Clin. Nutr.* 55:5385-5445.

Bray, G. and Ryan, D. (1997). Drugs used in the treatment of obesity. *Diabetes Rev.* 5:83-103.

Cahill, G.F., Herrera, M.G., Morgan, A.P., Soeldner, J.S., Levy, P.L., Reichard, G.A., and Kipnis, D.M. (1966). Hormone fuel relationships during fasting. *J. Clin. Invest.* 45:1751-1769.

Champigny, O. and Recquier, D. (1990). Effects of fasting and refeeding on the level of uncoupling protein mRNA in brown adipose tissue: Evidence for diet induced and cold induced responses. *J. Nutr.* 120:1730-1736.

Crenshaw, L.I. (1980). Temperature regulation in vertebrates. *Ann. Rev. Physiol.* 42:473-491.

de Quiroga, G.B. (1992). Brown fat thermogenesis and exercise: Two examples of physiological oxidative stress? *Free Radical Biology & Medicine* 13:325-340.

Frisch, R. (1991). Body weight, body fat, and ovulation. *Trends Endocrinol. Metab.* 2:191-197.

Geloen, A., Collet, A.J., Guay, G., and Bukowiecki, L.J. (1990). *In vivo* differentiation of brown adipocytes in adult mice: An electron microscopic study. *Am. J. Anat.* 188:366-372.

Geloen, A. and Trayhurn, P. (1990). Regulation of the level of uncoupling protein in brown adipose tissue by insulin requires mediation of the sympathetic nervous system. *FEBS* 267:265-267.

Giles, R.E., Blanc, H., Cann, H.M., and Wallace, D.C. (1980). Maternal inheritance of human mitochondrial DNA. *Proc. Natl. Acad. Sci. U.S.A.* 77:6715-6719.

Hamm, P., Shakelle, R.B., and Stamler, J. (1989). Large fluctuations in body weight during young adulthood and twenty-five year risk of coronary death in men. *Am. J. Epidemiol.* 129:312-318.

Harris, R.B.S. (1990). Role of set point theory in regulation of body weight. *FASEB J.* 4:3310-3318.

Hatefi, Y. (198)5. The mitochondrial electron transport and oxidative phosphorylation system. *Ann. Rev. Biochem.* 54:1015-1069.

Hervey, G.R. and Tobin, G. (1982). The part played by variation of energy expenditure in the regulation of energy balance. *Proc. Nutr. Soc.* 41:137-153.

Heusner, A.A. (1982). Energy metabolism and body size 1. Is the 0.75 mass exponent of Kleibers equation a statistical artifact. *Respiration Physiol.* 48:1-12.

Himms-Hagen, J. (1995). Brown adipose tissue thermogenesis in the control of thermoregulatory feeding in rats: A new hypothesis that links thermostatic and glucostatic hypothesis for control of food intake. *Proc. Soc. Exp. Biol. & Med.* 208:159-169.

Hirschberg, A.L. (1998). Hormonal regulation of appetite and food intake. *Ann. Med.* 30:7-20.

Ide, T. and Sugano, M. (1988). Effects of dietary fat types on the thermogenesis of brown adipocytes isolated from rat. *Agric. Biol. Chem.* 52:511-518.

Issartel, J.P., Dupuis, A., Garin, J., Lunardi, J., Michel, L., and Vignais, P.V. (1992). The ATP synthase F_0F_1 complex in oxidative phosphorylation. *Experientia* 48:351-362.

Jakobsen, K. and Thorbek, G. (1993). The respiratory quotient in relation to fat deposition in fattening-growing pigs. *Brit. J. Nutr.* 69:333-343.

Jeanrenaud, J. (1985). A hypothesis on the aetiology of obesity: dysfunction of the central nervous system. *Diabetologia* 28:502-513.

Kaul, R., Heldmaier, G., and Schmidt, I. (1990). Defective thermoregulatory thermogenesis does not cause onset of obesity in Zucker rats. *Am. J. Physiol.* 259:E11-E18.

Leibel, R. (1997). Single gene obesities in rodents: Possible relevance to human obesity. *J. Nutr.* 127:1908S.

Martin, R.J., White, D.B., and Hulsey, M.G. 1991. The regulation of body weight. *American Scientist* 79:528-541.

Miller, S.G., DeVos, P., Guerre-Millo, M., Wong, K., Hermann, T., Staels, B., Briggs, M.R., and Auwerx, J. (1996). The adipocyte specific transcription factor C/EBP modulates human gene expression. *Proc. Natl. Acad. Sci. U.S.A.* 93:5507-5511.

Prins, J.B. and O'Rahilly, S. (1997). Regulation of adipose cell number in man. *Clin. Sci.* 92:3-11.

Recquier, D., Casteilla, L., and Bouillaud, F. (1991). Molecular studies of the uncoupling protein. *FASEB J.* 5:2237-2242.

Roberts, S.B., Fuss, P., Evans, W.J., Heyman, M.B., and Young, V.R. (1993). Energy expenditure, aging and body composition. *J. Nutr.* 123:474-482.

Rohner-Jeanrenaud, F. (1995). A neuroendocrine reappraisal of the dual center hypothesis: Its implications for obesity and insulin resistance. *Internat. J. Obesity* 19:517-534.

Samec, S., Seydoux, J., and Dulloo, A.G. (1998). Role of UCP homologues in skeletal muscles and brown adipose tissue: Mediations of thermogenesis or regulators of lipids as fuel substrate? *FASEB J* 12:715-724.

Sjostrom, L.V. (1992). Morbidity of severely obese subjects. *Am. J. Clin. Nutr.* 55:508S-515S.

Stunkard, A.J., Harris, J.R., Pedersen, N.L., and McClearn, G.E. 1990. The body mass index of twins who have been reared apart. *N. Eng. J. Med.* 322:1483-1487.

Stunkard, A.J., Sorensen, T.I.A., Harris, C., Teasdale, T.W., Chakraborty, R., Schull, W.J., and Schulsinger, F. (1986). An adoption study of human obesity. *N. Eng. J. Med.* 314:193-198.

Trayhurn, P. and Jennings, G. (1986). Evidence that fasting can induce a selective loss of uncoupling protein from brown adipose tissue mitochondria of mice. *Bioscience Rep.* 6:805-810.

Truett, G., Bahary, N., Friedman, J., and Liebel, R. (199)1. Rat obesity gene fatty (fa). maps to chromosome 5: Evidence for homology with the mouse gene diabetes (db). *Proc. Natl. Acad. Sci. U.S.A.* 88:7806-7809.

Wallace, D.C. (1992). Diseases of the mitochondrial DNA. In: *Ann. Rev. Biochemistry* 61:1175-1212.

Webster, A.J.F. (1993). Energy partitioning, tissue growth and appetite control. *Proc. Nutr. Soc.* 52:69-76.

Welch, G.R. (1991). Thermodynamics and living systems: Problems and Paradigms. *J. Nutr.* 121:1902-1906.

Welle, S.L., Amatruda, J.M., Forbes, G.B., and Lockwood, D.H. (1984). Resting metabolic rates of obese women after rapid weight loss. *J. Clin. Endocrinol. Metab.* 59:41-44.

Westerteys, K.R. (1993). Food quotient, respiratory quotient and energy balance. *Am. J. Clin. Nutr.* 57:759S-765S.

Zhou, Y.T., Shimabukuro, M., Koyama, K., Lee, Y., Wang, M.Y., Trieu, F., Newgard, C.B., and Unger, R.H. (1997). Induction by leptin of UCP2 and fatty acid oxidation. *Proc. Natl. Acad. Sci. U.S.A.* 94:6386-6390.

Books

Bjorntorp, P. and Brodoff, B.N. (1992). *Obesity.* J.B. Lippincott, Philadelphia, 805 pps.

Bouchard, C. (1994). *The Genetics of Obesity*, CRC Press, Boca Raton, 245 pages.

Mitchell, P. (1986). *Chemiosmotic Coupling and Energy Transduction.* Glynn Research, Bodmin U.K.

Reichert, K. (1993). *Nutrition for Recovery*, CRC Press, Boca Raton, 128 pages.

Trayhurn, P. and Nicholls, D.G., (Eds.). (1986). *Brown Adipose Tissue.* Edward Arnold Publishers London, 299-338.

4 Proteins

CONTENTS

OVERVIEW

After the energy need is met, protein is the next most important macronutrient need. Proteins provide the amino acids that are needed to synthesize body protein. Protein, in its many forms, is an essential and universal constituent of all living cells. As much as one-half of the dry weight of the cell is protein. The human body is, on the average, 18% protein. Besides being plentiful, proteins serve a variety of functions. They serve as structural components, as biocatalysts (in the form of enzymes), as antibodies, as lubricants, as messengers (in the form of hormones), and as carriers. Proteins are composed of amino acids that must be provided in food. On the average, Americans consume about 100 g of protein per day. After digestion, the amino acids that compose food proteins are absorbed and used to synthesize body proteins. In this unit, the chemistry and physiology of the proteins are discussed.

AMINO ACIDS

CHEMISTRY

Amino acids consist of carbon, hydrogen, oxygen, nitrogen, and occasionally sulfur. All amino acids, with the exception of proline, have a terminal carboxyl group ($-C{\overset{\displaystyle O}{\underset{\displaystyle OH}{}}}$) and an unsubstituted amino (-NH$_2$) group attached to the carbon. Proline has a substituted amino group and a carboxyl group. Also attached to the carbon is a functional group identified as R; R differs for each amino acid (Table 4.1). The general structure of amino acids can be represented

as $R{-}\overset{\displaystyle H}{\underset{\displaystyle NH_2}{C}}{-}COOH$. While it is convenient to represent amino acids in this manner, in reality

$$
\begin{array}{c}
H \\
| \\
R\!\!-\!\!C\!\!-\!\!COO^- \\
| \\
NH_3{}^+
\end{array}
$$

the amino acids exist as the dipolar ion in the range of pH values (5.0-8.0) found within the body.

The student will find it useful to remember the basic structure of alanine and then remember that all of the rest of the amino acids have R groups that replace the terminal methyl group in alanine. For example, in valine, the methyl group is replaced with an isopropyl group; in phenylalanine, it is replaced with a phenyl group.

There are several ways to classify the amino acids. Protein chemists use the polarity of the R group as the basis for their classification of the amino acids. This classification system divides the amino acids into four groups: 1) nonpolar; 2) polar but not charged; 3) positively charged at pH 6.0–7.0; and 4) negatively charged at pH 6.0–7.0. The distribution of the amino acids into these groups is shown in Table 4.2. This classification system is considered more useful than others because it relates to the functions of the amino acids in protein structures. Another classification that is frequently useful is based on the chemical nature of the amino acids. This grouping is listed in Table 4.3

Nutritionists, while interested in the physical and chemical characteristics of the individual amino acids, classify the amino acids on the basis of whether the body can synthesize them in sufficient quantities to meet its need or whether the diet must provide them. For these purposes, then, amino acids are classified as essential or nonessential. The definition of essentiality rests with the species of animal in question and its physiological need. Felines, for example, require taurine, a metabolite of L-cysteine as a component of their diets. In the adult human, arginine need not be in the diet. However, during periods of high rates of protein synthesis, growth for example, not enough arginine can be synthesized. Additional supplies must then be provided in the diet. Table 4.4 lists the essential and nonessential amino acids for adults.

Occasionally, through a mutation in one or more genes that code for enzymes needed for amino acid interconversion or through a specific illness, certain of the nonessential amino acids cannot be synthesized. In these instances, the amino acid in question then becomes essential and must be provided in the diet. An example of the former is the mutation in the gene for phenylalanine hydroxylase, which results in phenylketonuria (PKU). This mutation is clinically characterized by severe mental retardation. Phenylalanine hydroxylase catalyzes the conversion of phenylalanine to tyrosine. In the patient with phenylketonuria, tyrosine cannot be synthesized and thus becomes an essential amino acid. Phenylalanine metabolites other than tyrosine are made and accumulated, and it is this accumulation of neurotoxic compounds that destroys cells in the brain, which in turn results in the characteristic symptom of phenylketonuria, mental retardation. Care must be taken in the above instance to provide the needed amino acids in the diet in sufficient quantities to maintain tissue protein synthesis without exceeding the body's capacity to utilize phenylalamine. If too much of the amino acid is provided to an individual unable to use it because of a genetic mutation in one or more steps in its metabolic pathway, some unusual metabolites of these amino acids may be formed and these metabolites can be toxic and destructive.

Stereochemistry

Amino acids, like the simple sugars, exist as stereoisomers. Their absolute configuration, similarly, is related to the configuration of glyceraldehyde. The Fischer projection of D-glyceraldehyde shows the hydroxyl function on the α carbon to the right. At a similar point in a D-amino acid, the amino function is to the right.

TABLE 4.1
Structures and Abbreviations of the Amino Acids. The Single Letter Abbreviations are Used as Shorthand in Delineating Large Protein Sequences

Name	Abbreviation	Structure
Glycine	Gly, G	$\begin{array}{c} H \\ | \\ H-C-COOH \\ | \\ NH_2 \end{array}$
Alanine	Ala, A	$\begin{array}{c} CH_3-CH-COOH \\ | \\ NH_2 \end{array}$
Valine	Val, V	$\begin{array}{c} CH_3 \\ \searrow \\ CH-CH-COOH \\ \nearrow \quad | \\ H_3C \quad NH_2 \end{array}$
Leucine	Leu, L	$\begin{array}{c} CH_3 \\ \searrow \\ CH-CH_2-CH-COOH \\ \nearrow \qquad\qquad | \\ H_3C \qquad\qquad NH_2 \end{array}$
Isoleucine	Ile, I	$\begin{array}{c} CH_3 \\ \searrow \\ CH_2 \\ \searrow \\ CH-CH-COOH \\ \nearrow \quad | \\ H_3C \quad NH_2 \end{array}$
Serine	Ser, S	$\begin{array}{c} CH_2-CH-COOH \\ | \qquad | \\ OH \quad NH_2 \end{array}$
Threonine	Thr, T	$\begin{array}{c} CH_3-CH-CH-COOH \\ | \quad | \\ OH \quad NH_2 \end{array}$

TABLE 4.1 (CONTINUED)

Cysteine (Cystein)	Cys, C	CH_2—CH—COOH, with SH and NH_2
Methionine	Met, M	CH_2—CH_2—CH—COOH, with S—CH_3 and NH_2
Aspartic Acid	Asp, D	HOOC—CH_2—CH—COOH, with NH_2
Asparagine	Asn, N	H_2N—C(=O)—CH_2—CH—COOH, with NH_2
Glutamic Acid	Glu, E	HOOC—CH_2—CH_2—CH—COOH, with NH_2
Glutamine	Gln, Q	H_2N—C(=O)—CH_2—CH_2—CH—COOH, with NH_2
Arginine	Arg, R	H_2N—C(=NH)—N(H)—CH_2—CH_2—CH_2—CH—COOH, with NH_2
Lysine	Lys, K	CH_2—CH_2—CH_2—CH_2—CH—COOH, with NH_2 and NH_2
Hydroxylysine	Hyl	CH_2—CH—CH_2—CH_2—CH—COOH, with NH_2, OH and NH_2
Histidine	His, H	imidazole ring (HN, N)—CH_2—CH—COOH, with NH_2

TABLE 4.1 (CONTINUED)

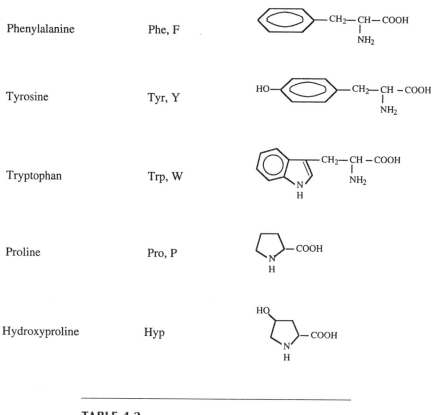

Phenylalanine	Phe, F
Tyrosine	Tyr, Y
Tryptophan	Trp, W
Proline	Pro, P
Hydroxyproline	Hyp

TABLE 4.2
Classification of Amino Acids Based on Polarity of the Functional Groups

Nonpolar R Groups

Alanine	Phenylalanine	Methionine
Valine	Tryptophan	Proline
	Leucine	Isoleucine

Polar Uncharged R Groups

| Serine | Asparagine | Cysteine | Glycine |
| Threonine | Glutamine | Hydroxyproline | Tyrosine |

Positively Charged R Groups

| Lysine | Hydroxylysine |
| Arginine | Histidine |

Negatively Charged R Groups

Aspartic acid
Glutamic acid

TABLE 4.3
Amino Acids Classified According to Chemical Nature

Monoamino monocarboxylic: glycines, alanine, valine, leucine, isoleucine
Diamino monocarboxylic (basic): arginine, lysine
Monoamino dicarboxylic (acidic): glutamic acid, aspartic acid
Sulfur containing: cystine (and cysteine), methionine
Aromatic: tyrosine, phenylalanine
Heterocyclic: proline, hydroxyproline, histidine, tryptophan

TABLE 4.4
Essential and
Nonessential Amino
Acids for Adult Mammals

Essential	Nonessential
Valine	Hydroxyproline
Leucine	Cysteine
Isoleucine	Glycine
Threonine	Alanine
Phenylalanine	Serine
Methionine	Proline
Tryptophan	Glutamic acid
Lysine	Aspartic acid
Histidine	Glutamine
*Arginine	Asparagine
	Hydroxylysine
	Tyrosine

*Not essential for maintenance of
most adult mammals.

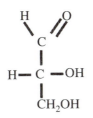

D -glyceraldehyde

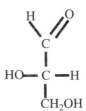

L-glyceraldehyde

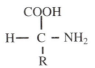

D-amino acid   L-amino acid

All of the amino acids except glycine (which has no asymmetric carbon atom) possess optical activity. The amino acids of nutritional importance are all L-amino acids, whereas the nutritionally important sugars are of the D-series. Species differences exist in the utilization of L vs. D amino acids. There are a number of D amino acids that are of use to single-cell organisms and, further, some D amino acids combine to form potent antibiotics. Gramicidin D and actinomycin D, for example, contain D-amino acids. Their utility as antibiotics rests with the fact that mammalian cells cannot absorb them as readily as microorganisms. Pathogenic organisms incorporate them into their intracellular material and these materials then become antimetabolites, successfully terminating the metabolic activity of the pathogen in question.

Acid-Base Properties

Because amino acids possess acidic carboxyl and basic amino groups, they can function as either hydrogen acceptors or donors. At low pH, amino acids can exist in the fully protonated form

$$
\begin{array}{c}
\text{H} \\
| \\
\text{R}-\text{C}-\text{COOH} \\
| \\
\text{NH}_3{}^+
\end{array}
$$

At higher pH levels, H+ from the carboxyl function will be released and the amino acid exists as the dipolar ion,

$$
\begin{array}{c}
\text{H} \\
| \\
\text{R}-\text{C}-\text{COO}^- \\
| \\
\text{NH}_3
\end{array}
$$

At even higher pH values, the amino function dissociates and the amino acid exists in the negatively charged form

$$
\begin{array}{c}
\text{H} \\
| \\
\text{R}-\text{C}-\text{COO}^- \\
| \\
\text{NH}_2
\end{array}
$$

If the amino acid has more than one amino or carboxyl group, further dissociation can occur and the range in pH over which this occurs is much broader. For example, aspartic acid exists at pH 1 as

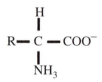
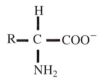

$$
\begin{array}{cc}
\text{COOH} & \\
| & \\
\text{CH}_2 & \\
| & \\
\text{CH-NH}_3{}^+ & \\
| & \text{at pH 3 as:} \\
\text{COOH} &
\end{array}
\qquad
\begin{array}{c}
\text{COOH} \\
| \\
\text{CH}_2 \\
| \\
\text{CH-NH}_3{}^+ \\
| \\
\text{COO}^-
\end{array}
\text{ at pH 6–8 as:}
\begin{array}{c}
\text{COO}^- \\
| \\
\text{CH}_2 \\
| \\
\text{CH-NH}_3{}^+ \\
| \\
\text{COO}^-
\end{array}
\text{ and at pH 11 as:}
\begin{array}{c}
\text{COO}^- \\
| \\
\text{CH}_2 \\
| \\
\text{CH-NH}_2 \\
| \\
\text{COO}^-
\end{array}
\text{ With each}
$$

change in the form of the amino acid that occurs, from the lowest to the highest pH, a hydrogen ion is released. The capacity to accept or release hydrogen ions is characteristic of all amino acids; however, only a few (glutamate, aspartate, histidine, and, perhaps, arginine) serve as buffers with respect to the regulation of hydrogen ion concentration in the body. Glutamine is especially important because its metabolism yields bicarbonate, which serves in the regulation of pH. However, because free amino acids are in low concentrations relative to the other buffering systems in the body, their buffering power is much less important than that of the carbonate and phosphate buffering system.

Reactions

The amino acids undergo characteristic chemical reactions at the -carboxyl group, at the α-amino group, and at the functional groups of the side chains. Such characteristic reactions are particularly useful to the biochemist, for they assist in the quantitative determination of the amino acid composition and sequence in a given protein. These reactions are summarized in Table 4.5.

TABLE 4.5
Characteristic Chemical Reactions of Amino Acids

Reaction Name	Reagent	Use
Ninhydrin reaction	Ninhydrin	To estimate amino acids quantitatively in small amounts
Sanger reaction	1-fluro-2,4-dinitrobenzene	To identify the amino terminal group of a peptide
Dansyl chloride reaction	1-dimethylamino-napthalene (also called dansylchloride)	To measure very small amounts of amino acids quantitatively
Edmann degradation	Phenylisothiocyanate	To identify the terminal NH2 group in a protein
Schiff base	Aldehydes	Labile intermediate in some enzymatic reactions involving α-amino acid substrates

Among the reactions that the functional groups on the side chains of the amino acids undergo, those that involve the thiol or sulfhydryl group of cysteine are important. This group is weakly acidic and quite reactive. It is very susceptible to oxidation by either oxygen in the presence of iron salts or by other oxidizing agents. When oxidized, cysteine is converted to cystine. In this conversion, two cysteine residues are joined together by a disulfide (–S–S–) bridge. Within the extracellular proteins, sulfhydryl groups react with one another to form disulfide bridges. These bridges stabilize the internal structure of the protein. Sulfhydryl groups also react with heavy metals to form mercaptides. This reaction is of great interest to the nutritionist since protein–mineral interactions, or more truly, mineral–sulfhydryl reactions, are important not only for an understanding of how minerals serve as cofactors in enzymatic reactions and for mineral transport into and out of cells, but also to an understanding of the mechanisms involved in heavy metal intoxication. Figure 4.1 illustrates this reaction.

No discussion of the chemical reactions of the amino acids would be complete without discussing the formation of the peptide bond (Figure 4.2). Without question, this is the most important reaction of these compounds. The formation of the peptide bond involves the removal of one molecule of water with the resultant linkage between the carbon of one amino acid to the amino group of a second amino acid. Water is formed when the hydroxyl ion of the carboxyl group of one amino acid combines with a hydrogen atom from the amino group of a second amino group. Peptide bonding is the basis for the formation of peptides, polypeptides, and proteins and is the linkage used in the primary structure of any sequence of amino acids.

The number of possible combinations of the 20 amino acids commonly found in proteins is almost limitless. In a dipeptide that contains two different amino acids (A and B), two combinations are available: A-B and B-A. In a tripeptide with three different amino acids, six combinations are available if all three amino acids are used and each used only one time: A-B-C; B-A-C; A-C-B;

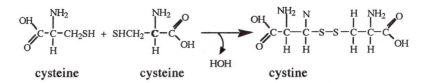

a) Formation of disulfide bridge

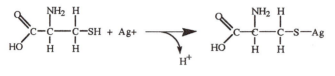

b) Formation of a mercaptide

FIGURE 4.1 Examples of sulfhydryl group reactions.

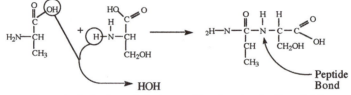

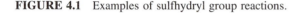

Example: L-alanine + L-Serine → Alanyl-serine (a dipeptide)

FIGURE 4.2 The formation of a peptide bond.

B-C-A; C-A-B; and C-B-A. The number of possible combinations of the sequential arrangement of different amino acids is determined by the expression n! (n factorial), when n is the number of different amino acids. If 20 amino acids are present in a protein, the number of possible combinations would be $20 \times 19 \times 18 \times 17 \ldots \times 1 = 2 \times 10^{18}$. The molecular weight of this molecule is about 2,400 (average molecular weight of an amino acid × number of amino acids = 120 × 20), a relatively small protein. If the molecule were larger, and if the amino acids were used more than once, the number of possible combinations is increased even more. That nature can consistently reproduce the same protein, when there are so many choices of amino acids and sequences, is due to its dependence on the codes for each of these proteins in the genetic material, DNA.

PEPTIDES

Two amino acids joined together form a dipeptide; three form a tripeptide and so on. Each amino acid in a chain is referred to as an amino acid residue. A chain of up to 100 amino acids joined together is called a polypeptide. If many amino acids are involved, then the compound is called a protein. Proteins have been identified that have as many as 300,000 amino acid residues and molecular weights in excess of 4×10^7.

The sequence of the amino acids that a given protein comprises is represented by a sequential arrangement of abbreviations for each. For example, the polypeptide bradykinin is represented in the following manner: Arg-Pro-Pro-Gly-Phe-Ser-Pro-Phe-Arg. The right-hand side of the chain represents the carboxyl terminal while the left-hand side represents the amino terminal. The systematic name for bradykinin is arginyldiprolylglyclyphenylalanyl-serylprolylphenylalanylargi-nine. This systematic name is seldom used except when one wishes to give the amino acid sequence of this peptide. The amino acid sequence of a given peptide or protein can vary and its variation is controlled genetically. Some of the proteins of importance in nutrition have been sequenced but these are few in number compared with the vast array of proteins in nature. Even if the proteins were sequenced, their systematic names would not be used because such a name would be very cumbersome.

PROTEIN STRUCTURE

Proteins are complex molecules having characteristic primary, secondary, tertiary, and quaternary structures. The primary structure is determined genetically as the particular sequence of amino acids in a given protein.

The genetic material, DNA (deoxyribonucleic acid), in the cell nucleus holds the code that dictates the amino acid sequence of the protein. A small amount of DNA is also found in the mitochondria (mtDNA). Should there be a change in the sequence of the nucleotides that compose the code, the sequence of amino acids in the resultant protein will be different. A change in the normal sequence of bases in the DNA is called a mutation. It can be a spontaneous mutation or one induced by drugs, a virus, or any one of a number of external variants that target the genetic material of the cell. Whether the substitution of one or more amino acids for another has an adverse effect on the activity of the protein being synthesized depends wholly on the amino acids in question. If these amino acids have functional groups in their R side chain that modify the three-dimensional structure and the function of the protein, then its activity will be abnormal. Throughout this text, examples of genetic mutations and their consequences are given to illustrate the importance of heredity in determining nutrient needs and tolerances.

Under normal pH and temperature conditions, a protein is characterized not only by its amino acid sequence but also by its three-dimensional structure; that is, how the chain of amino acids twists and turns and what shape this long chain of amino acids assumes. This three-dimensional shape, unique to each protein's particular amino acid sequence, is known as the native conformation of the protein. This assumption of shape may be spontaneous or may be catalyzed by enzymes and reflects the lowest energy state of the protein in its native environment. Protein conformation is usually divided into two categories: secondary and tertiary. The secondary and tertiary structures of a protein result from interactions between the reactive groups on the amino acids in the protein.

Secondary structure is the *local* conformation of the protein molecule. It is due to the formation of hydrogen bonds, disulfide bridges, and ionic bonds (in the case of the polar amino acids) between adjacent or nearby amino acids in an amino acid chain. As a result of these bonds, there is a regular recurring arrangement in space of the amino acids within the chain that can extend over the entire chain or only in small segments of it. Two kinds of periodic structures are found in proteins: the helix and the pleated sheet. In the helix, the amino acid chain can be viewed as wrapping itself around a long cylinder. The most common helical arrays are the α-helix and triple helix. The other periodic shape is the pleated sheet. It is essentially a linear array of the amino acid chain. These structures are shown in Figure 4.3. All of these structures are stabilized by hydrogen bonding.

Tertiary structure is the *regional* conformation a protein molecule possesses; it develops after the secondary structure is established. Tertiary structure refers to how the amino acid chain bends or folds in three dimensions to form a compact or tightly folded protein. Tertiary structure results from hydrogen bonding, disulfide cross-linkages, ionic bonds between polar amino acids, and interactions between hydrophobic R groups. This last feature tends to locate the hydrophobic R groups internally in the protein structure, away from the aqueous environment. A protein that clearly demonstrates tertiary structure is hemoglobin. Some parts of the amino acid chains in this molecule

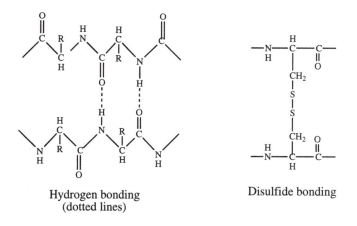

Hydrogen bonding
(dotted lines)

Disulfide bonding

Hydrogen and disulfide bonding between amino acids in a peptide chain.

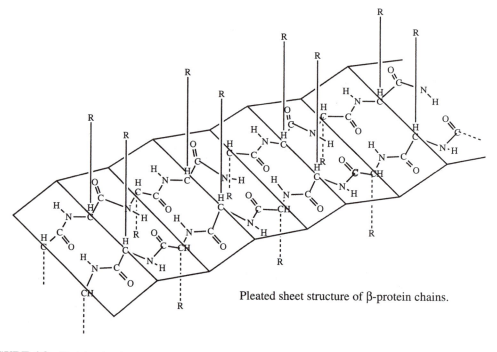

Pleated sheet structure of β-protein chains.

FIGURE 4.3 Protein structures.

can form helices; others cannot. This gives the molecule the fluidity to assume different three-dimensional shapes along the chain: It will bend back upon itself to accomplish the maximum number of hydrogen bonds and disulfide bridges.

As a result of the various bonds that can form within a protein molecule, essentially two kinds of proteins exist: fibrous protein and globular protein. Fibrous proteins resemble long ribbons or hairs. They tend to be insoluble in most solvents and include such tough, resilient protein structures as collagen and elastin. Fibrous protein can have either the helical or pleated-sheet structure. Collagen is an example of the triple helix; silk, a pleated-sheet structure. Where the fibrous proteins appear to have a long "stringy" shape, globular proteins are roughly spherical or elliptical. Many enzymes and antibodies have a globular structure.

The quaternary structure refers to how groups of individual amino acid chains are arranged in relation to each other within a given protein. It is the structure that results when two or more polypeptide chains combine. The chains (subunits) may be different or identical, yet each subunit still possesses its own primary, secondary, and tertiary structure. The number of subunits in a protein may vary; some proteins have only two subunits while others have as many as 2,130 subunits. The protein hemoglobin, for example, consists of four subunits and is one of the few proteins whose primary, secondary, tertiary, and quaternary structures are known. It contains four separate peptide chains: two chains that contain 141 amino acid residues and two chains that contain 146 amino acid residues. To each of these is bound a heme (iron) residue in a noncovalent linkage.

PROTEIN DENATURATION

One of the most striking characteristics of proteins is the response to heat, alcohol, and other treatments that affect their quaternary, tertiary, and secondary structures. This characteristic response is called *denaturation*. Denaturation results in the unfolding of a protein molecule, thus breaking its hydrogen bonds and the associations between functional groups; as a result, the three-dimensional structure is lost. Denaturation affects many of the properties of the protein molecule. Its physical shape is changed, its solubility in water is decreased, and its reactivity with other proteins may be lost. When denatured, the protein loses its biological activity. Heating will denature most proteins. As little as 15°C can denature some proteins, while the majority of food proteins are denatured at heats in excess of 60°C. Some proteins are very heat stable (those found in thermophillic bacteria for example), while others are quite labile. A very good example of protein denaturation is the coagulation of egg white when heated. Heat denaturation, unless extreme, does not affect the amino acid composition of protein and, indeed, may make these amino acids more available to the body because heating provokes the unfolding or uncoiling of the protein and exposes more of the amino acid chain to the action of the proteolytic digestive enzymes. For this reason, many cooked proteins are of higher biological value than those same proteins if consumed without heat treatment. If only mild denaturation occurs, it can be reversed. This process is called *renaturation*. If a protein is renatured, it will resume its original shape and biological activity.

CLASSIFICATION OF PROTEINS

CLASSIFICATION BY SOLUBILITY AND PROSTHETIC GROUPS

In addition to the conformational classification of proteins as described above, proteins have been classified on the basis of their solubility characteristics. As more and more information has been acquired about proteins, this classification system has become outmoded. However, because the vocabulary from this system has become so firmly entrenched in discussions of protein, it is necessary to be familiar with it. In this system, proteins are classed as simple or conjugated proteins. Simple proteins are those that contain only L-amino acids or their derivatives and no prosthetic group. Such proteins as albumin, histones, and protamines are examples of simple proteins.

Conjugated proteins contain some nonprotein substances linked by a bond other than an ionic bond. Since most proteins occur in cells in combination with prosthetic groups, conjugated proteins are the ones most nutritionists will recognize. Table 4.6 and the text below describe representative conjugated proteins.

Glycoproteins

A majority of the naturally occurring conjugated proteins are glycoproteins. Sugar molecules are covalently bound to proteins, especially those proteins that are secreted from cells (mucin, for example) and those that compose the proteins found in the outer surface of the plasma membrane. Different types of covalent linkages have been found. The most common are the N-glycosidic linkages formed

TABLE 4.6
Some Conjugated Proteins

Name	Prosthetic Group	Example
Glycoproteins and Mucoproteins	Nucleic acid carbohydrates which hydrolyze to amino acid sugars; mucoproteins contain 4% hexosamines and glycoproteins contain less	Serum alpha, beta, and gamma globulins; mucin
Lipoproteins	Neutral fats, phospholipids, cholesterol	Cell membranes; Blood lipid carrying proteins
Nucleoproteins	Nucleic acid	Chromosomes
Phosphoproteins	Phosphate joined in ester linkage	Milk casein
Hemoproteins	Iron	Catalase, Hemoglobin, the Cytochromes
Flavoproteins	Flavin adenine nucleotide (FAD)	FAD linked-succinate dehydrogenase
Metalloproteins	Metals (not part of a nonprotein prosthetic group)	Ferritin

between asparagine amide and the sugar. Another common linkage is the O-glycosidic linkage between either the serine or threonine hydroxyl group and a sugar. Glycoproteins include the mucin in saliva as well as the conjugated proteins of plasma, collagen, ovalbumin (the major protein of egg white), and plant agglutinins. The glycoproteins range in size from a molecular weight of 15,000 to more than one million; the carbohydrate component of these proteins varies from 1% to 85%. Some of these proteins have amino acids and uronic acids and are called *proteoglycans*.

Only 8 of the 100 or so carbohydrates that are known to occur in nature are found in glycoproteins (Table 4.7). These carbohydrates occur in chains containing no more than 15 saccharide units. Of the 20 amino acids in these proteins, only four (Table 4.8) actually bind to the carbohydrate moiety. The carbohydrates are linked to these amino acids by a nitrogen-oxygen glucosidic bond or through an oxygen bond. Some proteins contain small amounts of carbohydrate in loose association rather than as integral and characteristic parts of their structure. An example of this association is the glycosylated hemoglobin found in the blood of poorly controlled diabetics. In diabetes, blood glucose levels may fluctuate and exceed the normal range of 80-120 mg/dl. Some of this excess of glucose may be picked up by the hemoglobin and form glycosylated hemoglobin. Levels of glycosylated hemoglobin are used as indicators of the degree of control of the diabetic state.

TABLE 4.7
Components of Glycoproteins

Sugars Found in Glycoproteins		Amino Acids Which Bind to the Carbohydrates in Glycoproteins
Glucose	Acetylglucosamine	Asparagine
Galactose	Acetylgalactosamine	Serine
Mannose	Arabinose	Threonine
Fucose	Xylose	Hydroxylysine

The function of the carbohydrate moiety of glycoproteins is not well defined. Some of the glycoproteins, those located on the exterior aspect of the plasma membrane are part of the cell-recognition system. Others are essential to the immune mechanism as a component of globulin.

TABLE 4.8
Protein Content of Representative Foods in the Human Diet

Food	Protein, Grams
Milk 244 g (8 oz)	8
Cheddar cheese, 84 g (3 oz)	21.3
Egg, 50 g, (1 large)	6.1
Apple, 212 g (1–3 1/4" diameter)	0.4
Banana, 74 g (1–8 3/4" long)	.2
Potato, cooked, 136 g (1 potato)	2.5
Bread, white, slice, 25 g	2.1
Fish, cod, poached, 100 g (3 1/2 oz)	20.9
Oysters, 100 g (3 1/2 oz)	13.5
Beef, pot roast, 85 g (3 oz)	22
Liver, pan fried, 85 g (3 oz)	23
Pork chop, bone in, 87 g (3.1 oz)	23.9
Ham, boiled, 2 pieces, 114 g	20
Peanut butter, 16 g (1 tablespoon)	4.6
Pecans, 28 g (1 oz)	2.2
Snap beans, 125 g (1 cup)	2.4
Carrots, sliced, 78 g (1/2 cup)	0.8

Note: The composition of a wide variety of foods has been computerized and can be acquired on disc.

From Handbook #8, USDA, *Composition of Foods*. U.S. Government Printing Office, Washington, D.C.

Glycoproteins are essential components of membrane transport systems and are components of many receptors.

Lipoproteins

Lipoproteins are multicomponent complexes of lipids and protein that form distinct molecular aggregates with approximate stoichiometry between each of the components. In addition to protein, they contain polar and neutral lipids, cholesterol, or cholesterol esters. The protein and lipid are held together by noncovalent forces. The protein component (apolipoprotein) is located on the outer surface of the micellular lipid structure, where it serves a hydrophilic function. Lipids, primarily hydrophobic molecules, are not easily transported through an aqueous environment such as blood. However, when they combine with proteins, the resulting combination becomes hydrophilic and can be transported in the blood to tissue that can use or store these lipids. The importance of these lipoproteins as carriers is discussed later in Unit 6.

Membrane lipoproteins, like the glycoproteins, are essential components of membrane transport systems and, as such, are important in the overall regulation of cellular activity.

Nucleoproteins

Nucleoproteins are combinations of nucleic acids and simple proteins. The protein usually consists of a large number of the basic amino acids. Nucleoproteins are ubiquitous molecules that tend to have very complex structures and numerous functional activities. All living cells contain nucleoproteins. Some cells, such as viruses, seem to be entirely composed of nucleoprotein.

Other Conjugated Proteins

The phosphoproteins and the metalloproteins are associations of proteins with phosphate groups or such ions as zinc, copper, and iron. The association of protein with phosphate may be fairly loose, as with the phosphate-carrying protein, or tight as with the phosphate in casein and the iron in ferritin.

Heme proteins sometimes are grouped with the metalloproteins because of the iron they contain. Flavoproteins are primarily enzymes and have as their prosthetic group a phosphate containing adenine nucleotide, which functions as an acceptor or donor of reducing equivalents.

CLASSIFICATION BY FUNCTION

In addition to the system described above for the classification of proteins, the biochemist classifies these compounds on the basis of their function. Thus, proteins are classified as enzymes, storage proteins such as casein or ferritin, transport proteins such as hemoglobin, DNA-binding proteins such as the various transcription factors, contractile proteins such as myosin, immune proteins such as antibodies, toxin proteins such as the *Clostrodium botulinum* toxin, hormones such as insulin, receptor proteins such as the insulin receptor, intracellular transporters such as the mobile glucose transporters, and structural proteins such as elastin and collagen. Nutritionists might not use this system for classifying food proteins, yet will want to understand these functions as part of their knowledge about the protein nutrient class.

CLASSIFICATION BY NUTRITIVE VALUE

In nutrition, we are interested in food proteins as sources of needed amino acids. Those proteins that contain the essential amino acids in the proportions needed by the body are referred to as *complete* proteins. They are primarily of animal origin. Eggs, cheese, milk, meat, and fish are sources of complete protein. Proteins lacking in one or more essential amino acids or having a poor balance of amino acids relative to the body's need are *incomplete* or *imbalanced* proteins. These proteins are usually of plant origin, although some animal proteins are incomplete. The connective tissue protein called collagen, from which gelatin is prepared, lacks tryptophan; zein, the protein in corn, is low in lysine as well as tryptophan. Table 4.8 gives the protein and Table 4.9 gives amino acid content of several food proteins. When food selection is limited and there is a shortage of high quality protein-rich foods, incomplete proteins can be combined so that all of the essential amino acids are provided. For example, corn or wheat and soy or peanut proteins can be combined in the same meal so that all of the essential amino acids are provided. When these proteins are combined and consumed in sufficient amounts they will meet the amino acid needs of the consumer. This combination of incomplete proteins must be consumed within a relatively short time interval (less than 4 hours) to obtain the appropriate and needed amounts of amino acids. Maximum benefit is obtained when the combination is consumed at the same time. Supplementation of incomplete proteins with missing amino acids has been suggested for populations consuming diets having a single dietary item as its main protein source. This supplementation is not very practical over a long period of time due to the cost of the pure amino acid supplement. Such populations are also likely to develop other nutritional disorders when their food supply is so limited.

Through selected plant breeding and the use of biotechnology some of these plant foods can be improved to provide a better array of amino acids in their edible portions. A corn variety containing more lysine has been developed. This high-lysine corn shows promise for populations that have corn as a major food component. Other plant species have also been improved with respect to their amino acid content. However, some of these improved varieties may have special cultural requirements that economically challenged farmers cannot meet. Some of these cultivars may require added fertilizer, a very expensive item in such a farmer's budget. Agronomists, plant

TABLE 4.9
Average Amino Acid Content of Selected Foods (mg/100 g)

	Tryptophan	Threonine	Isoleucine	Leucine	Lysine	Methionine	Cystine	Phenylalanine	Tyrosine	Valine	Arginine	Histidine	Alanine	Aspartic Acid	Glutamic Acid	Glycine	Proline	Serine
Milk	90	294	407	626	496	156	57	309	325	438	233	168	220	465	1491	126	709	376
Cheddar Cheese	87	237	430	622	468	166	36	342	305	458	233	208	179	372	1745	98	731	384
Whole Egg	103	311	415	550	400	196	146	361	269	464	410	150	0	438	773	221	265	525
Beef	73	276	327	512	546	155	79	257	212	347	403	217	361	583	946	387	308	262
Lamb	81	286	324	484	506	150	82	254	217	308	407	174	349	576	948	365	289	250
Bacon	65	210	274	500	403	97	73	298	161	298	427	169	0	589	702	589	331	242
Chicken	76	266	330	452	549	163	84	246	220	307	395	180	0	614	1004	418	0	0
Fish	62	271	317	472	548	182	84	232	169	333	352	0	0	551	796	345	381	193
Baked Beans	61	295	314	524	381	64	19	359	179	336	270	20	0	0	0	0	0	0
Pecans	78	219	312	436	245	86	122	318	178	296	668	154	0	0	0	0	0	0
White Bread	61	189	288	448	151	95	134	312	163	292	228	129	180	286	1980	202	675	0
Corn Meal	38	249	289	810	180	116	81	284	382	319	220	129	622	776	1103	212	522	353
Rice	64	233	279	513	235	107	81	299	272	416	343	100	0	281	815	407	288	302
Banana	95	0	0	0	289	55	0	0	162	0	0	0	0	0	0	0	0	0
Oranges	39	0	0	0	221	33	0	0	0	0	0	0	0	0	0	0	0	0
Peas	52	229	287	390	295	50	68	240	152	256	555	102	183	596	442	202	0	0
Brussels Sprouts	63	218	264	276	280	66	0	210	0	274	396	150	0	0	0	0	0	0
Potatoes	67	246	274	311	333	78	60	276	112	334	308	90	292	0	625	0	208	250

From Handbook #8, Amino Acid Composition of Foods, USDA, U.S. Government Printing Office, Washington, D.C.

scientists and agricultural economists continue to work to improve the nutritional value of the crops raised as well as improve crop yield. With judicious planning of food choices, nonetheless, it is possible to meet the protein and amino acid needs of populations subsisting on plant foods with little food from animal sources.

In addition to the amino acid content, protein quality or rather the quality of the food containing the protein, is classed according to its total protein content. Potatoes, for example, contain a very good distribution of essential and nonessential amino acids, yet, because the potato contains so little protein (1.7%), it is not considered a good protein source. One would have to consume a lot of potatoes (3.18 kg or ~ 7 lb) to meet one's daily amino acid and total nitrogen requirements.

Protein Analysis

The total protein content of food is estimated from the total nitrogen content of the food as determined by the classical Kjeldahl method. This method also determines nonprotein nitrogen as well; however, the amount of error in the method due to the inclusion of these compounds is very small. Most proteins contain about 16 percent nitrogen. To convert the nitrogen content to protein, one uses the following formula:

$$P_G = N_G \times \frac{100}{16} = N_G \times 6.25$$

where P_G = grams of protein in 100 grams of food and
        N_G = grams of nitrogen in 100 grams of food

This conversion factor is an average factor. If more-exact figures are required, established conversion factors for each food category are available. For example, cereals generally have less protein nitrogen and more nonprotein nitrogen, thus, the conversion factor of 5.7 is used for cereal foods. On the other hand, milk has more protein nitrogen and the factor of 6.4 can be used. Generally speaking, because humans usually consume a mixed diet, the lower and higher factors tend to average out and the value of 6.25 is correct to use when the total protein content of a day's food is chemically determined.

The amino acid determination of a protein has two phases: qualitative identification and quantitative estimation of the residues. The peptide bond that connects the residues is cleaved by acid, base, or enzyme-catalyzed hydrolysis to give a mixture of amino acids. The free amino acids are separated from one another and identified using chromatographic or electrophoretic techniques. Once separated and identified, each amino acid present can be determined quantitatively. Several of the reactions given in Table 4.5 can be used. These assays do not establish the sequence of the amino acids or the protein's primary structure, but merely tell how much of each amino acid is present. The sequence of amino acids can be determined by cleaving one by one the amino acids in the chain and following this cleavage with an analysis of the individual amino acids. Usually high-performance liquid chromatography (HPLC) is used for this aspect of sequence analysis.

Biological Value of Dietary Protein (BV)

Although the total protein (nitrogen) content can be readily determined, as can the amino acid content of the food, albeit with greater difficulty, the determination of the BV of a given protein within a food is far more difficult. Biological value means how well the food is digested and absorbed and how well the component amino acids meet the amino acid needs of the consumer. The BV of a food protein depends not only on its amino acid content, but also on the needs of the consumer. For example, the BV of a food for a rapidly growing child is quite different from that for a non-growing adult. Growth carries with it a demand for particular amino acids as part of the total nitrogen requirement, whereas maintenance (as in the adult, nongrowing animal) has a total nitrogen requirement with less stringent demands for specific amino acids.

There is also a species dependence to BV. Chickens, because they grow feathers, need more sulfur-containing amino acids in their diets than humans. Thus, proteins having a higher proportion of sulfur-containing amino acids will have relatively higher biological values for chickens than for other species. Rats, the usual test animals in nutrition studies, grow fur, which contains a lot of arginine. This means that proteins rich in arginine will have a higher BV for rats than for humans. A number of methods for assessing BV have been used. Each has its advantages and disadvantages.

Using a *holistic* approach to assessing protein quality, H.H. Mitchell devised the nitrogen balance technique in 1924. This technique was based on Folin's definitions of endogenous and exogenous nitrogen excretion. By definition, the endogenous nitrogen comes from the nitrogen-containing excretory products synthesized in the body and not recycled. It is the unavoidable nitrogen loss. Exogenous nitrogen was defined as those nitrogen-containing products that are excreted in direct proportion to the amount of nitrogen consumed in the food. These are arbitrary definitions and there is some crossover between categories. They are, however, useful in the context of evaluating the biological usefulness of dietary protein. *Endogenous* nitrogen comes from the breakdown of body tissue and represents nitrogenous compounds produced as a result of one-way reactions. For example, when muscles contract, creatine phosphate breaks down to creatine and phosphate. While both the creatine and the phosphate can be recycled, some of the creatine is converted to creatinine and excreted in the urine. Its excretion is relatively constant, reflecting the muscle mass of an individual who is a normal healthy adult following a fairly regular daily routine. Other nitrogenous compounds considered to be in the endogenous category are uric acid, allantoin, 3-methyl histidine, and ammonia. Regardless of the dietary protein intake, excretion of these compounds by normal individuals with fairly uniform daily activity levels is relatively constant.

In contrast, *exogenous* nitrogen fluctuates in response to the dietary protein intake. The main compound providing this nitrogen is urea. Urea results when excess amino acids are deaminated. The body converts the $-NH_3$ to urea via the urea cycle and excretes the urea in the urine. Exogenous nitrogen is also found in the feces and represents undigested food protein. Fecal nitrogen represents not only the undigested-unabsorbed food but also the nitrogen of intestinal flora, desquamated intestinal cells, and intestinal enzymes. There are species differences in these excretory patterns. While mammals excrete primarily urea, birds excrete uric acid as their major nitrogenous excretory product. Figure 4.4 illustrates the principle of nitrogen balance.

These definitions, developed initially by Folin, were used by Thomas and Mitchell when they devised the nitrogen balance technique for evaluating protein quality. The method assumes that a given protein, when fed at maintenance levels, will completely replace the protein being catabolized during the normal course of metabolic events in the body. It also assumes that all nitrogen gain and loss can be measured. Thus, for good quality proteins, nitrogen balance (intake vs. excretion) should be zero for an adult individual and for poor quality proteins, nitrogen balance will be negative. For growing individuals, good quality proteins result in high nitrogen retentions while poor quality proteins result in low nitrogen retentions. The amount of protein retained can be determined by analyzing the total nitrogen content of the food, the feces, and the urine.

The BV was conceived as a ratio of the nitrogen retained to that absorbed multiplied by 100. In the original method, animals were fed a nitrogen-free diet for 7–10 days, then fed a diet containing the test protein at a level commensurate with their protein maintenance requirements for the same time interval. During each of these periods, the urine and feces were collected and analyzed for total nitrogen. Knowing the nitrogen intake and the nitrogen excretion during both the nitrogen-free and test periods, the biological value was calculated as follows:

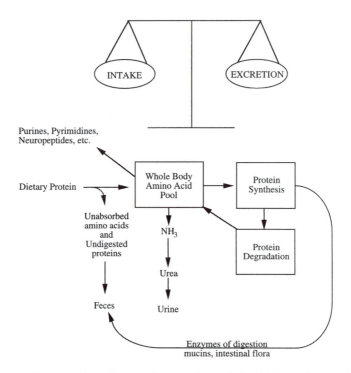

FIGURE 4.4 Nitrogen balance exists when the diet contains sufficient high-quality protein to provide amino acids for the synthesis of proteins lost through degradation.

$$BV = 100 \times \frac{N \text{ retained}}{N \text{ absorbed}} = 100 \times \frac{N_I - (N_{FT} - N_{FF}) - (N_{UT} - N_{UF})}{N_I - (N_{FT} - N_{FF})}$$

Where BV = Biological value
    N_I = Nitrogen intake
    N_{FT} = Fecal nitrogen during test period
    N_{FF} = Fecal nitrogen during nitrogen-free period
    N_{UT} = Urinary nitrogen during test period
    N_{UF} = Urinary nitrogen during nitrogen-free period

The method makes a lot of assumptions about overall protein metabolism and these assumptions can account for some of the error associated with evaluating the quality of the test protein in this way. The method is noninvasive and very useful for work with humans. However, nitrogen can be lost via routes other than urine and feces. In hot climates or in physically active subjects, significant nitrogen losses can occur through sweat. On an adequate protein intake, it has been estimated that up to 1 g N/dL can be lost. On an inadequate or low-protein diet, sweat losses can amount to 0.5 g N/dL. Hair, nail, and menstrual losses can also contribute error to the nitrogen balance technique. Usually sweat, hair, skin, and nail losses are ignored since they are minor in comparison with the urine and fecal losses but, as mentioned, they do contribute to the error term for the method. Other errors in the method include the possibility of daily cumulative errors in the collection and analysis of the food, urine, and feces and the effects of prior poor nutritional status on the responses of the subject to this procedure. Good subject cooperation is essential to insure quantitative ingestion of the food and quantitative collection of the urine and feces.

The main disadvantage of this method is theoretical in character. The basic assumption of "replaceability" of body protein by a food protein is valid only when comparing good quality proteins. When poor proteins such as zein, gelatin, or gluten are evaluated, unrealistically high values result. This overestimation results from the failure of the method to account for the mobilization of body protein to meet particular amino acid needs. If there is a deficiency of one or more of the essential amino acids in the test protein, the animal will catabolize body proteins in an effort to provide the missing amino acid to support the synthesis of vital short-lived proteins such as enzymes or hormones. There appears to be a hierarchy of body proteins — those that are most essential to the survival of the animal are synthesized in preference to those, such as muscle protein, that are not as essential. In any event, when the body proteins are mobilized, the needed amino acids they contain are utilized and the remaining ones are deaminated and used for energy. The amino group is then converted to urea and excreted, contributing to the urinary nitrogen level. The Mitchell nitrogen balance technique does not differentiate the source of the nitrogen in the excreta and, because of this, the technique is not as valid in evaluating incomplete proteins. Source differentiation could be accomplished through the use of isotopic markers that would allow the investigator to identify body protein as distinct from food protein. Heavy isotopes incorporated into the food protein as it is grown could identify the food nitrogen that was excreted. The use of heavy isotopes, however, is expensive as well as time consuming, so this variation in the Mitchell technique might not be frequently used. In efforts to circumvent the problem of overestimating the biological values of incomplete or imbalanced proteins, other methods, some of which are variations of the original nitrogen balance technique, have been proposed and used.

The nitrogen balance index (NBI) of Allison and coworkers relates the absorbed nitrogen to the nitrogen excretion of a separate but concurrent group of individuals fed a nitrogen-free diet. This technique requires less time than the Thomas-Mitchell method, but is subject to many of the same kinds of errors. Both methods suffer from the inaccuracies contributed by the methodological measure of the so-called endogenous nitrogen loss. Both methods assume that this loss is represented by the nitrogen excreted by the animal during the nitrogen-free period, when actually the feeding of such a diet accelerates protein loss rather than modeling the endogenous nitrogen excretion.

The dynamic state of the body proteins, that is, the constant need to synthesize proteins having a short half-life (see Unit 2 for discussion of half-life) must be considered. This synthesis must be accommodated by the catabolism of tissue protein, a catabolic process unlikely to occur extensively if good quality proteins are consumed. Because this overestimation of endogenous loss is more serious with proteins of poor quality, inconsistent biological values are obtained. This is particularly true when unrefined proteins or food mixtures are evaluated.

A more-accurate method for the evaluation of protein quality is one that actually measures the retention of nitrogen in the carcass from the ingested protein nitrogen. This is called the NPU-BV or NPU method. Using these methods that calculate BV from the change in carcass protein, groups of animals, usually rats, are fed diets containing graded amounts of the test protein or a nitrogen-free diet. After a period of 7–10 days, the animals are killed and the nitrogen content of the carcasses determined. Obviously, proteins of high quality will evoke a greater retention of nitrogen in the carcass than proteins of poor quality. Using this technique, biological value can be calculated as follows:

$$\text{NPU BV} = \frac{B_f - B_k + I_k}{I_f} \times 100$$

Where B_f = carcass nitrogen of animals fed test protein diet
B_k = carcass nitrogen of animals fed nitrogen free diet
I_k = absorbed nitrogen of animals fed nitrogen free diet
I_f = absorbed nitrogen of animals fed test-protein diet

While this method has the obvious advantage of actually measuring nitrogen retention, its disadvantages are also obvious. Feeding a protein-free diet induces an exaggerated body protein loss.

This method is inappropriate for large animals because of the technical difficulties associated with the determination of body composition and because of the excessive cost. Obviously, too, human studies would not be possible. However, conceptually, the method has merit and several investigators have devised variations that are useful in a variety of species.

One variation that is useful in man is to measure the changes in body composition indirectly using heavy or radioactive isotopes. The various methods for determining body composition changes (see Unit 2) can be used to evaluate proteins. For example, Steffee et al. used a stable isotope of nitrogen, ^{15}N, to study the rates of total body protein synthesis and breakdown as a response to variation in amounts of dietary protein. Constant infusions of ^{15}N-glycine allowed these investigators to assess the value of given proteins in the homeostatic situation where there is constant protein synthesis and breakdown. While a very useful technique, it is also very expensive and requires sophisticated techniques and equipment to make the appropriate measurements.

Another variation of the carcass retention method uses the naturally occurring radioactive isotope ^{40}K. The method measures the change in ^{40}K concentration in the adult body as a result of consuming a given protein for a period of 7–10 days. This method is based on the constancy of potassium as an intracellular ion. The concentration of potassium in the body can be directly related to the number of cells in the body and indirectly related to the protein in the body. Since a set percentage of this potassium exists as the naturally occurring radioactive isotope, measuring ^{40}K levels is a direct measure of body cell number and an indirect measure of body protein. If a poor quality protein is consumed, ^{40}K levels will fall. If a good quality protein is consumed, there will be no change. Again, while this method has the advantage of its applicability to the human, its disadvantage is one of cost and availability of the whole-body counters needed to determine the presence of the isotope.

By far the easiest variation of the carcass-retention method is the protein efficiency ratio (PER). In this method, carcass composition is not determined and it is assumed that the gain in body weight of a given animal is related to the quality of the protein fed. Thus, young growing animals are fed test protein-containing diets for a period of 28 days. The weight gain is computed and divided by the total protein intake.

The formula, $PER = \dfrac{\text{Weight gain in grams}}{\text{Protein intake in grams}}$ is easy to use and the method requires no specialized expensive equipment. This is the method used for protein quality evaluation by most food companies and has been adopted by the regulatory agencies of the U.S. and Canada as their method of choice in evaluating the nutritional quality of foods. The ease and simplicity of the method, however, should not lull the reader into thinking that it is a "choice" method. PER can vary from species to species and, within a given species, from strain to strain. Examples of within-species variation in the PER of a given protein is shown in Table 4.10. Seven different strains of rats were fed the same diet for 4 weeks. PER was calculated at the end of each week. As can be seen in this table, the PER varied from week to week and between the seven strains. Variation can be introduced if levels of protein intake higher or lower than 10% by weight are used. In addition, the methods make no allowance for the maintenance requirement of the animal. Values obtained from a variety of food proteins are nonlinear. That is, a protein having a PER of 2 may not have twice the nutritional value of a protein having a PER of 1. Examples of the PER for a variety of food proteins is shown in Table 4.11.

A modification of the PER is the net protein ratio. This method attempts to account for the maintenance needs of the animal. In this method, two groups of animals are used. One is fed a nitrogen-free diet, the other the test diet. This modification is accompanied by all the pitfalls of using the nitrogen-free diets that have been discussed.

A variety of methods employing the assay of enzymes concerned with protein metabolism have been devised. The determination of the activity of transaminase, xanthine dehydrogenase, renal

TABLE 4.10
The PER of a Test Protein as Calculated Using the Weight Gain
of Rats from Seven Different Strains

	PER			
RAT STRAIN	Week 1	Week 2	Week 3	Week 4
Holtzman	4.14	3.94	3.61	3.50
Charles River	4.29	3.64	3.54	3.60
ARS-Sprague Dawley	4.31	3.76	3.32	3.36
Osborne-Mendel	4.20	3.52	3.24	3.39
Wistar	4.47	3.59	3.33	3.37
Wistar Lewis	3.69	3.64	3.37	3.28
SSB/PL (NIH)	3.80	3.37	2.96	2.47

TABLE 4.11
PER of Various Foods

Eggs	3.9–4.0
Fish	3.5
Milk	3.0–3.1
Beef	2.3
Soybeans	2.3
Beans	1.4–1.9
Nuts	1.8
Peanuts	1.7
Gluten	1.0
Rice	2.0
Corn	1.2

arginase, and others have been reported as indicators of protein quality. Unfortunately, these methods have not been rigorously tested and compared with the presently available whole-body methods.

The holistic approach, while valuable and useful, is nonetheless time consuming, not particularly good for poor quality proteins, and expensive. The approaches discussed above do have the advantage of digestibility and amino acid availability being given due consideration.

Attempts to circumvent the time and expense of whole-animal work have resulted in a number of techniques. One method, the amino acid score or chemical score is a nonbiological method and requires the amino acid analysis of the test protein. The amount of the most limiting amino acid (only the essential amino acids are considered) is related to the content of that same amino acid in a reference protein. In most cases, this reference is egg protein, however, a theoretical protein based on the amino acid requirements of the species in question could also be used.

$$\text{Thus, Chemical Score} = \frac{\text{mg of limiting amino acid/g test protein}}{\text{mg of amino acid/g ideal protein}} \times 100$$

While this method is quick and does not use animals, it makes no allowance for digestibility or availability of the constituent amino acids. This is a rather important aspect of protein nutrition. Some protein foods are poorly digestible; others contain compounds that interfere with absorption. For example, some amino acids form sugar–amino acid complexes that render the amino acids less available to the body. This occurs with the browning of baked goods such as bread; while bread is not considered a prime protein source, evaluation of its protein quality using the amino acid score would be in error due to the browning reaction.

A variation on this chemical method tries to account for digestibility. In this method, test proteins are first digested *in vitro* using conditions resembling those in the gastrointestinal tract. The amino acid score is then determined on the products of this digestion. This is a promising approach to evaluating protein quality but will require considerably more work to validate it. At present, it represents an innovative approach to the problems associated with assessing protein quality.

PROTEIN USE

DIGESTION

The daily protein intake plus that protein that appears in the gut as enzymes, sloughed epithelial gut cells, and mucins, is almost completely digested and absorbed. This is a very efficient process that ensures a continuous supply of amino acids to the whole-body amino acid pool (see Figure 4.4). Less than 10% of the total protein that passes through the gastrointestinal tract appears in the feces. If the food contributes between 70 and 100 g of protein and the endogenous protein contributes another 100 g (range: 35 to 200 g) then about 1–2 g of nitrogen might be expected to be found in the feces. This is equivalent to 6–12 g protein. Of the dietary protein, the fecal protein might include the hard-to-chew or -digest, tough, fibrous, connective tissue of meat or nitrogen-containing indigestible kernel coats of grains or particles of nuts that are not attacked by the digestive enzymes. For example, whole peanuts have a structure that is difficult to broach by the digestive enzymes. Unless chewed very finely, much of the nutritive value of this food may be lost. Peanut butter, on the other hand, is very well digested because its preparation ensures that its particle size is *very* small and is thus quite digestible.

The purpose of protein digestion is to liberate the amino acids from the consumed proteins. Except for the period shortly after birth, the enterocyte cannot absorb intact proteins. Prior to gut closure, the neonate can absorb some proteins. Most of these proteins are immunoglobulins. The proteins found in the colostrum, or first milk, provide passive immunity to the newborn. After gut closure, only amino acids and small peptides can pass from the lumen of the gut into the blood stream. Thus, the food proteins must be hydrolyzed into their component amino acids, dipeptides, and tripeptides. This is accomplished through a series of enzymes that have specific target linkages as their point of action. These enzymes are summarized in Table 4.12. The protein hydrolases, called peptidases, fall into two categories. Those that attack internal peptide bonds and liberate large peptide fragments for subsequent attack by other enzymes are called the endopeptidases. Those that attack the terminal peptide bonds and liberate single amino acids from the protein structure are called exopeptidases. The exopeptidases are further subdivided according to whether they attack at the carboxy end of the amino acid chain (carboxypeptidases) or the amino end of the chain (aminopeptidases). The initial attack on an intact protein is catalyzed by endopeptidases, and the final digestive action is catalyzed by the exopeptidases. The final products of digestion are free amino acids and some di- and tripeptides that are absorbed by the intestinal epithelial cells.

In contrast to carbohydrate and lipid digestion, which is initiated in the mouth with the salivary amylase and the lingual lipase, protein digestion does not begin until the protein reaches the stomach and the food is acidified with the gastric hydrochloric acid. The HCl serves several functions. It acidifies the ingested food, killing potential pathogenic organisms. Unfortunately, not all pathogens are killed. Some are acid resistant or are so plentiful in the food that the amount of gastric acidification is insufficient to kill all of the pathogens.

Hydrochloric acid also serves to denature the food proteins, thus making them more vulnerable to attack by pepsin, an endopeptidase. Actually, pepsin is not a single enzyme. It consists of pepsin A, which attacks peptide bonds involving phenylalanine or tyrosine and several other enzymes that

TABLE 4.12
Digestive Enzymes and Their Target Linkages

Enzyme	Location	Target
Pepsin	Stomach	Peptide bonds involving the aromatic amino acids
Trypsin	Small intestine	Peptide bonds involving arginine and lysine
Chymotrypsin	Small intestine	Peptide bonds involving tyrosine, tryptophan, phenylalanine, methionine, and leucine
Elastase	Small intestine	Peptide bonds involving alanine, serine, and glycine
Carboxypeptidease A	Small intestine	Peptide bonds involving valine, leucine, isoleucine, alanine
Carboxypeptidase B	Small intestine	Peptide bonds involving lysine and arginine
Endopeptidase, Aminopeptidase, Dipeptidase	Cells of brush border	di- and tripeptides that enter the brush border of the absorptive cells

have specific attack points. The pepsins are released into the gastric cavity as pepsinogen. When the food entering the stomach stimulates HCl release and the pH of the gastric contents falls below 2, the pepsinogen loses a 44 amino acid sequence. The activation of the pepsins from pepsinogen occurs by one of two processes. The first, called *autoactivation,* occurs when the pH drops below 5. At low pH, the bond between the 44th and 45th amino acid residue falls apart and the 44 amino acid residue (from the amino terminus) is liberated. The liberated residue acts as an inhibitor of pepsin by binding to the catalytic site until pH 2 is achieved. The inhibition is relieved when this fragment is degraded, as happens at pH 2 or below or when it is attacked by pepsin. Since the fragment binds at the catalytic site of pepsin, this can happen. The other process is called *autocatalysis* and occurs when already active pepsin attacks the precursor pepsinogen. This is a self-repeating process that ensures ongoing catalysis of the resident protein. The cleavage of the 44 amino acid residue, in addition to providing activated pepsin, has another purpose. That is, it serves as a signal peptide for cholecystokinin release in the duodenum. This then sets the stage for the subsequent pancreatic phase of protein digestion. As described in the units on lipids and carbohydrates, cholecystokinin stimulates both the exocrine pancreas and the intestinal mucosal epithelial cell to release its digestive enzymes. The intestinal cell releases an enzyme, enteropeptidase or enterokinase, which activates the protease, trypsin, released as trypsinogen by the exocrine pancreas. This trypsin not only acts on food proteins, it also acts on other pre-proteases released by the exocrine pancreas and activating them. Thus, trypsin acts as an endoprotease on chymotrypsinogen, releasing chymotrypsin; on proelastase, releasing elastase; and on procarboxypeptidase, releasing carboxypeptidase. Trypsin, chymotrypsin and elastase are all endoproteases, each having specificity for particular peptide bonds as detailed in Table 4.13. Each of these three proteases have serine as part of their catalytic site so any compound that ties up the serine will inhibit the activity of these proteases. Such inhibitors as diisopropylphosphofluoridate react with this serine and in so doing bring a halt to protein digestion.

Through the action of pepsin, trypsin, chymotrypsin, and elastase, numerous oligopeptides are produced that then are attacked by the amino and carboxypeptidases of the pancreatic juice and those on the brush border of the absorptive cells. One by one, the amino acids are liberated from these chains and one by one, they are absorbed and appear in the portal blood.

ABSORPTION

Although single amino acids are liberated in the intestinal contents, there is insufficient power in the enzymes of the pancreatic juice to render all of the amino acids singly for absorption. The brush border of the absorptive cell therefore not only absorbs the single amino acid but also di- and tripeptides. In the process of absorbing these small peptides, it hydrolyzes them to their amino acid constituents. There is little evidence that peptides enter the blood stream. There are specific transport systems for each group of functionally similar amino acids, di- ,and tripeptides. Most of the biologically important L-amino acids are transported by an active carrier system against a concentration gradient (see Figure 4.5). This active transport involves the intracellular potassium ion and the extracellular sodium ion. As the amino acid is carried into the enterocyte, sodium also enters in exchange for potassium. This sodium must be returned (in exchange for potassium) to the extracellular medium. This return uses the sodium–potassium ATP pump. In several instances, the carrier is a shared carrier. That is, the carrier will transport more than one amino acid. Such is the case with the neutral amino acids and those with short or polar side chains (serine, threonine, and alanine). The mechanism whereby these carriers participate in amino acid absorption is similar to that described for glucose uptake (see the unit on carbohydrates). This mechanism is illustrated in Figure 4.5.

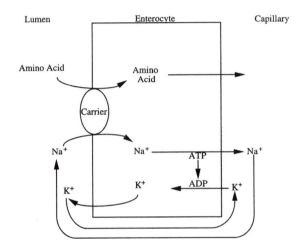

FIGURE 4.5 Carrier-mediated sodium-dependent amino acid transport. The amino acid enters the absorptive cell with sodium. The sodium is reirculated back to the lumen for reuse. The sodium is pumped out via Na$^+$K$^+$ ATPase system. As the sodium leaves the cell, potassium flows back in and the electrolyte balance is maintained.

METABOLISM

The amino acids leaving the absorptive cell enter a whole-body amino acid pool from which all cells withdraw amino acids for use in the synthesis of biologically important proteins, peptides, and amino acid derivatives. The peptides may be hormones or cytokines that the various signaling systems found in the body comprise. Amino acids not used for peptide or protein synthesis can be deaminated and the carbon unit used for energy or for the synthesis of glucose or fatty acids. In humans consuming a fat-rich diet, very little fatty acid synthesis occurs. Amino acids can also be decarboxylated to form amines. Amines are quite potent compounds that act as intracellular effectors such as the neurotransmitters or as high-energy compounds such as creatin phosphate.

Hormones: Regulators of Protein Metabolism

Hormones serve as internal messengers regulating the ebb and flow of a variety of cellular functions. As internal signals, hormones regulate such processes as heartbeat, vascular contraction, salt conservation, glucose uptake and utilization, glucose production, and oxygen consumption. Hormones can be viewed as system regulators.

TABLE 4.13
Some Protein and Peptide Hormones and their Function

Hormone	Source	Type	Function
Thyroid	Thyroid Gland	Dipeptide of tyrosine	Regulates oxygen consumption by tissues
Thyroid Stimulating Hormone (TSH)	Pituitary	Polypeptide	Stimulates synthesis and release of thyroid hormone by thyroid gland
Thyroid Releasing Factor	Hypothalamus	Tripeptide	Stimulates pituitary to release thyroid stimulating hormone
Calcitonin	Thyroid Gland	Polypeptide	Stimulates bone uptake of calcium
Parathyroid Hormone	Parathyroid Glands	Polypeptide	Raises serum calcium levels, lowers serum phosphorus levels; increases urinary phosphorus excretion, decreases urinary calcium excretion; activates vitamin D in renal tissue
Insulin	β cells of Islets of Langerhans (pancreas)	Protein	Regulates glucose utilization; stimulates glucose uptake; influences lipid and protein synthesis
Glucagon	α cells of Isles of Langerhans (pancreas)	Polypeptide	Rapid mobilization of hepatic glucose from glycoen; mobilizes fatty acids from adipose tissue stores; enhances hepatic glucose production from amino acids and glycerol
Somatostatin	D cells of Islets of Langerhans (pancreas)	Polypeptide	Inhibits food passage along gastrointestinal system, decreases gall bladder release of bile, slows uptake of nutrients from intestinal lumen; ihibit growth hormone release
Epinephrine	Adrenal Medulla	Tyrosine Derivative	Stimulates lipolysis, stimulates glycogen breakdown; increases vasodilation of arterioles of skeletal muscles, vasoconstriction of arteriolesin skin and viscera
Norepinephrine	Adrenal Medulla	Tyrosine Derivative	Exerts an overall vasoconstriction effect on vascular system
ACTH	Pituitary	Polypeptide	Stimulates production and release of adrenal corticoid hormones
Antidiuretic Hormone (ADH) (Vasopressin)	Pituitary	Polypeptide	Promotes water conservation; controls water resorption by kidney; raises blood pressure
Follicle stimulating Hormone (FSH)	Anterior Pituitary	Peptide	Controls testicular function; spermatogenesis; stimulates ovum production; enhances release of estrogen
Luteotropic Hormone (LH) (Prolactin)	Anterior Pituitary	Small Protein	Controls testicular function and spermatogenesis; stimulates ovum production; enhances release of estrogen
Growth Hormone	Anterior Pituitary	Small Protein	Stimualtes growth of long bones and muscles; stimulates production of somatomedin
Gastrin	Gastric Glands	Polypeptide	Stimulates acid and pepsin sescretion; stimulates growth of gastric mucosa
Cholecystokinin	Intestine, Pancreas	Polypeptide	Stimulates gall bladder contraction; stimulates pancreatic enzyme release
Secretin	Intestine, Pancreas	Polypeptide	Stimulates pancreatic secretion; augments action of cholecystokinin
Leptin	Adipose Tissue	Peptide (Cytokine)	Signals the satiety center of the brain; suppresses appetite; stimulates UCPs and apoptosis

Hormones are substances that are released into the bloodstream by a tissue or organ and have an action distal to that tissue. Not all hormones are proteins. Some are peptides, some are steroids, some are small polypeptides, and some are amino acid derivatives. All, however, serve as coordinators of activity in specific tissues.

The actions of many of these hormones are mediated by specific interactions with specific proteins in the membrane or cytosol, or certain of the organelles within the cell. These proteins are called receptors (See Unit 2). In turn, the hormones themselves are released via a cascade of sequential reactions that usually begin in the central nervous system, followed by signals generated in the hypothalamus, then the pituitary, and finally by the endocrine cell itself. This cascaded signaling system is a means to amplify the response to a specific stimulus. For example, an individual is suddenly exposed to a dangerous situation — perhaps an explosion or an oncoming car or a charging bull. The person perceives the danger and responds to it. The response involves the central nervous system as well as other systems that are involved in the fight-or-flight response to danger. Figure 4.6 illustrates this signal cascade system.

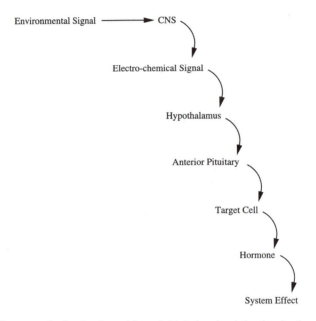

FIGURE 4.6 Signaling cascade that begins with an initial signal originating in the environment and ends with a whole-body systemic response.

Other stimuli may originate from the environment and likewise elicit a systemic response. Specific foods or nutrients can also evoke such cascades as discussed in Unit 3 with respect to food-intake regulation. This regulation involves a variety of signals from both the CNS and the gut. In summary, stimuli from the environment elicit specific electrical or chemical signals. These are generated by the hypothalamus which, either directly or indirectly (via releasing hormones) stimulates the anterior pituitary, which directly or indirectly signals the target endocrine cell to synthesize or release its hormone, which has the needed effect on metabolism. Not all hormone-release mechanisms use all steps in this cascade. Sometimes, short loops are used that bypass some of the initial steps in the cascade. In addition, there is some negative feedback involved that tells the target endocrine cell that enough hormone has been released.

Some of the peptide and protein hormones in the body are listed in Table 4.13. Others, notably the cytokines, are discussed in Units 2 and 3. The local hormones (the eicosanoids) are discussed in Unit 6. In general, hormones function through one of several mechanisms.

1. They induce enzyme synthesis by stimulating mRNA transcription. An increase in mRNA synthesis leads to an increase in enzyme protein synthesis. Hormones acting in this way are thought to be functioning as modifiers of gene expression.
2. Hormones stimulate enzyme synthesis through enhancing the translation of messenger RNA. Growth hormone, a small protein, appears to act in this fashion.
3. Hormones directly activate enzymes by either changing the phosphorylation state of the cell or one of its compartments or by changing the flux of ions as cofactors in the reactions.
4. Hormones activate membrane transport systems, which have G proteins as part of their structures.

In the cascade system illustrated in Figure 4.6, hormones or signals must emanate from one level of the cascade to the next for the system to work. The precision of the signaling system depends largely on the specificity of the signal for its target, and the specificity of the target for its signal. Some hormones are more specific than others. In general, the protein and peptide hormones are more specific than the steroid hormones. The polypeptide hormones bind to their cognate receptors lodged in the plasma membrane. These receptors generally penetrate the membrane and have a tyrosine-rich tail protruding into the cytosol (See Unit 2). Part of the hormone-receptor binding and subsequent cellular events involve G proteins. Not all of these hormone-receptor cascades use G proteins. The G proteins serve as the signal transducer for the hormone, stimulating a subsequent series of metabolic events that may involve the enzymes, adenyl cyclase, or phospholipase C and the calcium ion. The calcium ion plays a role in exocytosis, may be active in the exchange of metabolites across intracellular membranes, or may itself be a signal molecule.

While the details of the synthesis of all of these peptide and protein hormones have yet to be elucidated, some pathways are well known. The synthesis of thyroxine from tyrosine by the thyroid gland (Figure 4.7), and of dopamine, epinephrine, and norepinephrine, also from tyrosine, by the adrenal medulla and CNS is established. Note in Figure 4.7 that a cascade of signals is needed for the release of the hormone. The synthesis of the pancreatic hormones and of the more complicated protein hormones is not clear. The enzymes needed for some of these synthetic pathways have not been fully described nor have the control points in the synthetic pathways been fully elucidated. This is a very active area for research in endocrinology, as is the study of the signal transduction systems that explain the actions of each of these hormones. One of the more interesting observations is that many of the peptide hormones are encoded together in a single gene and that many copies of the same message can exist in this gene. For example, one gene has been found to encode ACTH (adrenocorticotropin hormone), β-lipotropin, α-lipotropin, α-MSH (melanocyte stimulating hormone), β-MSH, CLIP (corticotropin like peptide), β-endorphin and some of the enkephalins. This gene encodes for proopiomelanocortin as illustrated in Figure 4.8, which in turn can generate the above eight hormones.

Not all are generated by the same tissue or cell type but occur separately, generated by specific signals in specific cells. In the above example, one of the gene products, ACTH, is produced and released by the anterior pituitary under the control of the corticotrophin-releasing hormone. Enzymes are present in the corticotrophic cells that cleave the amino acid sequence of proopiomelanocortin at specific sites releasing ACTH and β-lipotropin into the circulation. These products can be cleaved further by cells of the pars intermedia to produce and release α-MSH, CLIP, α–lipotropin, and β-endorphin. CLIP is an abbreviation for corticotropin-like intermediary peptide. α-lipotropin and β-endorphin can be split further to produce β-MSH and met-enkephalin. The reason that all these gene products arise from the same initial compound has to do with the unique location in the different cell types of specific proteases that act on specific linkages and thus release these smaller peptides into the circulation. Only a few cell types possess these specific proteases.

Other hormones are also encoded together. Just as ACTH and β-lipotrophin are components of the proopiomelanocortin, so too are other hormones split off from prohormone molecules.

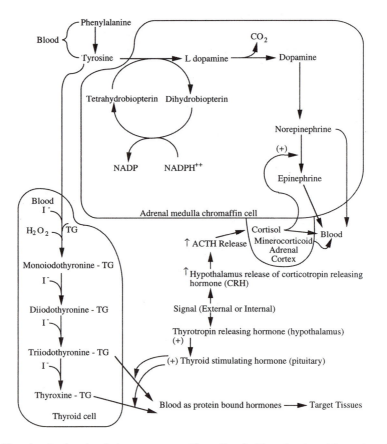

FIGURE 4.7 Tyrosine in the circulation enters specific cells of either the thyroid or adrenal glands. This tyrosine is used to make thyroid hormone and the catecholamines. These hormones are released into the circulation and are carried to their target cells, where they have their effects. Thyroxine synthesis occurs as a sequential iodination of tyrosine residues contained by the protein thyroglobulin (TG). At the target tissue, thyroxine is deiodinated to its active form, triiodothyronine.

Vasopressin and neurophysin II arise from the same molecule. Oxytocin and neurophysin I also have the same parent peptide. Although the above examples are all peptide hormones, no doubt we will find that nonhormone peptides can arise in similar fashion. Amino acids in the circulation enter a vast array of cell types, each of which has many uses for the amino acids brought to it by the circulation. As mentioned, small, medium, and large molecules can be made. The largest of these molecules are the proteins.

Protein synthesis

DNA

Protein synthesis is dependent on the simultaneous presence of all the amino acids necessary for the protein being synthesized and upon the provision of energy. If there is an insufficient supply of either, protein biosynthesis will not proceed at its normal pace. Chemically, the polymerization of amino acids into protein is a dehydration reaction between two amino acids.

The process whereby proteins are synthesized provides the basis for understanding genetic differences. It is also the basis for understanding how the unique properties of each cell type are maintained, since the properties that make cells unique are usually conferred by the proteins within

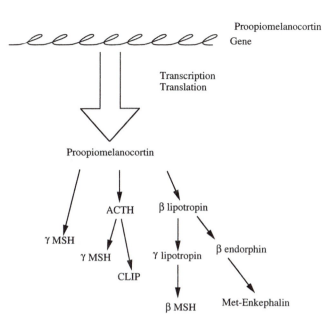

Gene Products

FIGURE 4.8   One gene encodes several signal peptides depending on the cell type and the signals generated to synthesize one or more of these products, ACTH and β-lipotropin gene products are under the control of corticotropin-releasing hormone (CRH), whereas αMSH, CLIP, γ-lipotropin, and β-endorphin gene products in the pituitary are under the control of dopamine. MSH = Melanocyte-stimulating hormone; CLIP = corticotropin-like intermediary peptide.

them. Some of these proteins are the structural elements of the cell. Others are enzymes that catalyze specific reactions and processes that characterize the cell in question. Still other proteins confer a particular biochemical function on the cell. The amino acid sequence of a particular protein is genetically controlled. This control is exerted through the polynucleotide, deoxyribonucleic acid (DNA). DNA is found in both the nucleus and the mitochondria. It is composed of four bases: adenine, guanine, thymine, and cytosine. These bases are condensed to form the DNA chain in a process analogous to the condensation of amino acids that compose the primary structure of a protein. Species vary in the percent distribution of these bases in their DNA. In mammals, the adenine-thymidine content varies from 45–53%. Small amounts of the base 5-methyl-cytosine, as well as methylated derivatives of the other bases, can also be found.

The chain of nucleotides that DNA comprises is formed by joining adenine, guanine, thymine, and cytosine through phosphodiester bonds. The phosphodiester linkage is between the 5′ phosphate group of one nucleotide and the 3′ OH group of the adjacent nucleotide. This provides a direction (5′ to 3′) to the chain. A typical segment of the chain is illustrated in Figure 4.9. The hydrophobic properties of the bases plus the strong charges of the polar groups within each of the component units are responsible for the helical conformation of the DNA chain. The bases themselves interact so that, in the nucleus, the two chains are intertwined. Hence, the term double helix applies to DNA. In the mitochondria, the DNA is circular, with connections between the light and heavy strands (see Unit 2). Hydrogen bonding between the bases stabilizes this conformation, as shown in Figure 4.10. Other factors as well serve to stabilize the structure of the DNA. Unwinding a small portion of the DNA, a necessary step in the initiation of transcription, occurs when these stabilizing factors are perturbed and signals are sent to the nucleus that transcription should begin. Unwinding

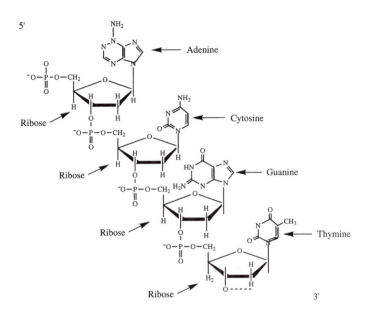

FIGURE 4.9 The bases that the DNA polynucleotide chain comprises are joined together by phosphodiester bonds using ribose as the common link between the bases.

exposes a small (~17 kb) segment of the DNA (the gene), allowing its base sequence to be available for complementary base pairing, as happens when messenger RNA is synthesized (transcription). The segment that is exposed contains not only the 600 to 1800 nucleotide-structural gene, but also a sequence called the promoter region. The promoter region precedes the start site of the structural gene and this is said to be upstream of the structural gene. Those bases following the start site are downstream. The nucleotides that code for a specific protein may not be adjacent to each other on the DNA strand but may be located nearby.

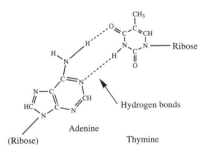

FIGURE 4.10 Hydrogen bonds form between complementary bases: adenine complements thymine; guanine complements cytosine. These bonds stabilize the double-helical array of the two DNA strands.

The DNA base sequence is unique for every protein that is synthesized in the body. While only a few bases are used for the DNA, the combinations and sequences of the combinations provide a specific code for each and every protein and peptide. The human genome project sponsored by the National Institutes of Health has as its goal the determination of the complete sequence and the mapping of subsequences. By mapping, we mean the identification, of each segment and the protein it encodes. Thus, the function of DNA is to determine the properties of the cell through the provision of a code that directs protein synthesis. It also functions to transmit genetic information from one generation to the next in a given species. Thus, DNA has a broad spectrum of function — it ensures the identity of both specific cell types and specific species.

The sequence of amino acids in each protein synthesized by the body is determined from a subunit of the DNA molecule known as the gene. It consists of several thousand bases (abbreviated as kb). The gene, through the sequence of bases that are found in its constituent nucleotides, codes for a polypeptide. The DNA in the nucleus is very stable with respect to the base sequence and content. It can be damaged by certain chemicals, free radicals, x rays, and other agents. However, nuclear DNA can self-repair; mitochondrial DNA has very limited repair capability. If a change in the base sequence does occur and is not repaired, a mutation is said to have occurred. Both base substitution and base deletion can occur as mutations. This mutation will then become part of the genetic information transmitted to the next generation. Some of the base substitutions have no effect on the gene product. This is because some amino acids have more than one combination of bases (codons) that stipulate a particular amino acid in the gene product (see Table 4.14). In addition, some mutations occur that have little effect on the functional or conformational characteristics of the resultant protein. For example, a mutation could occur that would result in an amino acid substitution of one neutral amino acid for another. This substitution might occur in a region outside of the active site(s) of the protein and with little effect on that protein's size and shape. Actually, such mutations and resultant amino acid substitutions are not mutations, per se, but polymorphisms. The resultant gene product retains its premutation function, yet has a slightly different amino acid sequence. Such polymorphisms are useful tools, however, because they allow population geneticists to track mutation and evolutionary events through related family members.

TABLE 4.14
Codons for the Amino Acids

Second Base	First Base			
	U	O	A	G
U	UUU }Phe UUC	CUU }leu CUC CUA CUG	AUU }Ile AUC AUA	GUU }Val GUC GUA GUG
	UUA }Leu UUG		AUG * MET	
O	UCU UCC }Ser UCA UCG	CCU CCC }Pr o CCA CCG	ACU ACC }Thr ACA ACT	GCU GCC }Ala GCA GCG
A	UAU }Tyr UAC	CAU }His CAC	AAU }Asn AAC	GAU }Asp GAC
	UAA STOP UAG STOP	CAA }G ln CAG	AAA }Lvs AAG	GAA }Glu GAG
G	UGU }Cys UGC	CGU CGC }Arg CGA CGG	AGU }Ser AGC	GGU GGC }Gly GGA GGG
	UGA STOP UGG Trp		AGA }Arg AGG	

*AUG also serves as a start codon

In the nucleus, the DNA is found in the chromosomal chromatin. Chromatin contains very long double strands of DNA and a nearly equal mass of histone and nonhistone proteins. Histones are highly basic proteins varying in molecular weight from ~ 11,000 to ~ 21,000. As a result of their high content of basic amino acids, histones serve to interact with the polyanionic phosphate backbone of the DNA so as to produce uncharged nucleoproteins. The histones also serve to keep the DNA in a very compact form and, as well, to protect this DNA from free radical attack. In mammals, the mitochondrial DNA does not have this protective histone coat. It is "naked" and much more vulnerable to damage. This damage can be quite severe, yet, because there are so many copies of the mitochondrial DNA and so many mitochondria in a cell, the effects of this damage might not be apparent.

During cell division, the nuclear DNA, as soon as its replication is completed, becomes highly condensed into distinct chromosomes of characteristic shapes. These chromosomes exist as pairs and are numbered. There are 46 chromosomes in the human. Included in this number are the sex chromosomes, the x and y chromosomes. If the individual has one X and one Y, he is a male; if two Xs are present, she is a female. The chromosomes are the result of a mixing of the nuclear DNA of the egg and sperm. Approximately half of each pair comes from each parent. If identical codes for a given protein are inherited from each parent, the resultant progeny will be a homozygote for that protein. If nonidentical codes are inherited, the progeny will be a heterozygote. Within the heterozygote population, there may be certain codes that are dominant — eye or hair color, for example. These are dominant traits and are expressed despite the fact that the individual has inherited two different codes for this trait. A mutation in a code that is not expressed is a recessive trait. If, by chance, two identical mutated genes are present that encode a certain protein, the expression of this mutated code will be observed. This is the basis for genetic diseases of the autosomal recessive or dominant type. Autosomal means a mutation in any of the chromosomal DNA except that which is in the X or Y chromosome. A mutation of the DNA in this chromosome is called a sex-linked mutation. If it results in a disease, it is called a sex-linked genetic disease. There is another inheritance pattern based on the mitochondrial genome. Because this genome is primarily of maternal origin, certain of the characteristics of the OXPHOS system will be inherited via maternal inheritance. A number of mitochondrial mutations result in a number of degenerative diseases (see Unit 2).

Having the codes in the nucleus for the synthesis of protein in the cytoplasm implies a communication between the cytoplasm and the nucleus and between the nucleus and the cytoplasm. Signals are sent to the nucleus that "inform" this organelle of the need to synthesize certain proteins. We do not know what all these signals are. Some are substrates for the needed proteins, some are nutrients, some are hormones, and some are signaling compounds that have yet to be identified. The communication between the nucleus and the cytoplasm is carried out by messenger RNA (mRNA).

Transcription

Messenger RNA is used to carry genetic information from the DNA of the chromosomes to the surface of the ribosomes (Figure 4.11). It is synthesized as a single strand in the nucleus by a process known as transcription. Chemically, RNA is similar to DNA. It is an unbranched linear polymer in which the monomeric subunits are the ribonucleoside-5'-monophosphates. The bases are the purines, adenine and guanine, and the prymidines, uracil and cytosine. Note that thymine is not used in RNA and that uracil is not present in DNA. RNA is single stranded rather than double stranded. It is held together by molecular base pairing and will contract if in a solution of high ionic strength. RNA, particularly the mRNA, is a much smaller molecule than DNA and is far less stable. It has a very short half-life (from minutes to hours) compared to that of nuclear DNA (years). Because it has a short half-life, the bases that compose it must be continually resynthesized. This synthesis requires a number of micronutrients as well as energy, which explains some of the symptoms of malnutrition. Among these symptoms are skin lesions. This is because the epithelial cells are among the shortest-lived cells and must be constantly renewed. This renewal depends on both adequate energy and amino acid supplies, and on the micronutrients that are involved in mRNA synthesis as well as cell renewal.

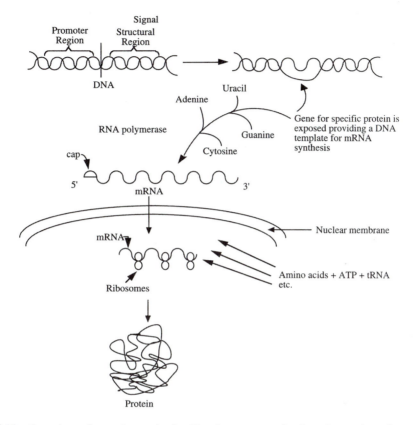

FIGURE 4.11 Overview of protein synthesis. Signals are transmitted to the nucleus that stimulate the exposure of a gene for a specific protein. A specific messenger RNA is synthesized. The mRNA moves out into the cytosol and attaches to the ribosome, whereupon tRNAs attached to amino acids dock at appropriate complementary bases and the amino acids are joined together to make protein.

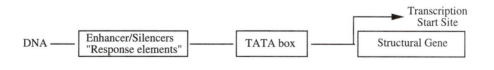

FIGURE 4.12 Detailed structure of the components of a gene that is to be transcribed.

The synthesis of mRNA from DNA is called transcription. The basic mechanism is known and involves three steps: initiation, elongation, and termination. Initiation is the process whereby basal transcription factors recognize and bind to DNA. These factors form a complex with RNA polymerase II. Most of gene expression can be defined as transacting factors (proteins) binding cis-acting elements (base sequences). Upstream of the transcription start site on DNA is a region called the promoter (Figure 4.12). Within the promoter, approximately 25 base pairs upstream of the start site, is a consensus sequence called the TATA box, which contain A-T base pairs. One of the basal transcription factors, the TATA binding protein (TBP), recognizes this sequence of DNA and binds there. This begins the process of transcription initiation as the transacting TBP binds the cis-acting TATA box and a large complex of basal transcription factors, RNA polymerase II, and DNA is formed. Elongation is the actual process of RNA formation through the use of a DNA template in the 5′ to 3′ direction. Shortly after elongation begins, the 5′ end of mRNA is capped by 7-methylguanosine triphospate. This cap stabilizes the mRNA and is necessary for processing and translation. The third step is the termination of the chain.

The regulation of transcription occurs at the initiation step. The promoter region contains many cis-acting elements, each named for the factor that controls them. In general, these regions are called enhancers, silencers, or more recently named, response elements. Examples include the retinoic acid response element (RARE), heat shock element (HSE), and cAMP response element (CRE). The transacting factors that bind these elements are in general called transcription factors. They are proteins with at least two domains, DNA binding and transcription activation. Recently it has been shown that coactivators are needed to bind transcription factors and increase transcription by both interacting with basal transcription factors and altering chromatin structure. Corepressors act to decrease transcription at both the level of basal transcription factors and chromatin structure. Coactivators and corepressors are proteins.

The true regulation of transcription occurs by the regulation of transcription factors. Transcription factors can be regulated by:

- their rates of synthesis or degradation
- phosphorylation or dephosphorylation
- ligand binding
- cleavage of a protranscription factor
- release of an inhibitor

One class of transcription factors important for nutrition is the nuclear hormone receptor super family, which is regulated by ligand binding. Ligands for these transcription factors include retinoic acid, fatty acids, vitamin D, thyroid hormone, and steroid hormones. All members of this super family contain two zinc fingers in their DNA-binding domains. Zinc is bound to histidine- and cysteine-rich regions of the protein that envelops the DNA in a shape that looks like a finger. The zinc finger is shown in Figure 4.13. The zinc ion plays an enormous role in gene expression because of its central use in the zinc finger. The nuclear hormone receptor super family is divided into four groups according to their dimerization potential, their site specificity and their localization (Table 4.15). Group I receptors bind the steroid hormones and bind DNA as homodimers. Group I response elements are palindromes of either AGAACA or AGGTCA spaced by 3 nucleotides. The specificity occurs by interactions between the specific nucleotide sequence and the protein sequence of the first zinc finger.

The RXRαβγ receptor that binds 9-cis retinoic acid binds to either the DR-1 or the IR-O response element. The DR1 response element also binds the PPARαβ(δ) receptor that in turn binds fatty acids, and the PPARγ that binds prostaglandin E 2. All three of these receptors bind to the same element. If only one were to bind, the process would be called homodimerization. If more than one receptor binds to the same element, we would have heterodimerization.

Group II receptors, also called the retinoid/thyroid subfamily, bind nutrients and metabolites such as retinoic acid, vitamin D, and fatty acids. Table 4.18 lists the nutrient receptors and their ligands. All of these receptors form heterodimers with the retinoid x receptor (RXR). 9-cis retinoic acid binds RXR and has a synergistic effect on transcription when dimerized with most receptors in this group. Generally, these receptors bind to direct repeats of degenerative AGGTCA sequences spaced by 1 (RXR, LXR, PPAR), 2 (alternative RAR, TR), 3 (VDR), 4 (TR, LXR), or 5 (RAR) nucleotides. Specificity occurs due to the spacing between the consensus sequence half sites. In

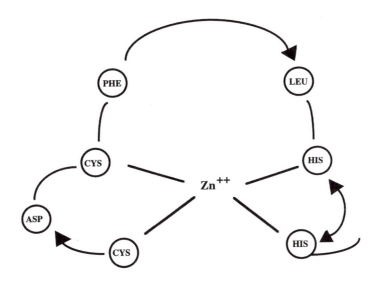

FIGURE 4.13   Zinc finger detail.

TABLE 4.15
Members of the Nuclear Hormone Receptor Super Family

Receptor Group[1]	Consensus Half Site	Binding Site	
Group 1			
GR, ER, PR, MR, AR	AGAACA or AGGTCA	→(3)←	Homodimers
Group 2			
RXR, RAR, TR, VDR, PPAR, MB67, RLD-1, ECR, USP, ARP-1, COUP-TF	AGGTCA	→(0-5)← →(0)←	Heterodimerize with RXR
Group 3			
NGF1-B, FTZ-F1 (ELP, SF-1) ROR, Rev-erb, BD73	(A,T)AAGGTCA	→	Monomers or heterodimerize with RXR
Group 4			
HNF-4	AGGTCA	→(1)←	Homodimers

[1] It may appear that the names of these receptors are in nonsense code. For ease in identifying specific protein ligand complexes, letter acronyms have been developed. Some of these codes are readily understood, but others appear more arcane. For example, TR means thyroid hormone binding receptor protein; RXR, a protein that binds 9-cis retinoic acid; VDR, a receptor that binds vitamin D (1,25(OH)$_2$ vitamin D), and so forth. Arrows indicate direction of consensus sequence (ex: →(3)← is an inverted repeat with three nucleotides spaces in between.

the case of the retinoic acid receptor (RAR) and thyroid receptor (TR), unliganded receptor can bind DNA and repress transcription.

There are numerous proteins, aside from those of the steroid receptor super family, that bind to specific base sequences in the promoter region. Some of these bind minerals, some bind other hormones, and some are, by themselves, transcription factors that have control properties.

In addition to these receptor proteins that bind to certain base sequences in the promoter region, we also have smaller molecules that similarly serve to stimulate or suppress transcription. One is

TABLE 4.16
Some Examples of Nutrient Effects on Transcription

Nutrient	Gene	Effect
Retinoic acid	Many genes	Increases transcription through its binding to RXR or RAR which in turn bind to the AGGTCA sequence in the promoter region
Vitamin B_6	Steroid hormone receptor	Suppresses transcription
Vitamin D	Many genes	Increases transcription of genes for calcium binding proteins
Glucose	Glucokinase	Increases transcription in pancreas and liver
Potassium	Aldosterone synthetase	Increases transcription in adrenal cortex
Fatty acids	Fatty acid synthetase	Suppresses transcription in liver
Selenium	Glutathione peroxidase, 5′ deiodinase	Increases transcription
Sodium	Endothelin 1	Increases transcription
Zinc	Zinc transporters	Increases transcription

the glucose molecule. It stimulates the transcription of glucokinase that has a glucose-sensitive promoter region. Only the β cell and the hepatocyte DNA have this region exposed and only these cell types express the glucokinase gene. Other cells have the gene but do not express it, probably because their glucose-promoter site is unexposed. Instead, these other cell types express a similar (but different) gene called hexokinase. There are a number of instances in the nutrition science literature where specific nutrients influence the transcription of genes that encode enzymes or receptors or carriers that are important to the use of that nutrient. Shown in Table 4.16 are examples of these influences. All of the above-mentioned serve to control transcription, a vital step in controlling gene expression.

Once the bases are joined together in the nucleus to form messenger RNA, the nucleus must edit and process it. Processing it includes capping, nucleolytic, and ligation reactions that shorten it, terminal additions of nucleosides and nucleoside modifications (Figure 4.14). Through this processing ,less than 25% of the original RNA migrates from the nucleus to the ribosomes, where it attaches prior to translation. The editing and processing is needed because immature RNA contains all those bases corresponding to the DNA introns. Introns are those groups of bases that are not part of the structural gene. Introns are intervening sequences that separate the exons or coding sequences of the structural gene. The removal of these segments is a cut-and-splice process whereby the intron is cut at its 5′ end, pulled out of the way, and cut again at its 3′ end; at the same time, the two exons are joined. This cut-and-splice routine is continued until all the introns are removed and the exons joined. Some editing of the RNA also occurs with base substitutions made as appropriate. Finally, there is a 3′ terminal poly A tail added.

The editing and processing step is now complete. This mature messenger RNA now leaves the nucleus and moves to the cytoplasm for translation. The nucleotides that have been removed during editing and processing are either reused or totally degraded. Of note is the fact that editing and processing also are mechanisms used to degrade the whole message unit. This serves to control the amount and half-life of this RNA. The endonucleases and exonucleases used in the cut-and-splice processing also come into play in the regulation of mRNA stability. Some mRNAs have very short half-lives (minutes) while other have longer half-lives (hours). This is important because some gene products are needed for only a short time. Hormones and cell signals must be short-lived and therefore the body needs to control or counterbalance their synthesis and action. One of the ways to do this is by regulating amount of mRNA (number of copies of mRNA for each gene product) that leaves the nucleus. Thus, this regulation is a key step in metabolic control.

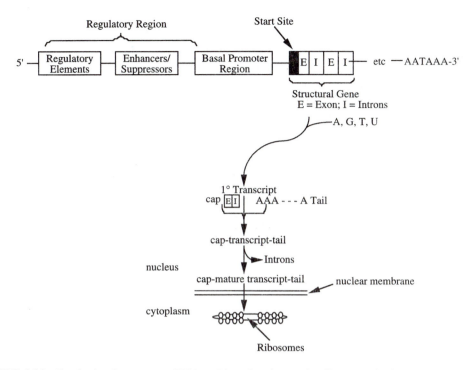

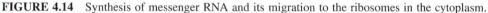

FIGURE 4.14 Synthesis of messenger RNA and its migration to the ribosomes in the cytoplasm.

Translation

Following transcription is translation. Translation is the synthesis of the protein using the order of the assemblage of constituent amino acids as dictated by the mRNA. This process is also influenced by specific nutrients. The translation of the ferritin gene, for example, is influenced by the amount of iron available in the cell. In iron deficiency, the messenger RNA start site for ferritin translation is covered up by an iron-responsive protein. This protein binds the 3′ UTR and inhibits the movement of the 40s ribosome from the cap to the translation start site. When iron status is improved, the start site is uncovered and translation can proceed. The actual site of translation is on the ribosomes; some ribosomes are located on the membrane of the endoplasmic reticulum and some are free in the cell matrix. Ribosomes consist almost entirely of ribosomal RNA and ribosomal protein. RNA is synthesized via RNA polymerase I in the cell nucleus as a large molecule; in this location, this RNA molecule is cleaved and leaves the nucleus as two subunits, a large one and a small one. The ribosome is reformed in the cytoplasm by the reassociation of the two subunits; the subunits, however, are not necessarily derived from the same precursor.

Ribosomal RNA makes up a large fraction of total cellular RNA. It serves as the "docking" point for the activated amino acids bound to the transfer RNA and the mRNA that dictates the amino acid polymerization sequence. Transfer RNA (tRNA) is used to bring an amino acid to the polysome (ribosome), the site of protein synthesis. Each amino acid has a specific tRNA. Each tRNA molecule is thought to have a cloverleaf arrangement of nucleotides. With this arrangement of nucleotides, there is the opportunity for the maximum number of hydrogen bonds to form between base pairs. A molecule that has many hydrogen bonds is very stable. Transfer RNA also contains a triplet of bases known, in this instance, as the anticodon. The amino acid carried by tRNA is identified by the codon of mRNA through its anticodon; the amino acid itself is not involved in this identification.

A few general statements can be made about the distribution of ribosomes in cells that have different capacities for the synthesis of proteins.

- Cells that synthesize large numbers of proteins have numerous ribosomes; conversely, cells that synthesize small numbers of proteins contain few.
- Of the proteins synthesized by a cell to be secreted from that cell for use elsewhere, most of the ribosomes are attached to the endoplasmic reticulum.
- Those cells that synthesize protein primarily for intracellular use have relatively few ribosomes attached to the endoplasmic reticulum membrane. Small groups of ribosomes called polysomes are involved in protein synthesis; under physiologic conditions polysomes are bound to the endoplasmic reticulum. The ribosome is bound to the membrane through its large subunit; the small subunit is involved in the binding of mRNA to the ribosome. The ribosomes have two binding sites used in protein synthesis: the amino-acyl site and the peptidyl site. These two sites have specific functions in protein synthesis.

Translation takes place in four stages, as illustrated in Figure 4.15. Each stage requires specific cofactors and enzymes. In the first stage, which occurs in the cytosol, the amino acids are activated by esterifying each one to its specific tRNA. This requires a molecule of ATP. In addition to a specific tRNA, each amino acid requires a specific enzyme for this reaction.

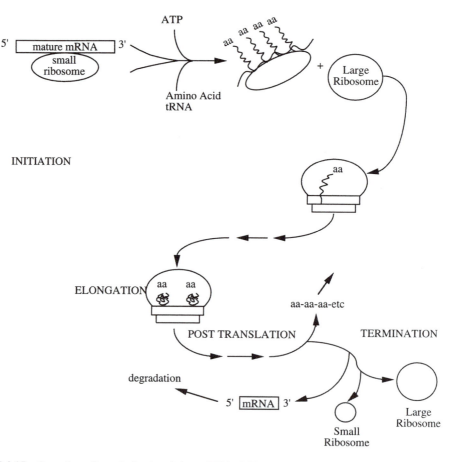

FIGURE 4.15   Overview of translation involving mRNA, tRNA-amino acids, small and large ribosomal units.

During the second stage, the initiation of the synthesis of the polypeptide chain occurs. Initiation requires that mRNA binds to the ribosome. An initiation complex is formed by the binding of mRNA cap and the first activated amino acid-tRNA complex to the small ribosomal subunit. The ribosome finds the correct reading frame on the mRNA by "scanning" for an AUG codon. The large ribosomal unit then attaches, thus forming a functional ribosome. A number of specific protein initiation factors (eIFs) are involved in this step.

In the third stage of protein synthesis, the peptide chain is elongated by the sequential addition of amino acids from the tRNA complexes. The amino acid is recognized by base pairing of the codon of mRNA to the bases found in the anticodon of tRNA and a peptide bond is formed between the peptide chain and the newly arrived amino acid. The ribosome then moves along the mRNA; this brings the next codon in the proper position for attachment of the next activated amino acyl-tRNA complex. The mRNA and nascent polypeptide appear to "track" through a groove in the ribosomal subunits. This protects them from attack by enzymes in the surrounding environment.

The final stage of protein synthesis is the termination of the chain. The termination is signaled by one of three special codons (stop codons) in the mRNA. After the carboxy terminal amino acid is attached to the peptide chain, it is still covalently attached to tRNA, which is, in turn, bonded to the ribosome. A protein-release factor promotes the hydrolysis of the ester link between the tRNA and the amino acid. Once the polypeptide chain is generated and free of the ribosome, it assumes its characteristic three-dimensional structure.

If, during the course of synthesis, there is any interference in the continuity of a supply of the needed amino acids, synthesis is stopped. Here lies the basis for the time factor of protein synthesis, a feature that nutritionists have recognized for several decades. It was established, on the basis of animal-feeding experiments, that protein synthesis would not occur if all the needed amino acids were not provided at the same time. In addition, since protein biosynthesis is very costly in terms of its energy requirement, synthesis is severely inhibited by starvation or energy restriction. In experimental animals, it has been shown that starvation inhibits the polymerization of mRNA units, thus significantly reducing the activity of the transcription process. Other studies have shown that animals starved and then refed "overcompensate" for this period of reduced mRNA synthesis by markedly increasing mRNA synthesis above normal during the period of realimentation after the starvation period. This starved–refed-induced increase in mRNA is manifested as an increase in the synthesis of enzymes necessary for the metabolism of the various ingredients in the diet used for realimentation. The signal(s) for the release of the starvation-induced inhibition of mRNA and enzyme synthesis include the macronutrients in the diet as well as the hormones glucocorticoid, thyroxine, insulin, and others.

If there is a mutation in the sequence of bases that the genetic code for a given protein comprises, the amino acid sequence generated in a protein will be incorrect. Whether this substitution of one amino acid for another in the protein being generated affects the functionality of the protein being generated depends entirely on the amino acid in question. Some amino acids can be replaced without affecting the secondary, tertiary, or quaternary structures of the protein (and hence, its chemical and physical properties) whereas others cannot. In addition, genetic errors in amino acid sequence may pose no threat to the individual if the protein in question is of little importance in the maintenance of health and well being, or it can have large effects on health if the protein is a critical one. In the synthesis of the important protein, hemoglobin, if the genetic code calls for the use of valine instead of the usual glutamic acid in the synthesis of the β chain in the hemoglobin molecule, the resulting protein is less able to carry oxygen. This amino acid substitution not only affects the oxygen-carrying capacity of the red blood cell but also affects the solubility of the hemoglobin in the red blood cell cytosol. This, in turn, affects the shape of the red blood cell, changing it from a dumbbell-shaped donut to a shape resembling a sickle, hence the name sickle cell anemia. The decreased solubility of the hemoglobin can be understood if one remembers the relative polarity of the glutamic acid and valine molecules. The glutamic acid side chain is more ionic and thus contributes more to the solubility of the protein than the nonpolar carbon chain of valine. This change in pH decreases its solubility in water, and, of course, a change in solubility leads to an increased viscosity of the blood as the red cells rupture spilling their contents into the blood stream.

The amino acid sequence within a given species for a given protein is usually similar. However, some individual variation does occur. An example of an "acceptable" amino acid substitution would be some of the ones that account for the species differences in the hormone insulin. As a hormone, insulin serves a variety of important functions in the regulation of carbohydrate, lipid, and protein metabolism. Yet, even though there are species differences in the amino acid sequence of this protein, insulin from one species can be given to another species and be functionally active. Obviously, the species differences in the amino acid sequence of this protein are not at locations in the chains that determine its biological function in promoting glucose use.

After translation is complete, the primary structure is complete. At this point, some post-translation modification can occur and specific nutrients can again influence the process. For example, after the translation of osteocalcin and prothrombin, two proteins that have glutamic acid-rich regions, these glutamate residues are carboxylated. This post-translational carboxylation requires vitamin K. Should vitamin K be in short supply, this carboxylation will not occur (or will occur in only a limited way) and these proteins will not be able to bind calcium. Both must bind calcium in order to function; osteocalcin in bone cannot bind calcium nor can prothrombin. Hence, bone will be more fragile and blood will not clot as needed.

As the chain of amino acid is produced the amino acids in that chain begin to interact; at first locally to form the protein's secondary structure. Then, as the chain twists and turns, more global interactions occur and the tertiary structure becomes apparent. All of these interactions, i.e., hydrogen bonding, disulfide bridges, etc. serve to stabilize the protein. Finally, as these tertiary structures are synthesized, they assemble as subunits of more-complex structures (quartenary structures) in the functional protein. Some very complex proteins have many subunits — for example, the cytochromes in the mitochondrial respiratory chain — whereas others have few.

Protein Turnover

Protein turnover consists of two processes: synthesis and degradation. Synthesis is described in the preceding section. The proteins synthesized by the body have a finite existence. They are subject to a variety of insults and modifications. Some of these modifications, touched upon as metabolic control processes, have been discussed — a prohormone is converted to an active hormone, an enzyme is activated or inactivated with the addition or removal of a substituent, and so forth. Thus, a dynamic state within the body exists with respect to its full complement of peptides and proteins. Some proteins have very short lifetimes and very rapid turnover times; other proteins are quite stable and long lived. Their turnover time is quite long. The estimate of the life of a protein, that is, how long it will exist in the body, is its half-life (see Unit 2). A half-life is that time interval that occurs when half of the amount of a compound synthesized at time X will have been degraded. Given the dynamic state of metabolism, some of these time estimates will be very short. Half-lives of biologically active compounds are very difficult to estimate, yet the concept is handy when one is trying to understand and quantitate the turnover of body protein. Hormones are examples of short-lived proteins. They may be released, serve their function, and be degraded within a very short period (seconds to minutes to hours) of time. The protein of the lens is an example of the latter; once synthesized, the lens protein is not degraded or recycled. Adult humans have a daily turnover of about 1–2% of their total body protein. Most of this is muscle protein because the largest group of body proteins comprises muscle.

Protein Degradation

Protein degradation ultimately results in amino acids that are usually recycled (Figure 4.4). There are some exceptions to this general rule; histidine in the muscle protein is methylated and excreted as 3-methyl histidine. This 3-methyl histidine cannot be reused and thus is an indication of muscle breakdown. Most of the products of protein degradation (the liberated amino acids) join the body's amino acid pool, from which the synthetic processes withdraw their needed supply. It is estimated that 75–80% of the liberated amino acids are reused.

Different proteins are degraded at different rates, which are determined not only by the physiological status of the individual but also by the amino acid composition of the protein in question. High rates of degradation of the structural proteins mean that considerable structural rearrangement is occurring. For example, during starvation, structural proteins are degraded at higher rates than during nonstarvation conditions. Prolonged trauma also elicits accelerated structural protein degradation. Short-lived proteins such as those mentioned above as proteins, enzymes, or receptors have in common regions rich in proline, glutamate, serine, and threonine. These amino acids, when clustered, provide a target for rapid degradation.

The process of degradation first reduces the protein to peptides and then reduces these peptides to their constituent amino acids. Two major pathways are used for this process. Extracellular, membrane, and long-lived intracellular proteins are degraded in the lysosomes by an ATP independent pathway. Short-lived proteins as well as abnormal proteins are degraded in the cytosol using ATP and ubiquitin. This pathway is illustrated in Figure 4.16.

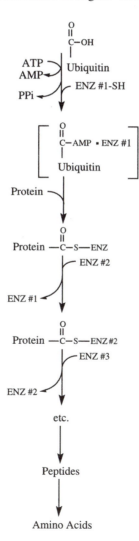

FIGURE 4.16 General pathway for intracellular protein degradation.

Protein degradation in the cytosol requires energy from ATP and the highly conserved 76 amino acid protein called ubiquitin. Proteins that are to be degraded via the ubiquitin-dependent pathway are derivatized by several molecules of ubiquitin. The ubiquitin is attached by non-peptide bonds between the carboxy terminus of ubiquitin and the δ amino groups of lysyl residues in the protein. This requires ATP.

Although the proteases of digestion are important to the degradation of dietary protein, they have no role in the intracellular protein degradation. Intracellular proteases hydrolyze internal peptide bonds. This is followed by the action of carboxy- and aminopeptidases, which remove single amino acids from the carboxy end or the amino end of the peptides.

Proteins in the extracellular environment are brought into the cell by endocytosis. This is a process similar to pinocytosis, where the cell membrane engulfs and encapsulates the extracellular material. Endocytosis occurs at indentations in the plasma membrane that are internally coated with a protein called *clathrin*. As in pinocytosis, the extracellular protein is surrounded by the plasma membrane to form an intracellular vesicle which, in turn, fuses with a lysosome. Degradation then occurs via calcium-dependent proteases called calpains or cathepsin. Both the Golgi and the endoplasmic reticulum are involved in providing proteases that degrade peptide fragments that arise during the maturation of proteins in the secretory pathway.

The rate of degradation varies from protein to protein and this rate is determined by the amino acid at the amino end of the protein amino acid chain. Proteins with short half-lives have regions rich in proline, glutamate, serine, and threonine. Proteins that are degraded slowly therefore have slower turnover times and longer half-lives.

Amino Acid Catabolism

Those amino acids in the body's amino acid pool that are neither used for peptide or protein synthesis nor to synthesize metabolically important intermediates are deaminated, and the carbon skeletons are either oxidized or used for the synthesis of glucose or fatty acids. Very little fatty acid synthesis occurs in humans consuming 20–30% of their energy as fat. There are three general reactions for the removal of NH_3 from the amino acids.

1. They can be transaminated with the amino group transferred to another carbon chain via amino transaminases.
2. They can be oxidatively deaminated to yield NH_3.
3. They can be deaminated through the activity of an amino acid oxidase.

Figure 4.17 illustrates these general reactions.

The amino acids can be loosely grouped in terms of their catabolism. Valine, leucine, and isoleucine, the branched chain amino acids, are similar in that each has a methyl group on its carbon chain. They can be transaminated with α ketoglutarate to form α keto acids. These acids are considered homologs of pyruvate and are oxidized by a series of enzymes that are similar to those that catalyze the oxidation of α ketoglutarate and pyruvate. The degradative steps are shown in Figure 4.18. Valine ultimately is converted to succinyl CoA, whereas isoleucine ends up as either acetyl CoA or propionyl CoA and leucine catabolism results in HMG CoA (ß-hydroxy ß-methyl-glutaryl coenzyme CoA). HMG CoA is split to acetyl CoA and acetoacetate. The HMG CoA produced in the catabolism of leucine is not used for cholesterol synthesis because it is produced in the mitochondria and does not travel to the cytosol, where cholesterol is synthesized. Instead, HMG CoA is further metabolized to acetoacetate and acetyl CoA.

Serine, threonine, and glycine are hydroxyamino acids. All three are gluconeogenic precursors (see Unit 5). Serine can be deaminated to pyruvate, which then can be transaminated to alanine. Serine can also be demethylated to form glycine, releasing a methyl group useful in one carbon metabolism. Threonine is degraded to acetyl CoA after deamination, as shown in Figure 4.19.

1. Transamination

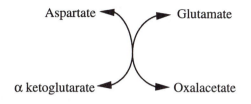

2. Oxidative deamination

$$\text{Glutamate} + \text{NAD(P)}^+ + \text{HOH} \longrightarrow \alpha \text{ ketoglutarate} + \text{NADPH}^+\text{H}^+$$
$$+ \text{NH}_3$$

3. Amino acid oxidase

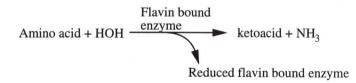

FIGURE 4.17 Amino acid reactions that result in the removal or transfer of the amino group.

Glutamate may be converted to glutamine via the enzyme glutamine synthetase. This enzyme is a mitochondrial enzyme and serves to fix the ammonia released in this compartment. Rat renal tissue is particularly rich in this enzyme, but human renal tissue is not. In birds and alligators, this enzyme is a cytosolic enzyme rather than a mitochondrial enzyme. Although the brain has some urea cycle activity, it uses glutamine formation primarily to reduce its ammonia level. To do this, it must also synthesize glutamate from α ketoglutarate. If it did not also convert pyruvate to oxalacetate, this synthesis of α ketglutarate would deplete the brain of citric acid cycle intermediates. Fortunately, carboxylation of pyruvate is very active in brain tissue.

Glutamate is converted to and formed from ornithine and arginine. These two amino acids are essential components of the urea cycle (Figure 4.20). The urea cycle consists of the synthesis of carbamyl phosphate, the synthesis of citrulline, then arginosuccinate, arginine, and, finally, urea. Ornithine and citrulline are shuttled back and forth as the cycle turns to get rid of the excess ammonia via urea release from arginine. The cycle functions to reduce the potentially toxic amounts of ammonia that arise when the ammonia group is removed from amino acids. Most of the ammonia released reflects the coupled action of the transaminases and L-glutamate dehydrogenase. The glutamate dehydrogenase is a bidirectional enzyme that plays a pivotal role in nitrogen metabolism.

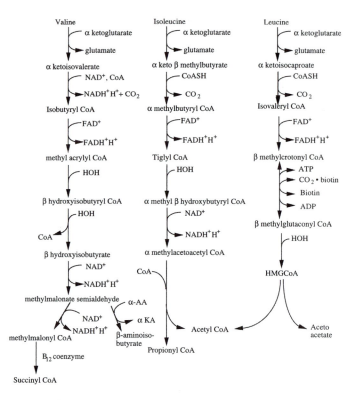

FIGURE 4.18 Catabolism of branched chain amino acids showing their use in the production of metabolites that are either lipid precursors or metabolites that can be oxidized via the Krebs cycle.

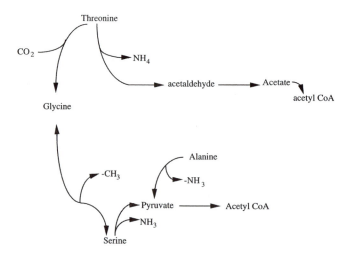

FIGURE 4.19 Catabolism of threonine showing its relationship to that of serine and glycine.

It is present in kidney, liver, and brain. It uses either NAD^+ or $NADP^+$ as a reducing equivalent receiver. It operates close to equilibrium using ATP, GTP, NADH, and ADP depending on the direction of the reaction. In catabolism, it channels NH_3 from glutamate to urea. In anabolism, it channels ammonia to α ketoglutarate to form glutamate. In the brain, glutamate can be decarboxylated to form γ-aminobutyrate (GABA), an important neurotransmitter. The decarboxylation is

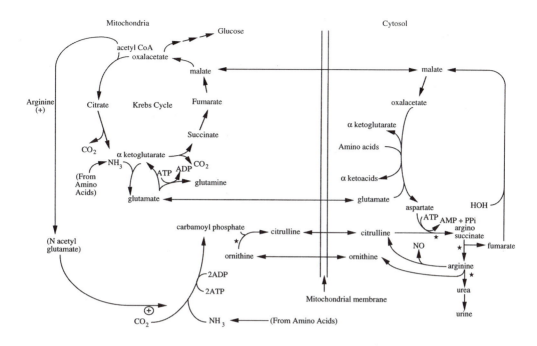

FIGURE 4.20   The urea cycle. Locations of mutations in the urea cycle enzymes are indicated with a star. Persons with these mutations have very short lives, with evidence of mental retardation, seizures, coma, and early death due to the toxic effects of ammonia accumulation. Rate controlling steps are indicated with a circled cross.

catalyzed by the enzyme, L-glutamate decarboxylase. Putrescine also can serve as a precursor of GABA either by deamination or via N-acetylated intermediates.

The urea cycle is, energetically speaking, a very expensive process. The synthesis of urea requires 3 moles of ATP for every mole of urea formed. The urea cycle is very elastic. That is, its enzymes are highly conserved, readily activated, and readily deactivated. Adaptation to a new level of activity is quickly achieved. While urea-cycle activity can be high when protein-rich diets are consumed and low when low-protein diets are consumed, the cycle never shuts down completely. The cycle, shown in Figure 4.21, is fine-tuned by the first reaction, the synthesis of carbamoyl phosphate. This reaction, which occurs in the mitochondria, is catalyzed by the enzyme carbamoyl phosphate synthetase. The enzyme is inactive in the absence of its allosteric activator, N-acetylglutamate, a compound synthesized from acetyl CoA and glutamate in the liver. As arginine levels increase in the liver, N-acetylglutamate synthetase is activated. This results in an increase in N-acetylglutamate. The urea cycle is initiated in the hepatic mitochondria and finished in the cytosol. The urea is then liberated from arginine via arginase and released into the circulation, whereupon it is excreted from the kidneys in the urine. Ornithine, the other product of the arginase reaction, is recyled back to the mitochondria only to be joined once again to carbamyl phosphate to make citrulline. Rising levels of arginine turn on mitochondrial N-acetylglutamate synthetase, which provides the N-acetylglutamate which, in turn, activates carbamoyl phosphate synthetase and the cycle goes on.

Arginine has many uses in metabolism. Not only is it an essential component of the urea cycle, it is a precursor for nitric oxide (NO), the polyamines, proline, glutamate, and creatine. Figure 4.21 shows how arginine is used in these pathways. When citrulline is produced from arginine, NO is produced. This occurs not only in the liver but also in other vital organs and the vascular tree. Nitric oxide production by endothelial cells is a vasodilator and thus plays a role in the regulation of smooth muscle tone. Many vasodilators such as the widely prescribed drug for angina pain, nitroglycerine, work by increasing the production of nitric oxide.

Phenylalanine is the precursor of tyrosine and the use of tyrosine as a hormone precursor has already been described (see Figure 4.7). Phenylalanine is converted to tyrosine via the hepatic enzyme phenylalanine hydroxylase. A number of mutations in the gene for this enzyme have been found and result in the disease phenylketonuria. This, if not diagnosed within the first few weeks of life, results in mental retardation. Tyrosine, if not used to make one of several hormones, is then deaminated and, through a series of reactions, ends up as fumarylacetate, which is split to provide acetoacetate and fumarate. Tryptophan catabolism shows no similarity to the catabolic pathways of any of the other amino acids. The pathway used by phenylalanine and tyrosine is outlined in Figure 4.21 and the pathway for tryptophan is shown in Figure 4.22. Tryptophan can be converted to niacin, one of the B vitamins. This conversion is not very efficient.

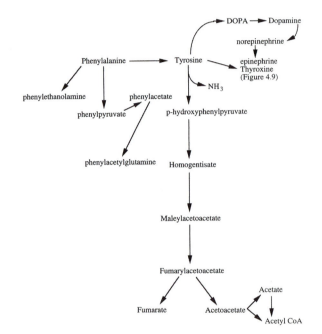

FIGURE 4.21 Phenylalanine and tyrosine catabolism. This pathway has a number of mutations that result in a variety of genetic diseases (see Table 4.17)

There is considerable product feedback inhibition of this reaction sequence by niacin. The metabolism of tryptophan is dependent on adequate intakes of vitamin B_6, pyridoxine. In pyridoxine deficiency, hydroxyanthranilate formation via the enzyme kynureninase is impaired, resulting in a characteristic increase in urinary levels of xanthurenic acid. This is used as a test of vitamin B_6 sufficiency. If subjects are deficient and are given a load dose of tryptophan, these subjects will excrete abnormal amounts of xanthurenate in their urine.

Tryptophan is the precursor of serotonin, an important neurotransmitter that serves a variety of functions in the regulation of smooth muscle tone, especially those smooth muscles of the vascular tree. In so doing, it plays an especially important role in the maintenance of blood pressure and the control of blood supply to the brain and vital organs. Several important drugs that address the problem of clinical depression alter the synthesis of serotonin from tryptophan or alter the action of serotonin once formed. Some of these drugs alter food intake as well (see Unit 3).

Histidine, an amino acid especially important for muscle protein biosynthesis is also of great importance in one-carbon metabolism. The principal pathway of histidine catabolism leads to glutamate formation and is shown in Figure 4.23 (as well as in other figures where glutamate and α ketoglutarate act in transamination). Glutamate is an important component of the urea cycle

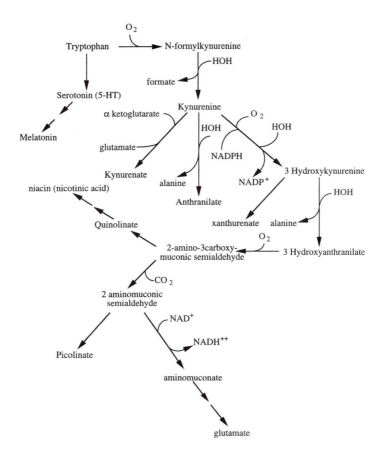

FIGURE 4.22 Catabolism of tryptophan showing conversion to the vitamin niacin. This conversion is not very efficient. Tryptophan catabolism also results in picolinate, which is believed by some to play a role in trace-mineral conservation.

(Figure 4.20). The decarboxylation of histidine yields histamine. This amine serves to stimulate gastric hydrochloric acid production and to stimulate vasoconstriction. A number of cold remedies and sinus remedies contain substances known as antihistamines that interfere with the vasoconstrictor action of histamine. Histidine in muscle can be methylated and the end product 3 methyl histidine can be measured in the urine and used as a measure of muscle protein turnover.

Lysine is one of the two essential amino acids whose amino group does not contribute to the total body amino group pool; the other is threonine. Although lysine can donate its amino group to other carbon chains, the reverse does not occur. Lysine is catabolized to acetoacetyl CoA, which then enters the Krebs cycle as acetyl CoA.

Methionine, cysteine, and cystine are important sulfur group donors. The importance of disulfide bridges in the structure of proteins has been described in the sections on protein structure and synthesis. Methionine is important for carnitine synthesis (see Unit 6). The pathway for methionine and cysteine is shown in Figure 4.24. Propionate is also the result of methionine catabolism. Should there be a defect in propionyl CoA carboxylase, propionate will accumulate. This is not the usual situation, for propionate is usually carboxylated to form succinyl CoA. Accumulation of methyl malonate is characteristic of vitamin B_{12} deficiency. Propionate can serve as the substrate for long-chain, odd-numbered fatty acids that are incorporated into myelin, the fatty covering of nerves. For some unknown reason, this myelin is abnormal in its function and fails to protect the peripheral nerve endings, which then die. This might explain the peripheral paresia that characterizes B_{12} deficiency. Just as mutations in the genes that encode proteins important to the regulation of energy

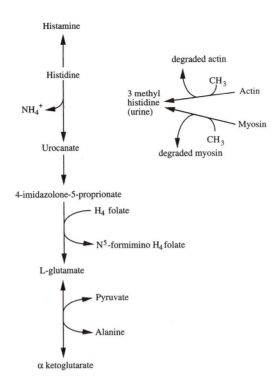

FIGURE 4.23 Catabolism of histidine. Note that 3-methyl histidine is not part of the pathway. This metabolite is formed in the muscle when the contractile proteins actin and myosin are methylated.

balance can occur with sometimes-serious, life-threatening effects, so too are there mutations in the genes that encode components of the metabolism of amino acids. Some of these are shown in Table 4.17.

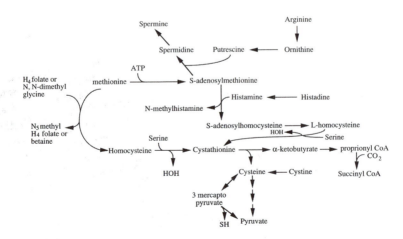

FIGURE 4.24 Conservation of SH groups via methionine–cysteine interconversion. Spermine, putrescine, and spermidine are polyamines that are important in cell and tissue growth.

TABLE 4.17
Genetic Mutations in Enzymes of Amino Acid Metabolism

Disease	Mutation	Characteristics
Maple syrup urine disease	Branched chain keto acid dehydrogenase (Several variants)	Elevated levels of α ketoacids and their metabolites in blood and urine; mental retardation, ketoacidosis, early death
Methylmalonuria	Methylmalonyl CoA mutase (Several variants) Inability to use vitamin B_{12}	High blood levels of methylmalonate; pernicious anemia, early death
Nonketotic hyperglycinemia	Glycine cleavage enzyme	Severe mental retardation, early death, high blood glycine levels
Hypermethioninemia	Methionine adenosyltransferase ($\uparrow$Km not deficiency per se)	Accumulation of methionine in blood (condition is benign)
Homocysteinemia	Cystathionine synthase	Elevated blood levels of methionine, homocysteine; abnormal collagen (no cross linking); dislocated lenses and other ocular malformations; osteoporosis; mental retardation, thromboembolism and vascular occlusions; short lifespan
Cystathioninuria	Cystathionase	Elevated levels of cystathionine in urine (condition is benign)
Phenylketonuria	Phenylalanine hydroxylase (several variants)	Increased levels of phenylalanine and deaminated metabolites in blood and urine; mental retardation; decreased neurotransmitter synthesis; shortened lifespan
Tyrosinemia	Tyrosine transaminase	Eye and skin lesions, mental retardation
	Fumarylacetoacetate hydrolase	Liver failure, renal failure
	p-hydroxylphenylpyruvate oxidase	Increased need for ascorbic acid
Albinism	Tyrosinase	Lack of melanin (skin pigment) formation; increased sensitivity to sunlight; lack of eye pigment
Alcaptonuria	Homogentisate oxidase	Elevated urine levels of homogentisate; slow deposits of homogentisate in bones, connective tissue and internal organs resulting in gradual darkening of these structures. Increased susceptibility to arthritis
Histidenemia	Histidase	Elevated levels of histidine in blood and urine. Can give false positive result in test for phenylketonuria. Elevated urocanase levels in sweat. Decreased histamine formation.

Amino Acid Derivatives

Creatine phosphate

The energy needed to drive the energy-dependent reactions of the body is provided by the high-energy bonds of the adenine nucleotides, the guanine nucleotides, and the uridylnucleotides. The concentrations of these nucleotides are carefully regulated and their energy is metered out as needed. Short, quick bursts of energy from these nucleotides are not possible. However, Mother Nature has devised another compound, creatine phosphate, that can do just this. Creatine is formed from glycine, arginine, and S-adenyl methionine in a reaction sequence as shown in Figure 4.25. The creatine circulates in the blood and can be found in measurable quantities in brain and muscle. The

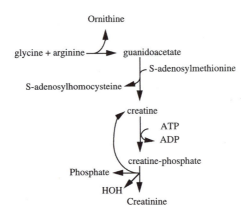

FIGURE 4.25   Formation of creatine phosphate.

creatine is phosphorylated to form creatine phosphate via the enzyme creatine kinase. Creatine can be converted to creatinine by irreversible nonenzymatic dehydration. Upon hydrolysis, creatine phosphate will provide sufficient energy for muscle contraction. This hydrolysis yields creatine and inorganic phosphate. Some of the creatine can be rephosphorylated, while the remainder is converted to creatinine that then is excreted in the urine. Creatine phosphate has the same free energy of hydrolysis as ATP. Creatine phosphate is found primarily in the muscle and provides the quick burst of energy needed each time a muscle contracts. Since the muscle activity produces the end product, creatinine, measuring creatinine allows for the estimation of the muscle mass (see Unit 2).

Because creatinine excretion is reasonably constant from day to day, researchers use the amount of creatinine in a 24-hour urine collection as an assurance of the completeness of the urine sample. Variations can occur if the generally sedentary subject has an unusually active day. A dramatic increase in muscle use will result in an increase in creatine-phosphate breakdown and an increase in creatinine excretion.

Choline

Choline is a highly methylated compound synthesized from serine. It is an essential component of the neurotransmitter acetylcholine, as well as an essential ingredient of the phospholipid, phosphatidylcholine.

Polyamines

Certain amino acids can be decarboxylated to form the polyamines (See Figure 4.24). Some polyamines are very short-lived compounds that are neurotransmitters. They are quickly broken down so as to limit their effects. The catecholamines fall into this category of polyamines. Other polyamines, putrescine and spermine, bind nucleic acids and other polyanions. They have a role in cell division.

FUNCTIONS OF PROTEINS

A variety of proteins are found in the body. Each serves a specific function in the maintenance of life. Any loss in body protein, in effect, means a loss in cellular function. In contrast to lipids and carbohydrates, which have a body reserve to be used in times of need, the functioning body has no true protein reserve. Humans, when they are deprived of or insufficiently supplied with protein, will compensate for this dietary deficiency by catabolizing some, but not all, of their tissue protein with a consequent loss in tissue functionality. Cells, tissues, organs, and whole systems cannot exist without the proteins serving their various functions.

PROTEINS AS ENZYMES

From conception to death, living cells use oxygen and metabolize fuel. Cells synthesize new products, degrade others, and generally are in a state of metabolic flux. For these processes to occur, catalysts are needed to enhance each of the many thousands of reactions occurring in the cell. These catalysts, called enzymes, are proteins. Enzymes make up the largest and most specialized class of proteins. Each enzyme is unique and catalyzes a specific kind of reaction. In the cell, enzymes are found in all the cellular compartments (cytoplasm, nucleus, mitochondria, etc.) as well as the membranes within and around the cell. The membrane-associated enzymes are part of the protein component of the cell wall. The location of an enzyme is one of its characteristics and dictates, in part, its role in metabolism.

Enzymes consist of specific sequences of amino acids. Should the sequence deviate, alterations in enzyme activity can be anticipated, unless, of course, the change in amino acid does not affect the active site of the enzyme or its molecular shape. The importance of the amino acid sequence is obvious and is related to the availability of R groups (on the amino acids) that will complement reactive groups on the substrate, the molecule on which the enzyme exerts its catalytic action. The catalytic function of the enzyme is intimately related to its amino acid sequence. Enzymes must possess a shape that will complement the molecular shape of the substrate in much the same way as a key fits into a lock. This shape, of course, is a function of the enzyme protein's primary, secondary, tertiary, and quaternary structure. Just as enzymes must have a specific shape, substrates must also have specific shapes to be catalyzed by their respective enzymes. This is the reason that only D-sugars or only L-amino acids can be metabolized by mammalian cells. These sterioisomers conform to the shape required by the enzyme that serves as its catalyst. While enzymes show absolute specificity, the specificity generally applies to only a portion of the substrate molecule. If the substrate is a small compound, this specificity applies to the entire molecule. If, however, the substrate is large and complex, the structural requirements are less stringent in that only that part of the substrate involved in the enzyme–substrate complex must have the appropriate molecular arrangement. The portion of the substrate not involved in the reaction (i.e., the nature of the R group) need not be the appropriate conformation. How does this specificity work? Many substrate–enzyme complexes form with a three-point attachment that leaves a fourth atom or R group free. If the attachment site can be approached from only one direction and only complementary atoms can attach, the substrate molecule can bind in only one way.

Some enzymes are specific for only one substrate; others may catalyze several related reactions. While some are specific for a particular substrate, others are specific for certain bonds. This is called *group specificity.* For example, glycosidases act on glycosides (any glycoside), pepsin and trypsin act on peptide bonds, and esterases act on ester linkages. Within these groups, certain enzymes exhibit greater specificity than others. Chymotrypsin preferentially acts on peptide bonds in which the carboxyl group is a part of the aromatic amino acids (phenylalanine, tyrosine, or tryptophan). Enzymes such as carboxypeptidase or aminopeptidase catalyze the hydrolysis of the carboxy-terminal or amino-terminal amino acid of a polypeptide chain. This bond specificity rather than molecular specificity is useful to the animal in that it reduces the number of enzymes needed within the organism. Incidentally, the above enzymes are very useful to protein chemists in their determination of the amino acid sequence of a given protein.

Cells synthesize enzymes in much the same fashion as they synthesize other proteins, yet enzymes are relatively short lived. Cells must continually synthesize their enzymes if they are to survive. A variety of signals serve as stimulants or inhibitors of this synthesis. One of these signals is the substrate. An excess of substrate will not only activate any preexisting enzyme in the cell, but will also serve to stimulate enzyme synthesis. The substrate may act at the level of mRNA transcription or at the level of translation or protein assembly. Hormones such as insulin, thyroid hormone, and glucocorticoid may also serve in this way to stimulate enzyme synthesis and/or activation. Hormonal inhibition of enzyme synthesis also occurs and serves as an internal regulator of the synthetic process.

PROTEINS AS CARRIERS AND RECEPTORS

A wide variety of compounds is carried in the blood between tissues and organs of the body. Some of the compounds require a specific protein for their transport. Not only is this protein necessary for the transport of compounds insoluble in blood, but it is also necessary to protect these compounds from further reactions during the transport process. Some of the membrane proteins are carriers, some are both carriers and enzymes, and still others are receptors. Both intracellular and extracellular carriers and receptors have been identified. Receptors were discussed in Unit 2.

The plasma proteins that can have a carrier function are the albumin and the α and ß globulins. Perhaps the best studied of the plasma proteins are those associated with the transport of lipid, since these lipoproteins (carriers plus lipids), when elevated, appear to be related to the development of cardiovascular disease (see Unit 6). These lipoproteins make up about 3% of the plasma proteins. They are loose associations of such lipids as phospholipids, triacylglycerols, and cholesterols, and represent an example of how proteins function as carriers.

In addition to serving as carriers of lipids, some of the globulins in the plasma can combine stoichiometrically with iron and copper as well as with other divalent cations. These combinations are called metalloproteins. The globulins serve to transport these cations from the gut to the tissues where they are used. The monovalent cations, sodium and potassium, do not need carriers, but many minerals do.

Many hormones and vitamins require transport or carrier proteins to take them from their point of origin to their active site. In addition, there are intracellular transport proteins, such as those in the mitochondrial membrane, that are responsible for the transfer of metabolites between the mitochondrial and cytosolic compartments. Finally, there are transport proteins that carry single molecules. The classic example is, of course, hemoglobin, the red cell protein responsible for the transport of oxygen from the lungs to every oxygen-using cell in the body.

PROTEINS AS REGULATORS OF WATER BALANCE

As substrates and solutes are transferred or exchanged across membranes, water has a tendency to follow in order to maintain equal osmotic pressure on each side of the membrane. If osmotic pressure is not maintained, the individual cells either shrink from lack of internal water or burst from too much. The balance of water between the intracellular and extracellular compartments is closely regulated (see Unit 2).

One of the most carefully controlled points of water balance is across the capillary membrane, where a close balance is maintained between the osmotic pressure of the blood plasma, the interstitial fluids, and the cells and the hydrostatic pressure exerted by the pumping action of the heart. The total osmotic pressure of the plasma and of the intra- and extracellular fluids is the result of its content of inorganic electrolytes, its organic solutes, and its proteins. The concentrations of the electrolytes and organic solutes in plasma, interstitial fluid, and cells are substantially the same, so that the contribution to the osmotic pressure by these substances is practically equal. However, since there are more proteins in plasma than in the cells, plasma exerts an osmotic pressure on the tissue fluids. The result of this inequity of solutes is the drawing of fluids from the tissue spaces and from the cells into the blood. Opposing this force is the hydrostatic pressure exerted by the pumping action of the heart, which moves fluids from the blood into the tissue spaces and into the cells. The hydrostatic pressure is greater on the arterial side of the capillary loop than on the venous side. There is an interplay among these four kinds of pressure — blood osmotic pressure, tissue osmotic pressure, blood hydrostatic pressure, and tissue hydrostatic pressure. This interplay results in a filtration of solutes and metabolites and the transfer of oxygen from the arterial blood into the tissues and cells it supplies and on the venous side, a resorption from the tissue space of CO_2, metabolites and solutes back into the blood supply.

Albumin plays a more significant role in maintaining the osmotic pressure than the other blood proteins because of its size and abundance. In the blood, there are more albumin molecules than other serum proteins and thus, albumin has considerable influence on osmotic pressure. Malnourished individuals are characterized by a reduction in serum proteins. With fewer proteins in the serum, water leaks out into the interstitial space and accumulates. The condition known as edema results. The edema of protein deficiency may also be the result of the body's inability to synthesize the protein hormones, particularly ADH (see Unit 2), which plays a role in controlling water balance. Edema not involving protein deficiency can also result from other factors such as increased blood pressure or renal disease, but the edema that results in these situations is a result of factors other than the plasma proteins. The effect of protein is on the distribution of water among the various body compartments, rather than on the total body water.

PROTEINS AS BIOLOGICAL BUFFERS

Proteins have the ability to accept or donate hydrogen ions and by so doing they serve as biological buffers. In blood, there are three important buffering systems: plasma proteins, hemoglobin, and carbonic acid–bicarbonate. The equilibrium reactions for each of these buffering systems follows:

$$H\,Protein \Leftrightarrow H^+ + Protein^-$$

$$H_2CO_3 \Leftrightarrow H^+ + HCO_3^-$$

$$HHb \Leftrightarrow H^+ + Hb^-$$

The first of these buffering systems, the plasma proteins, can function as a weak acid/salt buffer when the free carboxyl groups on the protein dissociate or as a weak base/salt buffer when the free amino groups dissociate. Although the buffering ability of the plasma protein is extremely important in maintaining blood pH, it is not as important as the other two systems.

The second buffering system, carbonic acid–bicarbonate, is extremely effective because there are reactions that follow this equilibrium that will regulate either acids or bases. The H_2CO_3 level in plasma never goes too high because it is in equilibrium with CO_2 ($H_2CO_3 \Leftrightarrow CO_2 + H_2O$), which is expelled by the lungs. In blood, this equilibrium proceeds very quickly because of the presence of carbonic anhydrase, an enzyme found in red blood cells that catalyzes it. If the carbonic acid–bicarbonate reaction goes in the opposite direction, the concentration of the HCO_3^- so formed will be regulated by the kidneys.

The third important buffering system in blood results from hemoglobin. Hemoglobin has six times the buffering power of the plasma proteins. It functions well as a buffer for three reasons. First, it is present in large amounts. Second, it contains 38 histidine residues, which are good buffers because they can dissociate to H^+ and the imidazole group. Third, hemoglobin exists in blood in two forms, reduced hemoglobin and oxyhemoglobin. The imidozole groups of reduced hemoglobin dissociate less than those of oxyhemoglobin; thus, it is a weaker acid and a better buffer.

Hemoglobin's role in maintaining blood pH is extremely important and is best appreciated by understanding the transport of oxygen and carbon dioxide during respiration through the blood. Oxyhemoglobin is formed when each of the four ferrous ions in hemoglobin reversibly combines with one O_2 molecule. The reaction between oxygen and hemoglobin is written as Hb + O_2 → HbO_2. The combination is not an oxygenation reaction because iron stays in the positive two-oxidation state. Instead, there is a loose association that exists between the oxygen and hemoglobin molecules.

At an oxygen tension of at least 100 mm Hg, hemoglobin is almost completely saturated with oxygen. This curve (Figure 4.26) has a sigmoid shape rather than linear, because after the first oxygen molecule is added to the hemoglobin, the affinity for the second is increased; the second increases the affinity for the third, etc. This increase in affinity results because, as the O_2 is taken up, the two ß chains move closer together. As O_2 is given up, they move farther apart. When fully saturated, as it is at normal physiologic conditions, each gram of hemoglobin contains 1.34 mL of oxygen. In a normal 100 mL of blood, there are about 15 g of hemoglobin and, hence, 20 mL of oxygen.

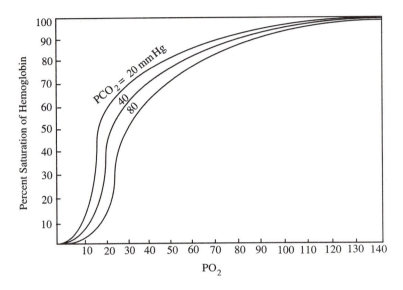

FIGURE 4.26   The dissociation curves of hemoglobin are 38 C and at partial pressures of CO_2 equal to 20, 40, and 80 mmHg. (Redrawn from Davenport: *The ABC of Acid-Base Chemistry*, 4th ed., University of Chicago Press, 1958.)

In addition to the oxygen carried in the blood in association with hemoglobin, there is additional oxygen present that is dissolved in the blood. Henry's law states that this concentration is a linear function of the pressure of the oxygen. Only 0.4 ml of oxygen is in blood by being dissolved there and, thus, the major source of oxygen in the blood is hemoglobin.

As the cells consume the oxygen carried to them by hemoglobin, the oxygen tension falls, the oxyhemoglobin more readily dissociates, and the saturation of the hemoglobin falls. At about 50 mm Hg, hemoglobin rapidly "unloads" its oxygen. In the tissues, oxygen tension is about 40 mm Hg. This tension is below that necessary for unloading to occur and a gradient of high to low oxygen tension exists that facilitates the passage of oxygen to the tissues. This gradual change in oxygen content of the blood can be followed visually. Leaving the lungs, the blood is bright red. As it moves through the vascular system toward the periphery, the blood gradually darkens and, by the time it returns to the lungs, it has a bluish hue, a color characteristic of deoxygenated hemoglobin and the reason that persons lacking good respiratory exchange have a bluish tinge to their skin.

The CO_2 that is expired by the cells is transported in three forms. That which diffuses into the red blood cells is rapidly hydrated to H_2CO_3 by the presence of the carbonic anhydrase. The H_2CO_3 then dissociates into H+ and HCO_3^-. The H+ is neutralized primarily by hemoglobin and the bicarbonate diffuses into the plasma. This is the form in which most expired CO_2 is carried. The hemoglobin is present primarily in the blood in the reduced form by the time significant quantities of carbon dioxide are present so it can better function as a buffer.

Some CO_2 that diffuses into red blood cells is not converted into bicarbonate ion but instead reacts with the amino groups of proteins, principally hemoglobin, to form carbamino compounds.

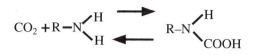

Reduced hemoglobin forms the carbamino compounds more readily than does oxyhemoglobin. The third form of CO_2 is that which is dissolved; it will exist as carbonic acid. It makes up only a small fraction of the total amount of CO_2 present. CO_2 present as carbonic acid will lower the blood pH.

That CO_2 that diffuses into the plasma also exists in these three forms. The carbamino compounds will form with the plasma proteins. Much less CO_2 is hydrated to form carbonic acid in plasma than in red blood cells because the carbonic anhydrase enzyme is located only in red blood cells. And, finally, a small amount of dissolved CO_2 is present in blood.

There is a much greater rise in the HCO_3^- concentration in red blood cells than in plasma. As a result, HCO_3^- will diffuse into the plasma. This represents the problem of maintaining electrochemical neutrality. It is accompanied by a diffusion of chloride ions from the plasma to the red blood cells. This phenomenon is known as the chloride shift. Since CO_2 transport will occur primarily in venous blood, the chloride content of venous blood is higher than that of arterial blood. At the lungs, when venous blood becomes arterial, all these reactions are reversed. Occasionally, these reactions are perturbed and the acid–base balance is not maintained. Under normal conditions, the carbonic acid:bicarbonate ratio is maintained at 1:20. When the CO_2 levels rise, carbonic acid levels rise and respiratory acidosis occurs. Conversely, when CO_2 levels fall, respiratory alkalosis occurs. By adjusting inspiration and expiration, respectively, small rises and falls in CO_2 levels can be adjusted, and the ratio of carbonic acid to bicarbonate remains constant. The kidney, through increasing its resorption of bicarbonate, can also assist in the regulation of this buffer system.

Large shifts in the acid–base balance that originate not in the respiratory system but rather as a result of metabolic alterations also occur. The prime example is the metabolic acidosis that occurs in the severe, uncontrolled diabetic. As a result of the lack of insulin, the metabolic fuel, glucose, cannot be used. The body then uses the alternate fuel, fatty acids. Fatty acid oxidation in the diabetic results in an accumulation of ketone bodies — acetone, acetoacetate, and ß-hydroxybutyrate. Normally, these substances are further oxidized to produce CO_2 and water. However, because so much fatty acid is being oxidized, its completion to CO_2 and water does not occur and the ketone bodies accumulate. These are acidic, and must be neutralized. All of the buffering systems are mobilized, but eventually they will not be able to compensate for this gradual increase in ketone bodies. The pH will fall, the enzymes that work at pH 7.4 will be appreciably less active, and the hemoglobin will become less able to carry oxygen. Unless treated with insulin, the patient will become comatose (lack of oxygen to the brain) and die.

Metabolic alkalosis is not nearly as common as metabolic acidosis. However, it can occur in persons having prolonged bouts of both diarrhea and vomiting. This is a result of the loss of the stomach acid, hydrochloric acid (the chloride ion), and the loss of potassium ions. Alkalosis can also occur in individuals who consume large quantities of alkali, as might occur in persons with peptic ulcers who self medicate with antacids. In any event, the elevated blood pH may result in slow and shallow breathing, lowered serum calcium and potassium levels, and muscle tetany (prolonged contractions). Buffering activity is not limited to the blood. The carbonic acid–bicarbonate buffering system is active in interstitial fluids. Intracellular buffers include the proteins and organic phosphates.

While the blood pH is maintained within a fairly narrow range through the systems just described, the urine pH can vary considerably depending on the metabolic state of the individual. The kidney and the urinary tract can tolerate a greater fluctuation in pH than can other tissues. Nonetheless, a number of buffer systems are also active in this tissue. In the kidney, although little buffering is done by the proteins, the bicarbonate buffer system is particularly active in the extracellular fluid. Once urine is produced, little effort is made to buffer its pH; it can vary from 4.7–8.0. The bladder and urinary tract are constructed so that this broad pH range is tolerated with little effect on the metabolism that occurs in these tissues.

PROTEINS AS STRUCTURAL ELEMENTS AND STRUCTURAL UNITS

The lipid component of the membrane is discussed in Unit 6. Analysis of the liver cell membrane has shown that this membrane contains 50–60% protein, 35% lipid, and 5% carbohydrate. The carbohydrate present is joined primarily to the protein-forming glycoproteins, compounds that constitute the receptors as well as the cell-recognition proteins. The protein portion of the membrane is so oriented that its hydrophilic aspects are also in proximity to the intracellular and extracellular fluids. The protein molecules are interspersed within the lipids and lend both structural stability and fluidity to the membrane.

Membrane function depends on how the proteins are placed in the membrane and on the fluidity that results from the combination of proteins in a lipid mixture. As indicated earlier, the lipid portion of the membrane needs to be fairly unsaturated. If saturated, a more rigid crystalline structure will form. By being fluid and less rigid, these lipids can allow the proteins to change their shape in response to ionic changes and thus these proteins can function as enzymes, carriers, or receptors, for the large variety of materials binding, entering, or leaving the cell.

How can these proteins serve in this fashion? Recall the protein conformation. The R groups of the amino acids project both in and out from the conformation and interact to form hydrogen bonds and disulfide bridges, however briefly, with compounds in proximity to them. Proteins that react with materials external to the cell may change their conformation and, in so doing, change their position within the membrane structure so that the reactive site changes from facing outward to the extracellular environment to facing inward toward the intracellular environment. Once facing inward, the material temporarily attracted to the membrane protein might be more attracted to another protein within the cell and "let go" of the membrane protein. Of course, this explanation is very simplistic. Transport into and out of cells probably involves many other reactions, a source of energy, and cations and/or anions for exchange. Yet this simplified explanation may be sufficient to explain the passage of a number of materials through the cell membrane. The reactive groups of the amino acid side chains, the R groups of the "structural" membrane proteins may also serve as identifiers or facilitators of reactive sites. Proteins serve as receptors for materials, such as insulin, that do not usually enter the cell. Insulin, also a protein, has reactive side chains protruding from it just as reactive side chains protrude from the proteins in the membrane. These two reactive groups interact and the binding of the insulin to the receptor occurs. Again, this is a very simplistic explanation of receptor action. In the instance of insulin, the receptor is probably a glycoprotein.

In addition to the function of proteins in the cell membrane as a structural element and as functional units, proteins are important intracellular structural units. Muscle is 20% protein, 75% water, and 5% inorganic material, glycogen, and other organic compounds. The major proteins in muscle are myosin, a large globular protein, and actin, a smaller globular protein. These two proteins plus the filamentous tropomyosin and troponin are the structural proteins of the muscles. The muscle proteins are characterized by their elasticity, which in turn contributes to the contractile power of this tissue.

Perhaps one of the most important structural functions of protein is that related to skin and connective tissue. The skin is composed of epithelial tissue that covers not only the exterior of the body but lines the gastrointestinal tract, the respiratory tract, and the urinary tract. One of the proteins found in the skin is melanin. Melanin is a tyrosine derivative and provides the pigmentation or color to the skin. Persons unable to form this pigment are albinos and their disease is called albinism. Three separate genetic errors have been identified as causes for albinism.

Another of the proteins found in skin is keratin, which is the protein that forms hair, nails, hooves, feathers, or horns. Each of these structures is slightly different from the others, but all contain keratin. This protein is insoluble in water and is resistant to most digestive enzymes. It has a high percentage of cystine.

Connective tissue holds all of the various cells and tissues together. It contains two distinct types of proteins: collagen and elastin. Collagen is the principal solid substance in white connective tissue. It contains a high percentage of proline, hydroxyproline, and glycine. It is difficult to degrade this protein and, like hair, it is relatively inert metabolically. Even in protein-deficient states, the body will synthesize collagen and elastin and these proteins will not be catabolized for needed amino acids. Incidentally, although the body does not readily catabolize collagen, this protein can be degraded to a limited degree by boiling in acid. It is then converted to gelatin. The collagen of bone, skin, cartilage, and ligaments differs in chemical composition from that of the white fibrous tissue that holds individual cells together within muscle, liver, and other organs. Elastin and chondroalbumoid are two other proteins in the connective tissue. They are present in small amounts and serve as part of the structural protein. Finally, bones and teeth belong to the structural protein class because they start out with a matrix protein ("ground substance") into which various amounts of minerals are deposited.

PROTEINS AS LUBRICANTS

The mucus of the respiratory tract, the oral cavity, the vaginal tract, and the rectal cavity reduces the irritation that might be caused by materials moving through these passages. This mucus is a mucoprotein, a conjugated protein that contains hexosamine. Proteins as lubricants also surround the joints and facilitate their movement. Should these lubricants be absent, or present but with substantial decreases in their fluidity through the deposition of minerals, skeletal movement may be difficult and painful.

PROTEINS IN THE IMMUNE SYSTEM

Proteins such as γ-globulin serve to protect the body against foreign cells. The immunoglobins produced by lymphocytes are large polypeptides having more than one basic monomeric unit. These proteins differ in their amino acid structure, which affects their secondary, tertiary, and quaternary structures. Just as the amino acid sequence of an enzyme determines substrate specificity, the amino acid sequence of the immunoprotein assures antigen–antibody specificity. The synthesis of particular immunoglobulins has been much studied. It is now well accepted that initiation of synthesis by the lymphocyte requires the binding of an antigen (a foreign protein) to the cell surface at particular locations called antigen receptors. As with other receptors on other cells, there must be a good conformational "fit" between the site and the antigen. Once the immunoglobulin is synthesized, it will bind with the foreign protein, immobilizing it, and the complex antigen–antibody will be formed.

PROTEIN INTAKE RECOMMENDATIONS

Human protein and amino acid requirements have been studied for well over 100 years using a variety of techniques. Nutrition scientists have collected data on the quantity of protein foods consumed vs. health, growth, and weight gain of various populations. The assumption was made that whatever "healthy" people ate was probably what kept them healthy and should, therefore, be used as a standard of comparison for other diets. These standards, with respect to protein, were invariably high for populations having an abundance of meat, milk, poultry, and fish in their diets. Voit and Atwater, around the turn of the century, found intakes of 118 and 125 g of protein per day, respectively, for adult men and termed these intakes as desirable.

As nutrition developed as a science, more-accurate methods for assessing nutrient needs were developed. Among these methods were those for assessing the intake and excretion of nitrogen compounds. The Kjeldahl method described in an earlier section as well as methods for determining the nitrogenous end products of metabolism were devised. These methods made possible the development of the concepts that today's scientists use to determine the nutrient requirements of humans as well as other species. In protein nutrition, it was realized that the body consists of two pools of protein, one with a short half-life that must be constantly renewed and one that is long lived, slowly broken down, and replaced. If one assumes that over a short period of time the pool having the long half-life contributes almost nothing to the nitrogenous metabolic end products, then a measure of the amount of nitrogen excreted will reflect only the turnover of the short-lived proteins. These proteins must be replaced by proteins newly synthesized from the amino acids provided by the diet. Hence, the term protein requirement (or the requirement for any nutrient) means that amount of protein that must be consumed to provide the amino acids for the synthesis of those body proteins irreversibly catabolized in the course of the body's metabolism. The intake of nitrogen from protein must be sufficient to balance that excreted; this basic concept is called nitrogen balance and has been discussed in the section that deals with the biological value of protein. While this concept is useful in understanding why we have a minimal need for protein in the diet, its application is fraught with difficulty. In the section on the biological value of protein, the possible sources of error in the nitrogen balance technique were discussed in terms of their contribution to the accuracy and precision of the methods available for comparing various food proteins. These same sources of errors also apply when using the nitrogen balance technique for assessing protein and amino acid requirements. Finally, the need for dietary protein is influenced by age, environmental temperature, energy intake, gender, micronutrient intake, infection, activity, previous diet, trauma, pregnancy, and lactation.

AGE

A protein intake in excess of maintenance needs is required when new tissue is being formed. Certain age periods, when growth is rapid, require more dietary protein than other periods. Age differences in protein turnover (protein flux) as well as protein synthesis explain some of the effect of age on protein need. Table 4.18 gives figures for humans at different ages. Premature infants (those infants born before their 10-lunar-month incubation time) grow at a very rapid rate and require between 2.5–5 g/protein/kg/day if they are to survive.

TABLE 4.18
Age Effects on Nitrogen Flux that Reflects Protein Flux and Protein Synthesis Rate Per Day

Age	Protein (N) Flux mg (N/kg/hr)	Total Body Protein Synthesis (g/kg/day)
Newborn	124 ± 46	17.4 ± 9.9
Infant	65 ± 7	6.9 ± 1.1
Young Adult	26 ± 2	3.0 ± 0.2
Elderly	19 ± 2	1.9 ± 0.15

Studies of full-term infants have indicated that a protein intake of 2–2.5 g/kg per day resulted in a satisfactory weight gain and that further increases in protein intake did not measurably improve growth. Older infants and children whose growth rate is not as rapid as the premature or newborn infant require considerably less protein (~ 1.25 g/kg/day). As growth rate increases during adolescence, the need for protein increases. Again, this can be related to the demands for dietary amino acids to support the growth process. As humans complete their growth, the need for protein decreases until it arrives at a level that is called the maintenance level. It is at this level that the concept of body protein replacement by dietary protein applies. During the growth period, it is very difficult to separate the requirements for maintenance from those of growth. The impulse for growth is so strong that it will occur in many instances at the *expense* of the maintenance of body tissues. For example, protein-malnourished children will continue to grow taller *even though* their muscles, as well as other tissues, show evidence of wastage due to dietary protein deficiency.

Growth carries with it not only a total nitrogen requirement but also a particular amino acid requirement. Maintenance, on the other hand, appears to have only a total protein requirement. Adults can make a number of short-term adjustments in their protein metabolism that can compensate for possible inequities or imbalances in amino acid intake as long as the total protein requirement is met. The young growing animal is not that flexible. The essential amino acid requirements are age-dependent. Histidine, although it can be synthesized in sufficient quantities by the adult to meet maintenance needs, is not synthesized in great enough amounts to support growth. Thus, histidine is an essential amino acid for the infant and growing child. This is due to the nature of the growth process.

At the other end of the life span, there are effects on protein need and metabolism. In part, this is due to the gradual accumulation of errors in the genetic code of the aging individual. Studies of humans from newborn to 80 years of age have shown that there is a graduate increase in the number of base deletions in the mitochondrial genome (see Unit 3). This may be due to the wide variety of genomic insults that occur over a lifespan. Exposure to ultraviolet light, noxious chemicals, drugs, or changes in the food supply can all affect the fidelity of the genome. These insults inflict their damage randomly so no one instance is responsible for the age effect, yet altogether there can be subtle and cumulative effects on gene expression and these, in turn, can affect the efficiency and fidelity of the gene products. Thus, metabolic processing of food materials loses its efficiency. The elderly person, although synthesizing less protein than the young growing person, may not synthesize this protein accurately. This, in turn, means a decline in function. Does this mean that the elderly may have an increase in protein need? We don't know. Until recently (see Unit 1), this portion of the population had not been well studied vis à vis protein need.

ENVIRONMENTAL TEMPERATURE

As environmental temperatures rise or fall above or below the range of thermic neutrality, animals begin to increase their energy expenditure to maintain their body temperature. In environments that are too warm, vasodilation occurs along with sweating and increased respiration. All of these mechanisms are designed to cool the body and all require an increase in the basal energy requirement as expressed per unit of body surface area. In cool environments, vasoconstriction and shivering occur in an effort to warm the body and prevent undue heat loss. Again, an increase in basal energy requirement is observed. Smuts, in 1934, found that nitrogen requirements were related to basal energy requirements. Through the study of a large number of species, he concluded that 2 mg nitrogen was required for every basal kcalorie required when the energy requirement was expressed on a surface area basis. Thus, any increase in basal energy needs due to change in environmental temperature will, because of the relationship between protein and energy, be accompanied by an increase in the protein requirement for maintenance. In addition, profuse sweating, as it occurs in very warm environments, carries with it a nitrogen loss that must be accounted for in the determination of minimal protein needs.

PREVIOUS DIET

The effects of previous diet on the determination of protein requirements may be rather profound. If, for example, the subjects selected for studies on protein needs have been poorly nourished prior to the initiation of the study, their retention of the protein during the study will be greater than would be observed in subjects who have been well nourished prior to the initiation of the study. In other words, malnourished subjects have a higher protein requirement than well-nourished subjects. This, of course, raises the issue of whether there are body protein reserves. Voit, Wilson, Cuthbertson, Fisher and others observed that animals fed a protein-free diet exhibit a "lag" before their nitrogen excretion level is minimized; during this phase, the animal is metabolizing his protein reserve. Other investigators maintain that there is no such thing as a protein reserve or store. These investigators maintain that every protein in the body has a function and if some of these proteins are lost, there is a loss in body function. Support for this concept is seen in the reduced ability of protein-depleted animals to fight infection or respond to the metabolic effects of trauma. Whether one believes that there is such an entity as a protein reserve may depend upon whether one perceives a difference between an optimal protein intake and a minimum protein intake. This difference may relate more to a personal opinion on how nutrient requirements should be defined. Some nutritionists believe in stating the absolute minimum requirement to sustain life and then adding on increments for each body function above mere survival; this is known as the particulate approach. Other nutritionists believe that one cannot separate and quantitate the individual requirements of each function beyond survival. They advocate a protein intake sufficient for optimal function of the animal; this is known as the integrative approach. The particulate and integrative approaches each have their merits when argued intellectually. However, since man does not merely exist, many human nutritionists tend to take the integrative approach to human nutrition requirements in their determination of protein needs.

PHYSICAL ACTIVITY

Research on protein needs for muscular work had its beginning in 1863 when Von Leiberg postulated that muscle as protein was destroyed with each contraction of the muscle. On this basis, he recommended that heavy muscular work required a heavy protein diet. This theory has been amply disproved, yet even today, many believe that a protein-rich diet will contribute to athletic prowess. Today, we know that muscle contraction does not result in destruction of the muscle. It does, however, require energy in the form of ATP, glucose, and fatty acids, and does result in the breakdown of creatine-phosphate to creatine, some of which is then converted to creatinine, a nitrogenous waste product excreted in the urine.

As the energy requirement is increased to support the increase in muscular activity, so too is the protein requirement in much the same manner as described above for the effects of temperature. In a number of studies, the athletic performance of subjects could not be directly related to the quantity of protein consumed above that determined to be the requirement for those subjects. When subjects were fed less than their respective protein requirements, their muscular efficiencies were reduced unless a vigorous training program was included as part of the experiment's protocol. Since most of the studies were of short duration and since muscle protein has a relatively long half-life, the lack of any demonstrable effect of protein intake on muscle performance (aside from the energy/protein relationship) is not surprising.

Other factors such as *sex, pregnancy, lactation,* and *trauma* affecting the protein requirement have been studied. As can be anticipated, males, due to their greater physical activity and larger body size, have a larger protein requirement than females; pregnancy, lactation, and trauma all increase the protein requirement.

RECOMMENDED DIETARY ALLOWANCES

For many years, the RDA for protein was set at 1 g/kg body weight for the average adult male. He was assumed to weigh 70 kg (about 155 pounds) so the RDA was 70 g/day. With an ever-increasing database that the Nutrition Board of the National Research Council can use for its recommendations, the RDA for protein has been adjusted downward every 5 years. At present, the protein RDA for an adult male is set at 63 g/day. This presumes that the dietary protein is coming from a mixed diet containing a reasonable amount of good-quality proteins. For persons subsisting on mixtures of poor-quality proteins, this RDA may not be adequate. Tables 1.11 and 1.12 give the current RDA for protein for different age groups (see Unit 1).

PROTEIN DEFICIENCY

One of the most common nutritional disorders in the world today is the deficiency of protein. Both adults and children are affected as the populations in the less-developed nations of the world exceed their food supply. Instances of deficiency in the U.S. have also been observed. Due to the ubiquitous nature of protein and its role in bodily function, protein deficiency is characterized by a number of symptoms. In many situations, not only is protein lacking in the diet but the energy intake is also insufficient. For this reason, it is difficult to segregate symptoms due solely to protein deficiency from those due solely to energy deficit. In children, one can observe the different symptoms and visualize them all as parts of a continuum called protein-energy or protein-calorie malnutrition (PEM or PCM) rather than distinctly different nutritional disorders. Kwashiorkor, a disease initially observed in Africa, was first regarded as a dietary state where only protein was deficient, not energy. Marasmus, on the other hand, was regarded as a dietary state where both protein and energy were deficient. Today, as mild and moderate cases of these two diseases are treated, it has become apparent that the symptoms of one may intermingle with the other so that a clear-cut diagnosis is impossible. For every severe case of either kwashiorkor or marasmus that is identified, treated, and cured, there are probably another 99 people who are not diagnosed and treated and who will, if they survive, experience life-long effects from their early nutritional deprivation.

KWASHIORKOR

Kwashiorkor usually affects young children after they weaned from their mothers' breast. The children are usually between 1 and 3 years old; they are weaned because their mothers have given birth to another child or is pregnant and cannot support both children. If the children have no teeth, they are given a thin gruel. This may be a fruit, vegetable, or cereal product mixed with water; it is not usually a good protein source. Cultural food practices or taboos may further limit the kinds and amounts of protein given to the child. Concurrent infections, parasites, seasonal food shortages, and poor distribution of food among the family members may also contribute to the development of kwashiorkor. The deficiency develops not only because of inadequate intake but also because, at this age, the growth demands for protein and energy are high.

Growth failure is the single most outstanding feature of protein malnutrition. The child's height and weight for his age will be less than that of his well-nourished peer. *Tissue wastage* is present but may not be apparent if edema is also present. The *edema* begins with the feet and legs and gradually presents itself in the hands, face, and body. If edema is advanced, the child may not appear underweight but many appear "plump." This plumpness can be ascertained as edema by feel. If a thumb were to be pressed on the surface of the foot or ankle and then removed, the depression would remain for a short time. This is edema. It is thought to result from insufficient ADH production and insufficient serum and tissue proteins needed to maintain water balance.

Protein-deficient children are usually *apathetic*, have little interest in their surroundings, and are listless and dull. These children are usually "fussy" and irritable when moved. Mental retardation may or may not result. *Hair changes* are frequently observed. Texture, color, and strength are affected. Black, curly hair may become silkier, lusterless, and brown or reddish-brown in color. *Lesions of the skin* are not always present, but if present, they give the appearance of old flaky paint. Depigmentation or darkly pigmented areas may develop, with a tendency for these areas to appear in places of body friction such as the backs of legs, groins, elbows. *Diarrhea* is almost always present. The diarrhea may be a result of the inability of the body to synthesize the needed digestive enzymes so that the food that is consumed can be utilized, or it may be the result of concurrent infections and parasites. In rats fed protein-free diets, significantly less intestinal enzyme activity has been measured. *Anemia* due to an inability to synthesize hemoglobin as well as red blood cells is invariably present. *Hepatomegaly* (enlarged liver) is usually observed.

In children consuming energy-sufficient–protein-insufficient diets, the enlarged liver is usually fatty because the child is unable to synthesize the proteins needed to make the transport proteins which, in turn, are needed to transport the lipids out of the liver. Studies with rats and chickens have shown that protein deficiency also results in decreases in a variety of hepatic enzymes, a decrease in hepatic RNA and DNA content, a reduction in spleen size, a decrease in antibody formation, a decrease in urea cycle activity and urea production, and a decrease in the levels of plasma amino acids. All of the above symptoms can be related to the various functions of proteins as discussed in the earlier section.

MARASMUS

Although children of all ages and adults can suffer from a deficiency of both energy and protein, the marasmic child is usually less than one year old. In developing countries, a common cause for marasmus is a cessation of breast feeding. Milk production by the mother may have stopped because of the mother's poor health, or the mother may have died, or, there may be a desire on the part of the mother to bottle feed her infant rather than breast feed. This decision to bottle feed may be made for a variety of reasons. The mother may view bottle feeding as a status symbol, or she may be forced to work to earn a living and may be unable to have her baby with her, or she may not be able to lactate. While under optimal conditions of economics and sanitation, the bottle-fed child may be well fed, in emerging nations this is not always true. The mother may not be able to buy the milk formula in sufficient quantities to adequately nourish the child, she may over-dilute the milk, or she may use unsafe water and unsanitary conditions to prepare the formula for the child. This, plus the insufficient nutrient content, often precipitously leads to the development of marasmus, a form of starvation characterized by *growth failure* with prominent ribs, a characteristic monkey-like face, and matchstick limbs with little muscle or adipose-tissue development; *tissue wastage* but not edema is present. Whereas the kwashiorkor child has a poor appetite, the marasmus child is eager to eat. The child is mentally alert but not irritable. *Anemia* and *diarrhea* are present for the same reasons as in kwashiorkor. The skin and hair appear to be of normal color.

The treatment of both kwashiorkor and marasmic children must be approached with due care and caution. Because their enzymes for digestion and their protein absorption and transport systems are less active, feeding these children with large quantities of good-quality protein would be harmful. Their diets must be gradually enriched with these proteins to allow their bodies sufficient time to develop the appropriate metabolic pathways to handle a better diet. Giving these children solutions of either predigested proteins or solutions of amino acids may be of benefit initially, but these solutions, too, must be used with care. If the amino acids in excess of immediate use are deaminated, and if the pathway for synthesizing urea is not fully functional, ammonia can accumulate in the child and become lethal. Schimke has shown that, in the rat, up to 3 days are needed to increase the activities of the urea cycle enzymes. The rat has a much faster metabolic rate than the human, so one would anticipate that a much longer period of time would be necessary for a similar induction in humans.

Not only must one be concerned about the enzymes of the malnourished child, protein-depleted children are also unable to synthesize adequate amounts of the protein hormones that regulate and coordinate their use of dietary nutrients. In addition, protein deprivation affects the structures of the cell and hormone receptors, further dampening the effectiveness of those hormones produced. Children with marasmus or kwashiorkor have been shown to have decreased blood sugar levels, decreased serum insulin and growth hormone levels, and, in marasmus, decreased thyroid hormone levels. Additional hormonal changes have been observed, but their relevance to treatment has not been ascertained. Most likely these changes in the levels of the protein-, peptide-, or amino acid-derived hormones are reflective of reduced synthesis of them as a result of a shortage of incoming amino acids. Changes in the steroid hormones probably reflect the response of the child to the stress of deprivation.

INTEGRATION OF THE METABOLIC FEATURES OF PROTEIN NUTRITION

In the preceding section, protein malnutrition and protein-energy malnutrition or starvation have been characterized. Throughout this unit, the chemical and biochemical nature of proteins has been discussed in detail. Individual catabolic pathways for the amino acids have been given as well as the process by which new body proteins are synthesized. But how does the body "know" when to synthesize a new protein or degrade a resident one? What messages are sent and received that integrate these anabolic and catabolic processes? How does the body cope with its ever-changing environment — of which nutrition is but a part?

Recall that some of the amino acids that are contained by the dietary protein can be decarboxylated and converted to amines. These amines are potent neurotransmitters. That is, they are capable of eliciting system responses via activation of certain neurons or neuronal pathways. Some of these systemic responses include the release of hormones that have positive effects on protein synthesis. An example might be the signals to the pituitary to release growth hormone which, when bound to its cognate membrane receptor, elicits a cascade of intracellular signals which, in turn, migrate to the nucleus and serve as instigators of protein synthesis. Providing that sufficient ATP and amino acids are available, protein synthesis will be stimulated. Another example might be the chronic ingestion of a high-sugar diet that stimulates insulin release. The insulin plus the glucose plus several other factors instigates the synthesis of enzyme proteins needed to metabolize this sugar load. Initiation and cessation of feeding is an example of a system response to changing levels of the neurotransmitter serotonin. Likely, other neurotransmitters are involved as well (see Unit 3 and the section on the regulation of food intake). Through the action of neurotransmitters, other systems can be activated or suppressed and these systems might include sleep or voluntary activity or other such whole-body actions. These responses will have effects on the need for energy and, because the energy need is tightly linked to the protein need, effects on the latter should be expected.

The dietary protein, once consumed, stimulates the release of a variety of gut hormones. These hormones likewise elicit systemic responses as outlined in the section on digestion and absorption. Further, once amino acids are liberated through the action of the digestive enzymes, these amino acids, as substrates for enterocyte carriers (see section on absorption) stimulate not only the carrier activity (substrate activation) but also are involved in the synthesis of the carrier itself by the enterocyte. This is not an uncommon phenomenon. A number of high-turnover proteins, i.e., enzymes, carriers, and hormones, have their synthesis dictated by rising levels of the substrates upon which they act. Hence, rising levels of cytosolic citrate in the cell might be expected to instigate the transcription of the messenger RNA for ATP citrate lyase, the enzyme that catalyzes the formation of acetyl CoA and oxalacetate from citrate and CoA with a concomitant hydrolysis of ATP to ADP and phosphate. So, too, might one expect to find in the enterocyte an increase in the mRNAs for those proteins that are responsible for the transport of the amino acids into the enterocyte via carrier-mediated mechanisms. Thus, we see multiple roles for the amino acids found in the dietary proteins and these roles are not restricted to just the enterocyte. Other cells, tissues, and organs also are affected. The enzymes that are responsible for amino acid metabolism are likewise synthesized or degraded in response to the levels of those amino acids on which they work. The expression of the genes that encode these enzymes may be unique to a given cell type, tissue, or organ, or may be universal. Uniqueness of gene expression means that factors other than the substrate are operative in the regulation of that expression. For example, muscle cells cannot complete the oxidation of histidine, which is liberated as muscle protein is degraded during muscle contraction and relaxation. Even though the muscle cell contains the same DNA as every other cell type, the expression of those genes responsible for the complete deamination and oxidation of histidine (see Figure 4.23) does not occur despite the rising levels of histidine. Instead, this histidine is methylated and excreted in the urine. In few other cell types does this methylation occur; histidine is usually metabolized as shown in Figure 4.23. However, expression of the gene for the enzyme responsible for histidine methylation is "turned on" by its substrate, histidine, and its affinity for this substrate as well as its activity as a catalyst exceeds that of any other enzyme in the muscle cell that might use histidine. As the muscles are increased in activity and size, the amount of methylated histidine found in the urine also increases. Here, then, is a complete loop. The histidine in the food is transported to the muscle that uses it to synthesize myosin and actin, and when that muscle is actively working, myosin and actin are degraded, with 3-methyl histidine appearing in the urine. Histidine has acted as a signal for the expression of genes coded for its transport, for its incorporation into muscle protein, and for its methylation and excretion. It has also served as a substrate for all of these processes plus those outlined in Figure 4.23.

Each of the amino acids, as well as every other nutrient consumed as part of the diet, likewise has multiple roles. In and of themselves, amino acids serve as signals of metabolic processes, or they can serve as substrates for the synthesis of proteins that act as carriers, receptors, enzymes, hormones, or structural materials.

The complexity of these interacting roles of amino acids as neurotransmitters, as enzyme activators, as inducers of gene expression, and as substrates for a multitude of synthetic and degradative reactions is enormous. Yet the brain and other vital organs signal each other such that integration of function occurs and a comprehensive metabolic pattern emerges. When the body is without sufficient nutrient intake to sustain normal body function, it has a hierarchy in place that controls amino acid use so that more-important functions are maintained at the expense of less-important ones. Hence, in the protein-malnourished child, the symptoms of weight loss, skin lesions, and hair changes are observed, while the activity of metabolic enzymes and hormones is conserved.

Protein synthesis is energetically very expensive as well as being dependent on amino acid availability. Thus, protein synthesis is also suppressed in a hierarchial manner. Skin cells and hair cells are not replaced, due to this decreased protein synthesis, as rapidly as in the well-nourished individual. Hence, the skin lesions and hair changes that typify protein malnutrition. Energy conservation and protein conservation similarly are preserved. The synthesis and release of hormones that accelerate protein breakdown and use are suppressed via effects of diet deprivation on the brain, peptides that signal food-seeking behavior are maintained, gut motility is suppressed so as to retard the passage of food from mouth to anus and extract as much nourishment as possible from that food, body activity is diminished to reduce energy expenditure (the symptom of lethargy), and sleep time is increased for the same reason. All of these defenses against death due to starvation are directed by the central nervous system and executed by the secretions of the endocrine organs. In turn, these defenses are activated when the body senses, via the gut cells, that insufficient food has been consumed.

Some of these defenses can be compromised by additional problems in the environment. If the drinking water is contaminated, the reduction in gut passage time as a defense is negated by pathogen-induced diarrhea. This results in a loss of gut contents and abrasion of the cells lining the intestinal tract. In this instance, the person is less able to cope with an inadequate food supply. The coordination of the defense against death due to starvation is disrupted by the stress response (also coordinated by hormones) to the invading pathogens. Such stress elicits a signal from the pituitary that stimulates an outpouring of the catecholamines and steroidal hormones by the adrenals. These hormones mobilize muscle protein, body-fat stores, and glycogen stores needed for the synthesis of antibodies to the pathogens as well as for the synthesis of replacement enterocytes and the conservation of electrolytes and water. Because such syntheses require energy, amino acids, and a number of micronutrients — all of which may be in short supply — it is easy to understand why malnourished individuals are more vulnerable to environmental contaminants and why the resultant disease is far more severe.

The interaction of disease and nutritional state can have lasting effects on body function. Hence, it is not uncommon to observe short stature in populations whose food supply is inadequate. Growth, a reflection of protein synthesis that in turn is dependent on nutrient intake, is suppressed because growth is lower on the hierarchical scale of body functions that are preserved in times of need. When the food supply changes and becomes reliably abundant with a variety of foods, including sources of good-quality protein, then the genetic potential for body size is fully realized. The average height of the population increases from one generation to the next and the body-fat stores are maintained at capacity. The latter feature may not be deemed to be desirable (see section on body weight, Unit 3).

SUPPLEMENTAL READINGS

Aragon, J., Sols, A. (1991). Regulation of enzyme activity in the cell: effect of enzyme concentration. *FASEB J.* 5:2945-2950.

Bach, L.A., Rechler, M.M. (1992). Insulin-like growth factors and diabetes. *Diabetes/Metabolism Reviews* 8:229-257.

Benevenga, N.J., Gahl, M.J., Blemings, K.P. (1993). Role of protein synthesis in amino acid catabolism. *J. Nutr.* 123:332-336.

Baumann, G. (1993). Growth hormone binding proteins. *Proc. Soc. Exp. Biol. & Med.* 202:392-400.

Clarke, S.D., Abraham, S. (1992). Gene expression: nutrient control of pre and posttranscriptional events. *FASEB J.* 6:3146-3152.

Freedman, L.P., Luisi, B.F. (1993). One of the mechanisms of DNA binding by nuclear hormone receptors: A structural and functional perspective. *J. Cell. Biochem.* 51:140-150.

Gietzen, D.W. (1993). Neural mechanisms in the responses to amino acid deficiency. *J. Nutr.* 123:610-625.

Glenney, J.R. (1992). Tyrosine-phosphorylated proteins: mediators of signal transduction from tyrosine kinases. *Biochem. Biophys. Acta.*1134:113-127.

Greenberg, C.S., Birckbichler, P.J., Rice, R.H. (1991). Transglutaminases: multifunctional cross-linking enzymes that stabilize tissues. *FASEB J.* 5:3071-3077.

Harper, A.E., Yoshimura, N.N. (1993). Protein quality, amino acid balance, utilization and evaluation of diets containing amino acids as therapeutic agents. *Nutrition* 9:460-469.

Hartree, A.S., Renwick, A.G. (1992). Molecular structures of glycoprotein hormones and functions of their carbohydrate components. *Biochem. J.* 287:665-679.

Kilberg, M.S., Stevens, B.R., Novak, D.A. (1993). Recent advances in mammalian amino acid transport. *Ann. Rev. Nutrition.* 13:137-166.

Kollmar, R. and Farnham, P.J. (1993). Site specific utilization of transcription by RNA poymerase II. *P.S.E.B.M.* 203:127-139.

Lea, M.A. (1993). Regulation of gene expression in hepatomas. *Int. J. Biochem.* 25:457-469.

Lobley, G.E. (1993). Species comparisons of tissue protein metabolism: Effects of age and hormonal action. *J. Nutr.* 123:337-343.

Maltese, W.A. (1990). Post translational modifications of proteins by isoprenoids in mammalian cells. *FASEB J.* 4:3319-3328.

Muller, H. and Scott, R. (1992). Hereditary conditions in which the loss of heterozygosity may be important. *Mutation Res.* 284:15-24.

Olson, E.N. (1988). Modification of proteins with covalent lipids. *Prog. Lipid. Res.* 27:177-197.

Putney, J.W. and Bird, G. (1993). The inositol phosphate-calcium signaling system in non excitable cells. *Endocrine Rev.* 14:610-631.

Rapoport, T.A. (1991). Protein transport across the endoplasmic reticulum membrane: facts, models, mysteries. *FASEB J.* 5:2792-2798.

Reichel, R.R. and Jacob, S.T. (1993). Control of gene expression by lipophilic hormones. *FASEB J.* 7:427-436.

Van der Rest, M. and Garrone, R. (1991). Collagen family of proteins. *FASEB J.* 5:2814-2823.

Vedeckis, W.Y. (1992). Nuclear receptors, transcriptional regulation and oncogenesis. *Proc. Soc. Exp. Biol. & Med.* 199:1-12.

Wolfe, R.R., Jahoor, F., and Hartl, W.H. (1989). Protein and amino acid metabolism after injury. *Diabetes Metab. Rev.* 5:149-164.

Wu, G., and Morris, S.M. (1998). Arginine metabolism: Nitric oxide and beyond. *Biochem. J.* 336:1-17.

Young, V.R. and Marchini, J.S. (1990). Mechanisms and nutritional significance of metabolic responses to altered intakes of protein and amino acids with reference to nutritional adaptation in humans. *Am. J. Cli. Nutr.* 51:270-289.

Books

Berdanier, C.D., Hargrove, J.L., Eds.. (1993). *Nutrition and Gene Expression.* CRC Press, Boca Raton, 579 pages.

Strachan, T. and Read, A.P. (1996). *Human Molecular Genetics.* Wiley-Liss, New York, 632 pgs.

5 Carbohydrates

CONTENTS

OVERVIEW

Carbohydrates provide as much as 60% of the daily energy intake. The percentage of the diet that is carbohydrate varies inversely with economic conditions and with the percentage of the diet that is fat and protein. As a general rule, carbohydrate-rich foods are less expensive than fat- and protein-rich foods. Hence, as people have more disposable income, they tend to buy and consume fewer cereals, breads, fruits, and vegetables and buy more meat, butter (or margarine), milk, and eggs. This is not always true, however. Over the last decade, education about the possible health risks of high intakes of fatty foods and the health benefits of high fiber intakes, as well as the benefits of consuming fruits and vegetables, has altered the eating habits of many consumers. This, in turn, has had an impact on the percent of intake provided by this macronutrient class.

The term carbohydrate originated in the late 1800s with the idea that there existed naturally occurring compounds composed of carbon, hydrogen, and oxygen, which could be represented as hydrates of carbon. For instance, glucose ($C_6H_{12}O_6$), sucrose ($C_{12}H_{22}O_{11}$), and starch ($C_6H_{10}O_5)_n$ could all be represented by the general formula $C_x(H_2O)_y$. This definition proved to be too rigid because it excluded such common carbohydrate compounds as deoxyribose ($C_5H_{10}O_4$) and ascorbic acid ($C_6H_8O_6$) but included the compound acetic acid ($C_2H_4O_2$), which is not a carbohydrate. A more comprehensive definition evolved: carbohydrates are polyhydroxy aldehydes or ketones and their derivatives.

CLASSIFICATION

Carbohydrates are divided into three major classes: monosaccharides, oligosaccharides, and polysaccharides. A monosaccharide consists of a single polyhydroxy aldehyde or ketone unit. An oligosaccharide contains two to ten monosaccharide units. The upper limit on the number of monosaccharides in an oligosaccharide is not rigorously defined. Disaccharides, composed of two monosaccharides, are the most common oligosaccharides. A polysaccharide contains many monosaccharides.

STRUCTURE AND NOMENCLATURE

MONOSACCHARIDES

Monosaccharides, called simple sugars, have the empirical formula $(CH_2O)_n$, where n is 3 or more. Although monosaccharides may have as few as three or as many as nine carbon atoms, those of interest to the nutritionist have five or six. The carbon skeleton is unbranched, and each carbon atom, except one, has a hydroxyl group and a hydrogen atom. At the remaining carbon atom, there is a carbonyl group. If the carbonyl function is on the last carbon atom, the compound is an aldehyde and is called an *aldose*; if it occurs at any other carbon, the compound is a ketone and is called a *ketose*. These structures are illustrated in Figure 5.1.

The simplest monosaccharide is the three-carbon aldehyde or ketone, *triose*. Glyceraldehyde is an aldotriose; dihydroxyacetone is a ketotriose. Successive chain elongation of trioses yields *tetroses, pentoses, hexoses, heptoses*, and *octoses*. In the aldo-series. these are called aldotriose, aldotetrose, aldopentose, aldohexose, etc.; in the keto-series,they are ketotriose, ketotetrose, ketopentose, ketohexose, etc. Figure 5.2 shows the D-aldose monosaccharides that have three to six carbons.

Figure 5.3 illustrates the corresponding D-ketoses. Within a given series of the same number of carbon atoms, these molecules differ only in the arrangement of the hydrogen atom and the hydroxyl group about the carbon atoms. Compare, for example, glucose and mannose — the

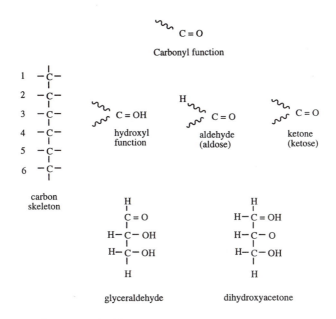

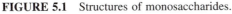

FIGURE 5.1   Structures of monosaccharides.

configuration of the hydrogen and hydroxyl group about each of the carbons is the same except for carbon two. In glucose, the hydroxyl function is to the right; in mannose, it is to the left. Two sugars that differ only in the configuration about one carbon atom are referred to as epimers. D-glucose and D-mannose are epimers with respect to the number-two carbon atom; D-mannose and D-talose are epimers with respect to the number-four carbon atom.

Configuration and conformation are two frequently used terms that are easily confused. Configuration is the arrangement in space of atoms or groups of atoms of a molecule that can be changed only by breaking and making bonds. Conformation is the arrangement in space of atoms or groups of atoms of a molecule that can arise by rotation about a single bond and that are capable of a finite existence.

Picture a one-legged pirate; his configuration is fixed. He can sit, stand, or lie down, but he still has one head, two arms, and one leg, and this has not changed. In other words, his conformation can change but his configuration cannot.

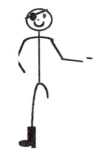

Configuration of a one-legged pirate

Hexoses are white crystalline compounds, freely soluble in water but insoluble in such nonpolar solvents as benzene and hexane. Most of them have a sweet taste and are by far the most abundant of the monosaccharides. Of these, glucose, fructose, and galactose are most often found in foods, frequently as compounds of disaccharides or polysaccharides. Mannose is occasionally found, but

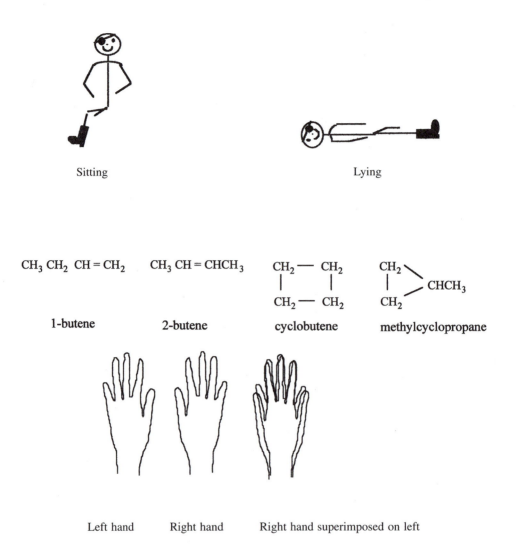

only in complexes that are poorly digested. Aldopentoses are important components of DNA and RNA; derivatives of triose and heptose are intermediates in carbohydrate metabolism.

Stereoisomeric Forms

All of the monosaccharides, except dihydroacetone, contain at least one asymmetric carbon atom, which, in the simplest sense, is one to which four different constituents are attached. Molecules that possess an asymmetric center can exist in *stereoisomeric* forms.

Stereoisomers have the same structural framework but differ in the spatial arrangement of the various substituent groups. Stereoisomers include *cis* and *trans* forms, (chair and boat forms) and epimers. They are different from *structural isomers*. Structural isomers have different structural frameworks; the bonding arrangements for the component atoms are different. C_4H_8 is the molecular formula for the four structural isomers that follow:

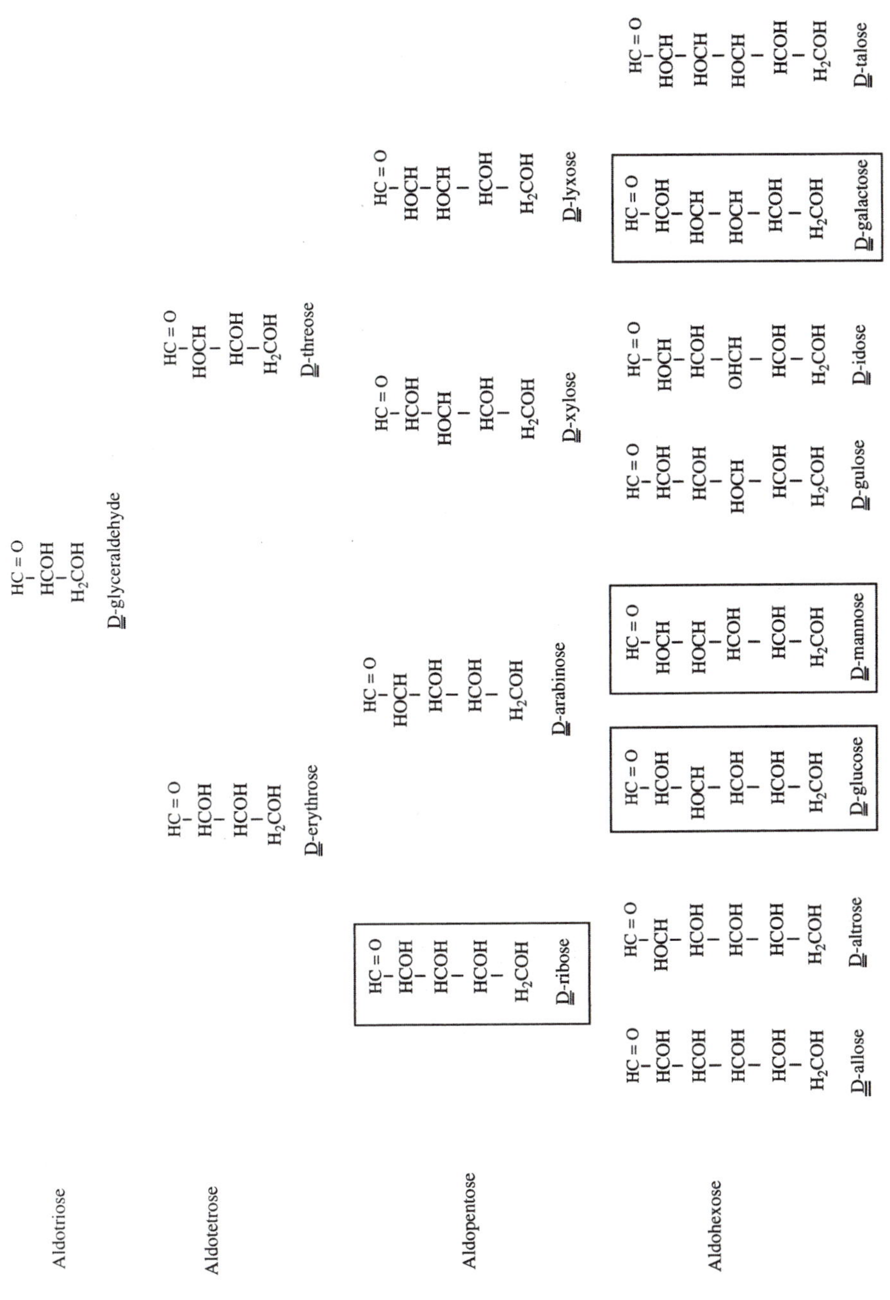

Aldotriose

```
HC = O
HCOH
H₂COH
D-glyceraldehyde
```

Aldotetrose

```
HC = O        HC = O
HCOH          HOCH
HCOH          HCOH
H₂COH         H₂COH
D-erythrose   D-threose
```

Aldopentose

```
HC = O     HC = O       HC = O      HC = O
HCOH       HOCH         HCOH        HOCH
HCOH       HCOH         HOCH        HOCH
HCOH       HCOH         HCOH        HCOH
H₂COH      H₂COH        H₂COH       H₂COH
D-ribose   D-arabinose  D-xylose    D-lyxose
```

Aldohexose

```
HC = O    HC = O    HC = O     HC = O     HC = O    HC = O    HC = O       HC = O
HCOH      HOCH      HCOH       HOCH       HCOH      HOCH      HCOH         HOCH
HCOH      HCOH      HOCH       HOCH       HCOH      HCOH      HOCH         HOCH
HCOH      HCOH      HCOH       HCOH       HOCH      OHCH      HOCH         HOCH
HCOH      HCOH      HCOH       HCOH       HCOH      HCOH      HCOH         HCOH
H₂COH     H₂COH     H₂COH      H₂COH      H₂COH     H₂COH     H₂COH        H₂COH
D-allose  D-altrose D-glucose  D-mannose  D-gulose  D-idose   D-galactose  D-talose
```

FIGURE 5.2 D-Aldoses having from three to six carbon atoms. Those of the greatest biological significance are enclosed in boxes.

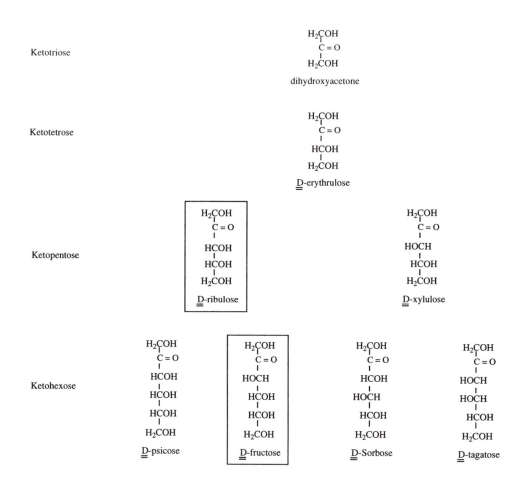

FIGURE 5.3 D-Ketoses having from three to six carbon atoms. Those of the greatest biological significance are enclosed in boxes. Ketoses are sometimes named by inserting an "-ul" into the name of the corresponding aldose. D-Ribulose is the ketopentose corresponding to the aldopentose D-ribose.

For example, glyceraldehyde may occur in either the D or the L stereoisomer. D and L stereoisomers bear the same relationship to each other as one's right and left hands; if both hands are laid flat on a table and the right hand slid on top of the left hand, the right hand does not cover the left (note that thumbs stick out in opposite directions). When the chemical structure for each of these molecules is written as projection formulas, their differences are obvious — the hydroxyl group and the hydrogen atom on the asymmetric carbon reverse positions; these two compounds are mirror images of each other. Mirror-image forms of the same compound are called enantiomers. Pairs of enantiomers (the D and L stereoisomers of a molecule) possess the same chemical and physical properties except for rotating plane-polarized light in opposite but equal directions; i.e., the values of their specific rotation have opposite signs. A note of caution, however, a D or an L used in the name of a sugar molecule does not refer to the sign of its optical rotation; these letters specify the absolute configuration of the molecule. If one desires to include the sign of optical rotation in the molecular name, a (+) for dextrorotary, rotation to the right, or (−) for levorotary, rotation to the left, is used. For example, the specific rotation of the D-glyceraldehyde is 14°; hence, its name is D-(+)-glyceraldehyde; D-lactic acid has a specific rotation of −3.8, and is called D-(−)-lactic acid.

By convention, a carbohydrate belongs to the D series if, when it is written in the projection formula with the aldehyde or hydroxyketone group at the top, the hydroxyl group on the next to the last carbon is to the right; conversely, if the molecule is written exactly as just described except for the fact that the hydroxyl group on the next to the last carbon is written to the left, it belongs to the L-series. A molecule which possesses n asymmetric carbons has 2n as the upper limit of the number of stereoisomers. The aldohexose series has four asymmetric carbon atoms; thus, it has 16 stereoisomers or eight pairs of enantiomers. One of these pairs is α-D-glucose and α-L-glucose.

In nature, D monosaccharides are much more abundant than L. Most mammalian cells require D sugar because they are unable to metabolize the L form. However, a few L monosaccharides can be found; among the most important are L-rhamnose and L-sorbose. Glucose is often called dextrose because the stereoisomer almost always rotates plane-polarized light to the right; it is dextrorotary. Similarly, fructose is often called levulose because its most common natural form is levorotary.

Anomeric Forms

In the section on stereoisomeric forms, glucose was referred to as α-D-glucose instead of D-glucose. The presence of the Greek letter alpha (α) adds another dimension to the structure of carbohydrates. This new feature can be more readily understood if one realizes that aldehydes and ketones can

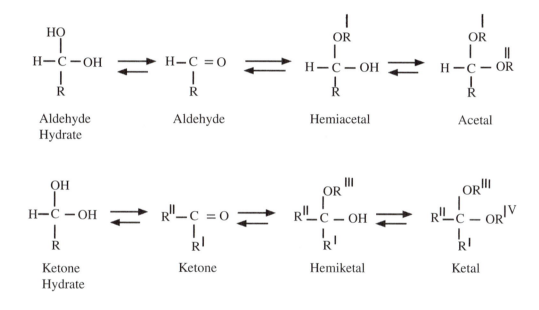

add hydroxyl groups at the carbonyl function. If water is added, the unstable hydrate of the aldehyde is formed. If alcohol is added, a *hemiacetal* is formed. If alcohol is added to the hemiacetal, a full *acetal* (or simple acetal) is formed by the elimination of water.

Ketones undergo similar reactions but form hemiketals or ketals. The hemiketal, having four different constituents, is an asymmetric carbon atom; it exists in one of two stereoisomeric forms.

In the case of carbohydrates, the same hemiacetal formation can occur but it will be an intramolecular reaction and a ring is produced. A six-membered ring, containing five carbon atoms and one oxygen atom is called pyranose (after pyran). A five-membered ring, containing four carbons and one oxygen, is called a furnose (after furan). Figure 5.4 illustrates these two structures. As with aldehydes, this addition reaction in a carbohydrate produces an asymmetric carbon atom; it is referred to as the anomeric carbon. We now have two monosaccharides that differ only in their configuration about the anomeric carbon; they are called anomers and are referred to as α and β forms. In the α form, the hydroxyl group is below the plane of the ring to which it is attached. In the β form, it is above. This ring closure is illustrated for D-glucose and D-fructose in Figure 5.5.

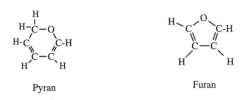

FIGURE 5.4   Structural representations of pyran and furan rings.

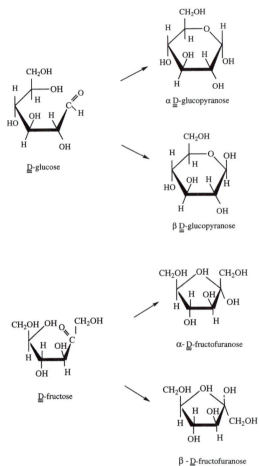

FIGURE 5.5   Ring closure of D-glucose and D-fructose to make the pyranose and furanose forms.

The monosaccharides in the body undergo a number of reactions that will be detailed in the section on metabolism. These reactions produce five general groups of products as shown in Table 5.1.

OLIGOSACCHARIDES

Oligosaccharides consist of two to ten monosaccharides joined with a glycosidic bond. The bond is formed between the anomeric carbon of one sugar and any hydroxyl function of another. If two monosaccharides are bonded in this manner, the resulting molecule is a disaccharide; if three, a trisaccharide; if four, a tetrasaccharide, etc.

TABLE 5.1

Product	Example
Phosphoric acid esters	Glucose-6-phosphate
Polyhydroxy alcohols	Sorbitol
Deoxy sugars	Deoxyribose
Sugar acids	Gluconic acid
Amino sugars	Glucosamine

Disaccharides

Of the oligosaccharides, by far the most prevalent in nature are the disaccharides. Of dietary significance are the disaccharides lactose, maltose, and sucrose.

Lactose, the sugar found in the milk of most mammals (it is lacking in the milk of the whale and the hippopotamus), consists of a D-galactose and D-glucose joined with a glycosidic linkage at carbon one of galactose and carbon four of glucose. The glucose residue of lactose possesses a free anomeric carbon; the α form is the most predominant. Lactose is a reducing sugar. The glycosidic linkage between galactose and glucose is symbolized by β (1→4).

An important characteristic of lactose is its ability to promote in the intestinal tract the growth of certain beneficial lactic acid-producing bacteria. These bacteria have a possible role in the displacement of undesirable putrefactive forms of bacteria. Lactose also appears to enhance the absorption of calcium.

Maltose, also known as malt sugar, contain two glucose residues. The glycosidic linkage is α (1→4).

Celliobiose, the repeating disaccharide unit of cellulose, and gentiobiose are two other disaccharides that have as their repeating units D-glucose. In celliobiose, the glycosidic linkage is β (1→4); in gentiobiose it is β (1→6). Since all have free anomeric carbons, they are reducing sugars.

Sucrose, also known as table sugar, cane sugar, beet sugar, and grape sugar, is a disaccharide of glucose and fructose linked through the anomeric carbon of each monosaccharide. Because neither anomeric carbon is free, sucrose is a nonreducing sugar. It is not a hemiacetal and does not undergo mutarotation. In dilute acid or in the presence of the enzyme invertase, sucrose hydrolyzes into its constituent monosaccharides. The hydrolysis of sucrose to ($[a]_D^{20} = -65.5°$) D-glucose ($[a]_D^{20} = +52.5°$) and D-fructose ($[a]_D^{20} = -92°$) is called inversion because it is accomplished by a change in the sign of specific rotation from dextro (+) to levo (-) as the equimolar mixture of glucose and fructose is formed; this mixture is called *invert sugar*. The development of an enzyme that will isomerize D-glucose to D-fructose has proven to be commercially valuable. It provides a method of obtaining a product known as high-fructose corn syrup, similar to invert sugar and containing no sucrose.

Invert sugar syrups are available commercially at varied levels of inversion. They are sweeter than sucrose at comparable concentrations. This greater sweetness reflects the D-fructose component of the syrup and is an important and critical feature. When sucrose is used in the preparation of acidic foods, some inversion invariably takes place. For instance, if it is used to sweeten fruit drinks, it is completely inverted within a few hours. In soft drinks, there is also a considerable amount of inversion. Honey is largely invert sugar. Bees collect primarily sucrose from flowers, and enzymes invert sucrose in their bodies. Honey, however, is not pure glucose and fructose; its other major constituents are sucrose, water, and small quantities of flavor extract peculiar to the flower from which it is obtained. In general, the disaccharides, while of importance as dietary sources of carbohydrates, have few metabolic functions. They are hydrolyzed into their component monosaccharides in the enterocyte and converted to glucose, which is the body's primary metabolic fuel.

A few oligosaccharides with more than two monosaccharide moieties are of nutritional significance. Stachyose, a tetrasaccharide composed of two molecules of D-galactose, one of D-glucose, and one of D-fructose, is found in certain foods, particularly those of legume origin. It is usually found with raffinose (fructose, glucose, and galactose) and sucrose. The human digestive tract does not possess an enzyme that can hydrolyze stachyose or raffinose. Evidently, however, these sugars are fermented in the lower intestinal tract by the intestinal flora. This further metabolism is thought to be responsible for the unwanted flatus (gas produced and released by the intestinal tract) that frequently follows the ingestion of many legumes.

Polysaccharides

Polysaccharides (also known as glycans) are compounds consisting of large numbers of monosaccharides linked by glycosidic bonds; they are analogous in structure to oligosaccharides. Some have as few as 30 monosaccharides. However, most of the polysaccharides found in nature have a high molecular weight; they may contain several hundred or even thousands of monosaccharide units. Polysaccharides differ from one another in the nature of their repeating monosaccharide units, in the number of such units in their chain, and in the degree of branching.

The polysaccharides that contain only a single kind of monosaccharide or monosaccharide derivative are called *homopolysaccharides*; those with two or more different monomeric units are called *heteropolysaccharides*. Often homopolysaccharides are given names that indicate the nature of the building blocks: for example, those that contain mannose units are mannans; those that contain fructose units are called fructans. The important biological polysaccharides are the *storage polysaccharides*, the *structural polysaccharides*, and the *mucopolysaccharides*.

Storage polysaccharides

Among plants, the most abundant storage polysaccharide is starch. It is deposited abundantly in grains, fruits, and tubers in the form of large granules in the cytoplasm of cells; each plant deposits a starch characteristic of its species. Starch exists in two forms: α-amylose and amylopectin. α-Amylose makes up 20–30% of most starches and consists of 250–300 unbranched glucose residues bonded by α (1→4) linkages. The chains vary in molecular weight from a few thousand to 500,000. The molecule is twisted into a helical coil. Amylopectin, which the remainder of the starch in a plant comprises, is highly branched. Its backbone consists of glucose residues with α (1→4) glycosidic linkages; its branch points are α (1→6) glycosidic bonds. Although the structure of amylopectin is shown in Figure 5.6 as being linear, it too exists as a helical coil.

When amylose is broken down in successive stages by either the enzyme amylase or by the action of dry heat, as in toasting, the resulting polysaccharides of intermediate chain length are called *dextrin*. Amylopectin, when broken down by the same methods, does not cleave at its branch points. This end product is a large, highly branched product called *limit dextrin*.

Other homopolysaccharides are found in plants, bacteria, yeast, and mold as storage polysaccharides. Dextrans, found in yeast and bacteria, are branched polysaccharides of D-glucose with their major backbone linkage α (1→6). Inulin, found in artichokes, consists of D-fructose monomers with β (2→1) glycosidic linkages. Mannans are composed of mannose residues and are found in bacteria, yeasts, mold, and higher plants.

Among animals, the storage polysaccharide is glycogen. Glycogen is stored primarily in the liver and muscles. Like amylopectin, glycogen is a branched polysaccharide of D-glucose with a backbone glycosidic linkage of α (1→4) and branch points of α (1→6). However, its branches occur every 8 to 10 residues, as compared with every 12 for amylopectin. Glycogen is of no importance as a dietary source of carbohydrate. The small amount of glycogen in an animal's body when it is slaughtered is quickly degraded during the postmortem period.

The helical coil of amylose.

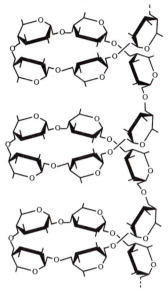

An α (1→6) branch point in amylopectin

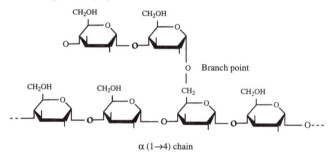

FIGURE 5.6 Structures of storage polysaccharides.

Structural polysaccharides

Cellulose is the most abundant structural polysaccharide in the plant world. Fifty percent of the carbon in vegetables is cellulose; wood is about one-half cellulose and cotton is nearly pure cellulose. It is a straight chain polymer of D-glucose with β (1→4) glycosidic linkages between the monosaccharides. Cellobiose, a disaccharide, is obtained on partial hydrolysis of cellulose. The molecular weight of cellulose has been estimated to range from 50,000 to 500,000 (equivalent to 300 to 3000 glucose residues). Cellulose molecules are organized in bundles of parallel chains, called fibrils, which are cross-linked by hydrogen bonding; these chains of glucose units are relatively rigid and are cemented together with hemicelluloses, pectin, and lignin.

Hemicellulose bears no relation structurally to cellulose. It is composed of polymers of D-xylose having β (1→4) glycosidic linkages with side chains of arabinose and other sugars. Pectin is a polymer of methyl D-galacturonate. Pectin is found in fruit and is the substance needed to make jelly out of cooked fruit. The juice plus sucrose plus the pectin form a gel that is stable for many months at room temperature. Pectin is a nonabsorbable carbohydrate that has pharmacological use as well. It is a key component, together with kaolin (clay), of an antidiarrheal remedy.

There are other structural polysaccharides found in nature. Chitin is a polysaccharide that forms the hard skeleton of insects and crustaceans and is a homopolymer of N-acetyl-D-glucosamine.

Agar, derived from sea algae, contains D- and L-galactose residues, some esterified with sulfuric acid, primarily with 1→3 bonds; alginic acid, derived from algae and kelp, contains monomers of D-mannuronic acid; and vegetable gum (gum guar) contains D-galactose, D-glucuronic acid, rhamnose, and arabinose. These are used as food stabilizers by the food-processing industry. Algin derivatives, for example, are used to stabilize the emulsions of salad dressings; gum guar is frequently used to stabilize processed cheese products. It acts to retard the separation of the solids from the fluid component in such products.

Mucopolysaccharides

The mucopolysaccharides are heteropolysaccharides that are components of the structural polysaccharides found at various places in the body. Mucopolysaccharides consist of disaccharide units in which glucuronic acid is bound to acetylated or sulfurated amino sugars with glycosidic β (1→3) linkages. Each disaccharide unit is bound to the next by a β (1→4) glycosidic linkage. Thus, they are linear polymers with alternating β (1→3) and β (1→4) linkages.

Hyaluronic acid is the most abundant mucopolysaccharide. It is the principal component of the ground substance of connective tissue and is also abundant in the synovial fluid in joints and the vitreous humor of the eye. The repeating unit of hyaluronic acid is a disaccharide composed of D-glucuronic acid and N-acetyl-D-glucosamine; it has alternating β (1→3) and β (1→4) glycosidic linkages. The molecular weight is several million.

Another mucopolysaccharide that forms part of the structure of connective tissue is chondroitin. It differs from hyaluronic acid only in that it contains N-acetyl-D-galactosamine residues rather than N-acetyl-D-glucosamine ones. The sulfate ester derivatives of chondroitin, chondroitin sulfate A and chondroitin sulfate C, are major structural components of cartilage, bone, cornea, and other connective tissue. Types A and C have the same structure as chondroitin, except for a sulfate ester at carbon atom 4 of the N-acetyl-D-galactosamine residue on type A and one at carbon atom 6 of type C.

Heparin (β-heparin) is a mucopolysaccharide that is similar in structure to hyaluronic acid, in that it contains residues of D-glucuronic acid. However, in heparin, these residues contain varying portions of both sulfate and acetyl groups. Its structure is not entirely known. It is a blood anticoagulant.

SOURCES OF CARBOHYDRATE

Carbohydrates are constituents of all living cells. As such, one could anticipate finding one or more carbohydrates in almost all foods of importance to man. Practically speaking, however, foods from animal sources contain few carbohydrates. Milk, with its high lactose content, is the only animal source of any significance. Cow's milk contains 4.8% lactose; human milk, 7%. Eggs, scallops, and oysters contain small amounts of carbohydrate. The percentage of carbohydrate in several common foods can be seen in Table 5.2.

Foods from plant sources, on the other hand, contain large amounts of carbohydrates. Oranges, bananas, and apples are good sources of fructose. Potatoes and cereal grains are good sources of starch.

The sugar content of several fresh fruits and vegetables is given in Table 5.3. The starch content is not shown. Canned and frozen fruits contain additional sugar, which is added as part of the syrup needed to preserve the structure of the fruit. This syrup may be either a sucrose syrup or a high-fructose syrup made using an enzymatic process that starts with cornstarch. This syrup varies in its fructose and glucose content and is used because of its intense sweetness and low cost. Thus, canned and frozen fruits may have more sugar in them than when eaten fresh and unprocessed. These high-fructose corn syrup solutions are also used in soft drinks to add body without affecting or masking flavors. Canners and preservers choose these syrups because they penetrate the fruit easily and preserve its natural form, flavor, and color.

**TABLE 5.2
Percent Carbohydrates in
Common Foods**

	% CHO
Fruits and Vegetables	5–20%
Milk	5%
Shellfish	<1%
Fish	<1%
Lean pork	<1%
Ice cream, cake, pie	40–50%
Lunch meat	<5%
Cheese, roast beef	<1%
Peanut butter, bacon	<10%
Nuts	<10%
Butter, margarine	0%
Salad oil	0%
Sugar	100%

**TABLE 5.3
Free Sugar Content (gram/100 gram fresh weight) in Fruits and
Vegetables**

Item	Glucose	Fructose	Sucrose	Maltose	Raffinose	Stachyose
Apple	1.17	6.04	3.78	Trace		
Beans, Lima	0.04	0.08	2.59		0.20	0.59
Beans, Pole Snap	0.48	1.30	0.28		0.26	
Broccoli	0.73	0.67	4.24			
Peach	0.91	1.18	6.92	0.12		
Strawberry	2.09	2.40	1.03	0.07		

(Adapted from R.S. Shallenberger, in *Sugars in Nutrition*, H.L. Sipple and K.W. McNutt, Eds.,
New York: Academic Press, 1974, 112–126.)

In addition to the sugars and starches, plants contain cellulose, hemicellulose, pectin, and lignin (a noncarbohydrate). These carbohydrates provide fiber, or indigestible residue. Table 5.4 gives the amounts of crude fiber in many common foods. By definition, crude fiber is the residue of plant food left after extraction by dilute acid and alkali. The exact amount of fiber that a food can provide is the subject of some dispute. In the past, chemical analyses of foods have given their crude fiber. However, the term "crude fiber" does not include all the undigested material that may prove to have nutritional value to man. While cellulose, plant fibers, and other so-called nondigestible carbohydrates are not digestible by the enzymes located in the upper portion of the intestine, the intestine contains flora that can partially degrade some of these food components. This degradation provides fatty acids and other useful compounds that are then absorbed by the lower small intestine and colon.

Data on the dietary fiber content of foods are needed; the values for dietary fiber are not identical to those for crude fiber. Several methods of analysis for dietary fiber are being investigated. One obtains a value of the fiber content of food by difference. The amount of fiber is estimated to be that part of the food left in the fat-free, alcohol-insoluble residue after subtraction of available carbohydrate and protein. Southgate has developed a detailed and time-consuming method for the

TABLE 5.4
Fiber Content in
Common Foods

Item	Fiber (g/100 g)
Almonds	2.6
Apples	0.9
Beans, Lima	1.8
Beans, string	1.0
Broccoli	1.5
Carrots	1.0
Flour, whole wheat	2.3
Flour, white wheat	0.3
Noodles, dry	0.4
Oat flakes	1.4
Pears	1.5
Pecans	2.3
Popcorn	2.2
Strawberries	1.3
Walnuts	2.1
Wheat germ	2.5

(Adapted from Tables of Food Composition, *Scientific Tables*, K. Diem and C. Letner, Eds., 7th ed., Ardsley, New York: CIBA-Geigy, 1974.)

determination of cellulose, hemicellulose, and lignin in foods consumed by humans. Van Soest and Goering have developed a simpler method, but theirs was originally designed for animal feeds. Table 5.5 lists values of fiber in foods obtained by these different methods. They indicate that only one-fifth to one-half of the total dietary fiber is crude fiber. Fruits and vegetables have higher values of the total dietary fiber determined as crude fiber than do cereals and legumes.

TABLE 5.5
Extraction Method Effects on the Fiber Content of Food. Fiber content of food (g/100 gm)

Food	Crude Fiber	Southgate Method Cellulose	Hemicellulose	Lignin	Van Soest Method Acid-Detergent Fiber	Lignin	Indigestible Residue Enzymatic	By Difference
Apple	0.66–1.0	0.47	0.66	0.18	0.18	0.18	1.15	1.7–2.4
Carrots	1.0	0.81	0.29	0.08			1.64	2.9–3.1
Peas	0.57–2.0	3.06	1.42	0.33			3.29	5.2
Wheat Bran	9.1	9.3	21.7	4.3	12.2	2.8	48.8	

(Adapted from J. L. Kelsay, A review of research on effects of fiber intake on man. *American Journal of Clinical Nutrition* 31(1978):142.)

DIGESTION AND ABSORPTION

Once a carbohydrate-rich food is consumed, digestion begins. As the food is chewed, it is mixed with saliva, which contains α amylase. This amylase begins the digestion of starch by attacking the internal α 1,4-glucosidic bonds. It will not attack the branch points having α 1,4, or α 1,6-glucosidic bonds, hence the salivary α amylase will produce molecules of glucose, maltose, α-limit dextrin, and maltotriose. The α-amylase in saliva has an isozyme with the same function in the pancreatic juice. The salivary α-amylase is denatured in the stomach as the food is mixed and acidified with the gastric hydrochloric acid. As the stomach contents move into the duodenum, it is called chyme. The movement of chyme into the duodenum stimulates pancreazymin release. This gut hormone acts on the exocrine pancreas stimulating it to release pancreatic juice into the duodenum. Pancreazymin has another name, cholecystokinin. The two names were given before it was realized that the two different functions, the stimulation of the release of pancreatic juice from the exocrine pancreas and bile from the gall bladder, were performed by the same hormone. This hormone is secreted by the epithelial endocrine cells of the small intestine, particularly the duodenum. Its release is stimulated by amino acids in the lumen and by the acid pH of the stomach contents as it passes into the duodenum. The low pH of the chyme also stimulates the release of secretin which, in turn, stimulates the exocrine pancreas to release bicarbonate and water so as to raise the pH of the chyle. This is necessary so as to maximize the activity of the digestive enzymes located on the surface of the luminal cell.

As mentioned, starch digestion begins in the mouth with salivary amylase. It pauses in the stomach as the stomach contents are acidified, but resumes when the chyme enters the duodenum and the pH is raised. The amylase of the pancreatic juice is the same as that of the saliva. It attacks the same bonds in the same locations and produces the same products — maltose, maltotriose, and the small polysaccharides (average of eight glucose molecules) called α-limit dextrins. The limit dextrins are further hydrolyzed by α-glucosidases on the surface of the luminal cells. The hydrolysis of the bonds not attacked by α-amylase or α-glucosidase, or the disaccharidases, maltase, lactase or sucrase, are passed to the lower part of the intestine, where they are attacked by the enzymes of the intestinal flora. Most of the products of this digestion are used by the flora themselves; however, the microbial metabolic products may be of use. The flora can produce useful amounts of short-chain fatty acids and lactate as well as methane gas, carbon dioxide, water, and hydrogen gas. The carbohydrates of legumes typify the substrates these flora use. Raffinose, which is an α-galactose 1→6 glucose 1→2 β- fructose and trehalose, and α-glucose 1→1 α-glucose are the typical substrates from legumes for these flora. The flora will also attack portions of the fibers and celluloses that are the structural elements in fruits and vegetables. Again, some useful products may be produced, but the bulk of these complex polysaccharides having β linkages and perhaps other substituent groups as part of their structure, are largely untouched by both intestinal and bacterial enzymes. These undigested, unavailable carbohydrates serve very useful functions:

1. They provide bulk to the diet, which in turn helps to regulate the rate of food passage from mouth to anus.
2. They act as adsorbants of noxious or potentially noxious materials in the food.
3. They assist in the excretion of cholesterol and several minerals, thereby protecting the body from overload.

Populations consuming high-fiber diets have a lower incidence of colon cancer, fewer problems with constipation, and, as a general rule, lower serum cholesterol levels.

The disaccharides in the diet are hydrolyzed to their component monosaccharides by enzymes also located on the surface of the luminal cell. Lactose is hydrolyzed to glucose and galactose by lactase; sucrose is hydrolyzed to fructose and glucose, and maltose is hydrolyzed to two molecules of glucose. Table 5.6 lists these enzymes together with their substrates and products. One of these enzymes, lactase, declines in activity after weaning. In rodents, this decline is regulated at the level of transcription by factors in addition to the cessation of milk consumption. This may also occur in the human, however, the identity of these regulatory substances has not been fully elucidated. Because the majority of humans in the world are lactose intolerant at adulthood and because milk contains so many essential nutrients in addition to lactose, it would be useful to understand the regulation of lactase gene expression. If one could prevent the age-related decline in lactase activity, milk and milk products could be used by more people to improve their nutritional status. Therapy for lactose-intolerant individuals consists simply of restricting lactose intakes. Some individuals tolerate fermented products such as yogurt and cheese fairly well, while varying amounts of fresh milk induce the typical symptoms of diarrhea and flatulence.

TABLE 5.6
Enzymes of Importance to Carbohydrate Digestion

Enzyme	Substrate	Products
α Amylase	Starch, amylopectin, glycogen	Glucose, maltose, maltotriose, α limit dextrin
α Glucosidase	α limit dextrin	Glucose
Lactase	Lactose	Galactose, glucose
Maltase	Maltose	Glucose
Sucrase/isomaltase	Sucrose/α limit dextrin	Glucose, fructose

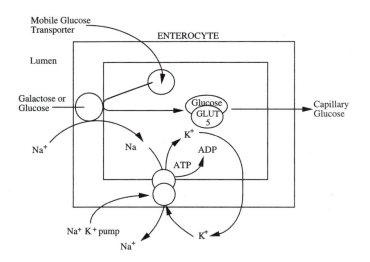

FIGURE 5.7   Two systems are used for glucose uptake by the enterocyte. One, the active transport of glucose from the lumen into the enterocyte uses the energy-dependent Na^+K^+ exchange to facilitate the movement of glucose across the cell membrane. The other uses a mobile glucose transporter (GLUT5) to move the glucose through the cell to the capillary side of the enterocyte.

Once the monosaccharides are released through the action of the above enzymes, they are absorbed by one of several mechanisms. Glucose and galactose are absorbed by an energy-dependent, sodium-dependent, carrier-mediated mechanism. This mechanism is termed active transport because glucose is transported against a concentration gradient. Because the transport is against a concentration gradient, energy is required to "push" the movement of glucose into the enterocyte. This transport is diagrammed in Figure 5.7. Glucose and galactose appear to compete for the same active transport system. They also compete for a secondary transporter, a sodium-independent transporter (the glucose transporter, GLUT 2) found in the basolateral surface of the enterocyte membrane. The two transporters differ in molecular weight. The sodium-dependent transporter has a molecular weight of 75 k Da, while the sodium-independent transporter weighs 57 k Da. This sodium-independent transporter is a member of a group of transporters called GLUT 1, 2, 3, or 4. Each of these transporters is specific to certain tissues. They are sometimes called mobile glucose transporters because, when not in use, they reside in the endoplasmic reticulum. Under the appropriate conditions they move from the endoplasmic reticulum to plasma membrane, where they fuse with the plasma membrane and bind glucose. Upon binding, the transporter and its associated glucose are released from the membrane. Through this mechanism, the glucose enters the intestinal absorptive cell.

Fructose is not absorbed via an energy-dependent, active-transport system, but by facilitated diffusion. This process is independent of the sodium ion and is specific for fructose. Once in the enterocyte, it too is transported by a carrier. In the enterocyte, much of the absorbed fructose is metabolized so that little fructose can be found in the portal blood even if the animal is given an intraluminal infusion of this sugar. On the other hand, an infusion of sucrose will sometimes result in measurable blood levels of fructose. The reason that this occurs may be due to the location of sucrase on the enterocyte. Rather than extending out into the lumen as do the other disaccharidases that are anchored to the enterocyte by a glycoprotein, sucrase is more intimately anchored. The sucrose molecule then is closely embraced by the enzyme, which, in turn, facilitates both the hydrolysis of sucrose and the subsequent transport of its constituent monosaccharides. Thus, both monosaccharides enter the enterocyte simultaneously. If the diet is particularly rich in sucrose, the rise in both glucose and fructose in the portal blood will be measurable. This has some interesting consequences, as will be discussed later in the section on metabolism.

Of the other monosaccharides present in the lumen, passive diffusion is the means for their entry into the enterocyte. Pentoses, such as those found in plums or cherries and other minor carbohydrates, will find their way into the system only to be passed out of the body via the urine if the carbohydrate cannot be used.

METABOLISM

OVERVIEW

Once absorbed by the intestinal cell, glucose passes into the portal blood and circulates first to the liver and then throughout the body. Glucose is the universal, and, in many cases, the preferred fuel for almost all cells. Even though man consumes almost as much energy from carbohydrate as from fat, the body prefers to oxidize the carbohydrate and store the fat. However, because man is not constantly consuming food, these fuel choices are not always possible. The body can protect itself from a lack of food energy by using stored energy. Some of this store (less than a day's need) can be provided by glycogen, a polymer of glucose. Hence, glucose in excess of immediate oxidative need is used to synthesize glycogen in the muscle and liver. Once the glycogen stores are filled, surplus glucose from the diet can be converted to fatty acids and stored as triacylglycerols in the adipose fat depots. In times of need, this fat can be oxidized, as can the stored glycogen. For those cells having an absolute requirement for glucose (certain brain cells), this important fuel can be provided through glycogenolysis or synthesized via gluconeogenesis in the liver and kidney. All of these processes (see Figure 5.8), including food intake regulation (see Unit 3), glucose oxidation, lipid oxidation, fatty acid synthesis glycogenesis, glycogenolysis, and gluconeogenesis are under genetic, dietary, and hormonal control. This control is carefully integrated so that normal blood-glucose levels are maintained at 100 ± 20 mg/dl (4-6mmol/L). Excursions below or above this range may occur. If the excursion is of short duration, there is no cause for alarm. However, if these excursions are of more than an hour, then, depending on the reason for these excursions,

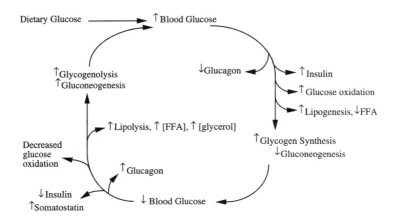

FIGURE 5.8 Overview of glucose metabolism. As blood-glucose levels rise due to the influx of dietary glucose, blood-insulin levels rise and glucagon levels fall. Glucose oxidation increases, as does glycogenesis and lipogenesis. Gluconeogenesis falls. As the blood-glucose levels fall, these processes reverse. Glucagon levels rise, insulin falls; glycogenolysis and gluconeogenesis rise, and peripheral glucose oxidation decreases.

medical assistance may be required. Before a discussion of the regulation of glucose homeostasis can be entered, it is first necessary to describe the various pathways involved in this regulation.

GLYCOLYSIS

The glycolytic pathway for the anaerobic catabolism of glucose can be found in all cells in the body. This cytosolic pathway begins with glucose, a 6-carbon unit, and through a series of reactions, produces 2 molecules of pyruvate. The pathway is shown in Figure 5.9. The pathway also produces ATP by substrate phosphorylation as well as through its contribution of reducing equivalents to the respiratory chain. Because two of the steps require ATP (the initial kinase step and the phospho-fructokinase step), the net ATP production of the glycolytic sequence is 8 ATPs. The control of glycolysis is vested in several key steps. The first step is the phosphorylation of glucose through the formation of glucose-6-phosphate. In the liver and pancreatic β cell this step is catalyzed by the enzyme glucokinase. A molecule of ATP is used and magnesium is required. Glucose-6-phosphate is a key metabolite. It can proceed down the glycolytic pathway, or move through the hexose monophosphate shunt (or "shunt"), or be used to make glycogen. How much glucose-6-phosphate is oxidized directly to pyruvate depends on the type of cells, the nutritional state of the animal, its genetics, and its hormonal state. Some cell types, the brain cell for example, do not make glycogen. Some people do not have shunt activity in the red cell because the code for glucose-6-phosphate dehydrogenase has mutated such that the enzyme is not functional. Insulin-deficient animals likewise might have little shunt activity due to the lack of insulin's effect on the synthesis of its enzymes. All these factors determine how much glucose-6-phosphate goes in which direction.

Two enzymes are used for the activation of glucose: glucokinase and hexokinase, both of which are present in the liver. While hexokinase activity is product inhibited, glucokinase is not. The hexokinase in the nonhepatic tissues must be product inhibited to prevent the hexokinase from tying up all the inorganic phosphate in the cells as glucose-6-phosphate. The Km for glucokinase is greater than that for hexokinase, so the former is the main enzyme for the conversion of glucose to glucose-6-phosphate in the liver. The other enzyme will phosphorylate not only glucose but other 6-carbon sugars as well. The amount of fructose phosphorylated to fructose-6-phosphate is small in comparison with the phosphorylation of fructose at the carbon 1 position catalyzed by fructokinase.

Glucose-6-phosphate is isomerized to fructose-6-phosphate and then is phosphorylated once again to form fructose-1,6-bisphosphate. Another molecule of ATP is used and again magnesium is an important cofactor. Both kinase reactions are rate controlling reactions in that their activity

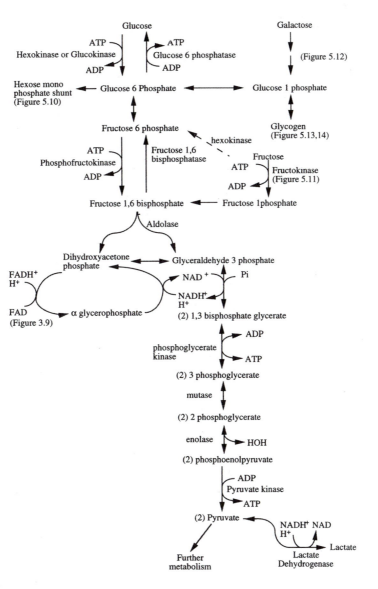

FIGURE 5.9   The glycolytic pathway.

determines the rate at which subsequent reactions proceed. The phosphofructokinase reaction is unique to the glycolytic sequence, while the glucokinase or hexokinase step is not. Thus, one could argue that the formation of fructose-1,6-bisphosphate is the first *committed* step in glycolysis. Glycolysis is inhibited when phosphofructokinase is inhibited. This occurs when levels of fatty acids in the cytosol rise, as in the instance of high rates of lipolysis and fatty acid oxidation. Phosphofructokinase activity is increased when levels of fructose-6-phosphate rise or when cAMP levels rise. Stimulation occurs also when fructose-2,6-bisphosphate levels rise. In any event, glycolysis then proceeds with the splitting of fructose-1,6-bisphosphate to dihydroxyacetone phosphate (DHAP) and glyceraldehyde-3-phosphate. At this point, another rate-controlling step occurs. This step is one that shuttles reducing equivalents into the mitochondria for use by the respiratory chain. This is the α-glycerophosphate shuttle (see Unit 3). This shuttle carries reducing equivalents from the cytosol to the mitochondria. DHAP picks up reducing equivalents when it is converted to α-glycerol phosphate. These reducing equivalents are produced when glyceraldehyde-3-phosphate is oxidized in the process of being phosphorylated to 1,3-diphosphate glyceraldehyde. The α-glyc-erophosphate enters the inner mitochondrial membrane, whereupon it is converted back to DHAP and releases its reducing equivalents to FAD, which in turn transfers the reducing equivalents to the mitochondrial respiratory chain. The reason that this shuttle is rate limiting is due to the need to regenerate NAD⁺ in the cytosol. Without NAD⁺, the glycolytic pathway ceases. NAD⁺ itself cannot pass through the mitochondrial membrane so substrate shuttles are necessary. Another means of producing NAD⁺ is by converting pyruvate to lactate. This is a non-mitochondrial reaction catalyzed by lactate dehydrogenase. It occurs when an oxygen debt is developed, as happens in exercising muscle. In these muscles, more oxygen is consumed than can be provided. Glycolysis is occurring at a rate faster than can be accommodated by the respiratory chain that joins the reducing equivalents transferred to it by the shuttles to molecular oxygen, making water. If more reducing equivalents are generated than can be used to make water, the excess is added to pyruvate to make lactate. Thus, rising lactate levels are indicative of oxygen debt.

There are other shuttles that also serve to transfer reducing equivalents into the mitosol (see Unit 3). These are the malate–aspartate shuttle and the malate–citrate shuttle. Neither of these are rate limiting with respect to glycolysis. The malate–aspartate shuttle has rate-controlling properties with respect to gluconeogenesis, while the malate–citrate shuttle is important to lipogenesis.

Once 1,3-bisphosphate glycerate is formed, it is converted to 3-phosphoglycerate with the formation of 1 ATP. The 3-phosphoglycerate then goes to 2-phosphoglycerate and then to phos-phoenolpyruvate. These are all bidirectional reactions that are also used in gluconeogenesis. The phosphoenolpyruvate is dephosphorylated to pyruvate with the formation of another ATP. Because of the great energy loss to ATP formation at this step, this reaction is not reversible. Gluconeogenesis uses another enzyme, phosphoenolpyruvate carboxykinase, to reverse this step. Glycolysis uses pyruvate kinase to catalyze the reaction. At any rate, pyruvate can now be activated to acetyl CoA, which can enter the mitochondrial citric acid cycle.

The glycolytic pathway is dependent on both ATP for the initial steps of the pathway, the formation of glucose-6-phosphate and fructose-1,6-bisphosphate, and on the ratio of ATP to ADP and inorganic phosphate, Pi. In working muscle, the continuance of work and the continuance of glycolysis depend on the cycling of the adenine nucleotides and the export of lactate. ATP must be provided at the beginning of the pathway, and ADP and Pi must be provided in the latter steps. If the tissue runs out of ATP, ADP or Pi, or accumulates lactate and H⁺, glycolysis will come to a halt and work cannot continue. This is what happens to the working skeletal muscle. Exhaustion sets in when glycolytic rate is down-regulated by an accumulation of lactate. An interesting clinical condition arises in some humans and in pigs that have a genetic error in the regulation of their lactate export and adenine nucleotide cycling. This error is unnoticed unless the individual is anesthetized with an anesthesia such as halothane. When anesthetized, body temperature rises precipitously, muscle rigor and acidosis quickly follow. This condition is known as malignant hyperthermia and occurs in one child in 15,000 and one adult in 50,000–100,000. Unless it is quickly recognized and measures are taken to reduce the body temperature and combat the acidosis, death will result. The biochemical explanation has to do with ATP, ADP, and Pi cycling and the export of lactate from the muscle cell. Apparently, the anesthesia affects several exchange mech-anisms in the membranes within and around the muscle cell. Affected is the coupling of respiration to ATP synthesis by the mitochondria, and the energy normally trapped in the high-energy bond of the ATP molecule is released as heat. Probably the ADP generated in the early ATP-dependent steps of glycolysis is not sent into the mitochondria for rephosphorylation into ATP, and instead is recycled through substrate phosphorylation. Since ADP is exchanged (via several different exchange mechanisms) for ATP, the cell must make some adjustments in its metabolism. Muscle tends to use the glycolytic pathway with the excess product, pyruvate, sent back to the liver as lactate. Although muscle does not lack mitochondria, its mitochondrial activity cannot keep pace with its glycolytic flux when the muscle is working hard and long, or in this instance, when the person (or pig) with the genetic disease of malignant hyperthermia is anesthetized with halothane, which acts as a mitochondrial uncoupler. Hence, the pyruvate/lactate spillover. The lactate must exit the cell via a lactate/H^+ symport. This requires a normal or accelerated blood flow. If the lactate and H^+ are not carried away by the blood, they accumulate. H^+ inhibits the activity of phosphofructokinase and lactate acts as a feedback inhibitor of glycolysis. When an anesthesia such as halothane is used on susceptible individuals, there is a further disruption in the control of glycolysis. There is an accelerated futile cycling between fructose-6-phosphate and fructose-1,6-phosphatase as well as a dramatic decrease in glycolytic flux. The decrease in flux is secondary to the lactate and H^+ accumulation. Under halothane anesthesia, blood flow is reduced. This, coupled with the genetic error(s) in the membranes, results in the phenotypic expression of the malignant hyperthermic genotype.

HEXOSE MONOPHOSPHATE SHUNT

The shunt provides an alternate pathway for the use of glucose-6-phosphate. It is an important pathway because it generates reducing equivalents carried by $NADP^+$ and because it generates a phosphorylated ribose for use in nucleotide synthesis. It is estimated that approximately 10% of the glucose-6-phosphate generated from glucose is metabolized by the shunt.

As can be seen in Figure 5.10, the shunt contains two NADP-linked dehydrogenases, glucose-6-phosphate dehydrogenase and 6-phosphogluconate dehydrogenase. The rate-limiting steps in the reaction sequence comprise these two enzymes. In the instance where there is an active lipogenic state, these reactions provide about 50% of the reducing equivalents needed by the lipogenic process (see Unit 6). In fact, if one wanted a quick assessment of the lipogenic response to a variety of treatments, one could measure the activity of these enzymes using an aliquot of a tissue homogenate plus enough substrate and magnesium to optimize the conditions of the assay. There is an excellent correlation between this dehydrogenase activity and lipogenesis.

Lipogenesis is not the only process that requires reducing equivalents carried by NADP. The microsomal P450 enzymes need them, as does the maintenance of glutathione in the reduced state. The glutathione system in the red cell maintains the redox state and integrity of the cell membrane. If sufficient reducing equivalents are not produced by the shunt dehydrogenase reactions to reduce glutathione the red-cell-membrane integrity is lost and hemolytic anemia results. Glutathione reduction is important to the red blood cells' function of carrying oxygen and exchanging it for carbon dioxide. There are a number of genetic mutations in the code for red cell glucose-6-phosphate dehydrogenase. The code is carried as a recessive trait on the X chromosome and thus only males are affected. These mutations are usually silent. That is, the male having a defective red cell glucose-6-phosphate dehydrogenase does not know he has the problem unless his cells are tested or unless he is given a drug such as quinine or one of the sulfur antibiotics that increase the oxidation of $NADPH^+H^+$.

When this happens, $NADPH^+H^+$ is depleted and is not available to reduce oxidized glutathione. In turn, the red cell ruptures. In almost all cases, the affected male has sufficient enzyme activity to meet the normal demands for $NADPH^+H^+$. It is only when stressed by these drugs that a problem develops.

In any event, as shown in Figure 5.10, glucose-6-phosphate proceeds to 6-phosphoglucolactone, a very unstable metabolite which is in turn reduced to 6-phosphogluconate. 6-phosphogluconate is decarboxylated and dehydrogenated to form ribulose-5-phosphate with an unstable intermediate (keto-6-phosphogluconate) forming between the 6-phosphogluconate and ribulose-5-phosphate. Ribulose-5-phosphate can be isomerized to ribose 5-phosphate or epimerized to xylulose 5-phosphate. Xylulose and ribose 5-phosphate can reversibly form sedoheptulose 7-phosphate with release of glyceraldehyde 3-phosphate. This, of course, will be recognized as a component of the glycolytic sequence.

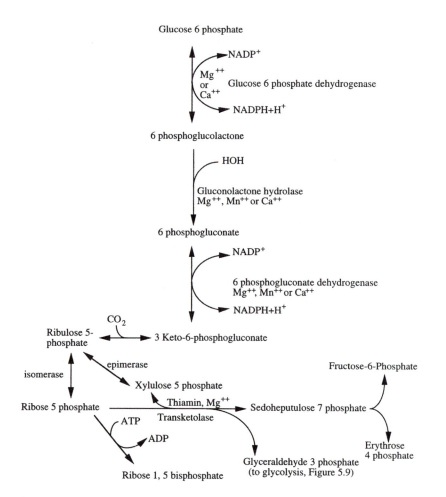

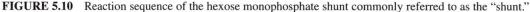

FIGURE 5.10 Reaction sequence of the hexose monophosphate shunt commonly referred to as the "shunt."

INTERCONVERSION OF DIETARY SUGARS

Fructose

In the course of digestion, the simple sugars glucose, fructose, and galactose are released from sucrose, maltose, and lactose. These sugars are usable by most cells after they have been converted to glucose. There are specific cells that have specific needs for these monosaccharides. The testes need fructose for sperm production and the mammary cells need galactose for lactose production. In each instance, there are reactions that are of interest to the nutrition scientist. Shown in Figure 5.11 is the metabolism of fructose. Although two enzymes are available for the phosphorylation of fructose, one of these, fructokinase, is present only in the liver. Just as hexokinase has a lower Km for glucose than glucokinase for the substrate glucose, so too does hexokinase with respect to fructose and fructokinase. The Km for fructokinase is so high that, in fact, most of the dietary fructose that enters the portal blood is metabolized in the liver. This is in contrast to glucose, which is metabolized by all the cells in the body. As a result, sucrose-rich, low-fat diets fed to rats or mice will result in a fatty liver. These diets contain ~65% total weight as sugar and only 5% as fat. The fatty liver occurs because the dietary overload of fructose from sucrose exceeds the capacity of the liver to completely oxidize it to CO_2 and HOH, so it uses the sugar metabolites as substrate for fatty acid and triacylglyceride synthesis. Until the hepatic lipid export system increases sufficiently to transport this lipid to the storage depots, the lipid accumulates, hence, the fatty liver.

Normal rodents adjust to this fructose intake so that after a few weeks the liver returns to its normal (~ 4%) fat content. Those rodents with diabetic tendencies do not adapt and the fatty liver persists throughout their lives. Humans are rarely fed this much sugar and so little fat. There are circumstances, however, that are analogous to this rodent paradigm. The human who is provided nutrition support via parenteral feeding is one such instance. The parenteral feeding solution is rich in sugar (glucose) and contains only enough fatty acid to meet the essential fatty acid requirement. There is concern that patients so treated will have metabolic consequences similar to that described for the rat fed a 65% sugar, 5% fat diet. Concern for the normal human also has developed because of the observed increase in consumption of beverages and foods containing high-fructose syrups. Nutrition scientists began to question whether this dietary change might have untoward effects. However, just as normal rats can adapt to such dietary change, so too can the normal human.

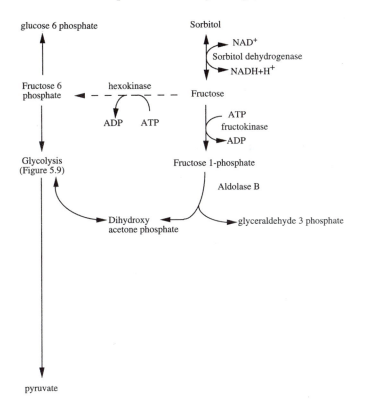

FIGURE 5.11 Metabolism of fructose.

The pathway for fructose metabolism shows three enzymes, any one of which, if mutated, results in a condition known as fructosemia. The first is relatively harmless; that is, a mutation in the gene for fructokinase. As discussed above, hexokinase will phosphorylate fructose and, if the dietary burden is light, the disease of fructosemia will be harmless. Its characteristics of elevated blood and urine levels of fructose are of little concern.

A second mutation has been identified in the gene for aldolase B. This is the enzyme that catalyzes the splitting of fructose-1-phosphate to glyceraldehyde phosphate and dihydroxyacetone phosphate. Recall that aldolase A catalyzes the splitting of fructose-1,6-bisphosphate. Aldolase A is found in all tissues, whereas aldolase B is located only in the liver. The mutation is such that the enzyme has a reduced affinity for its substrate, fructose-1-phosphate. The results of this reduced affinity include hypoglycemia, due to an inhibition of glycogenolysis by fructose-1-phosphate. This hypoglycemia is not responsive to glucagon stimulation. Prior to the identification of the aldolase

B gene mutation, this form of fructosemia was misdiagnosed as one of the glycogen-storage diseases because of the presence of hypoglycemia in the face of ample liver glycogen stores. In addition to the disturbance in glycogenolysis, patients with this disorder vomit after a fructose load, have elevated levels of urine and blood fructose, grow poorly with evidence of jaundice, hyperbiliru-binemia (high levels of bilirubin in the blood), albuminuria (albumin in the urine), amino aciduria (amino acids in the urine), and some patients may have damaged renal proximal convoluted tubules.

The third mutation involves only the liver enzyme fructose-1,6-bisphosphatase. The muscle enzyme is normal in activity. This enzyme is a key enzyme in the hepatic gluconeogenic pathway, so, as one might expect, hypoglycemia is one of the characteristics of a mutation in this enzyme. Other characteristics include an enlarged liver, poor muscle tone, and increased blood lactate levels. All of these mutations are uncommon and all are autosomal recessive traits. Heterozygotes are not detectable.

Galactose

Another monosaccharide of importance, especially to infants and children, is galactose, which is a component of the milk sugar, lactose. In the intestine, lactose is hydrolyzed to its component monosaccharides, glucose and galactose. Galactose is converted to glucose and eventually enters the glycolytic sequence as glucose-6-phosphate. This pathway is shown in Figure 5.12. Galactose is phosphorylated at carbon 1 in the first step of its conversion to glucose. It can be isomerized to glucose-1-phosphate or converted to UDP-galactose by exchanging its phos-phate group for a UDP group. This UDP-galactose can be joined with glucose to form lactose in the adult mammary tissue under the influence of the hormone prolactin. However, usually the UDP-galactose is converted to UDP-glucose and thence used to form glycogen. When glycogen is degraded, glucose-1-phosphate is released, which, in turn, is isomerized to glucose-6-phosphate and enters the glycolytic sequence.

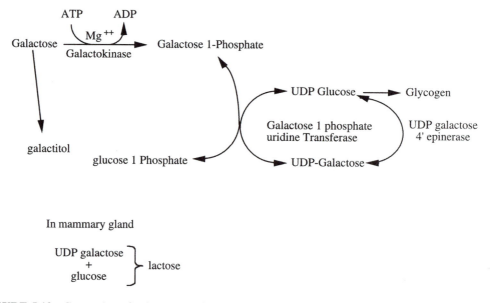

FIGURE 5.12   Conversion of galactose to glucose.

Three autosomal recessive mutations in the genes for enzymes involved in galactose conversion to glucose have been reported. Galactosemia results in each instance. One of these mutations involves the gene for galactose-1-phosphate uridyl transferase. Three variants have been described. One of these variants is fairly innocuous in that the mutation occurs only in the enzymes found in the red cell. This variant is called the Duarte variant, and affected individuals have 50% less red cell galactose-1-phosphate uridyl transferase activity than normal individuals. These people have no other discernible characteristics.

The second variant is far more severe in its effects on the patient. The enzyme in the liver is abnormal and does not function to convert galactose-1-phosphate to UDP galactose. As a result, galactose-1-phosphate accumulates, and some is converted to the sugar alcohol galactitol via NADH aldose reductase action. In this disease, cataracts in the eye form, accompanied by mental retardation and increased tissue levels of galactose-1-phosphate, galactitol, and galactonic acid. These last metabolites are excreted in the urine. Also characteristic of this mutation in galactose-1-phosphate uridyl transferase, are decreased blood-glucose levels, decreased glycogenesis, decreased mutase activity and decreased pyrophosphorylase activity. Since UDP-galactose is necessary for the formation of the galactoyl lipids, chondroitin sulfate formation is decreased. A mutation in the gene for galactokinase also results in accumulations of galactose and galactitol and cataracts. Two variants of this gene have been reported. The galactitol accumulation was found to be the causative agent in the formation of cataracts. Except for cataract formation due to galactitol accumulation, no other symptoms have been described for this form of galactosemia.

Finally, two mutations in the gene for UDP galactoepimerase have been reported. The defect is present only in the red blood cell and the patient is symptom free.

Mannose

Although the main dietary monosaccharides are glucose, fructose, and galactose, mannose is also present in small amounts. Mannose found in food is converted to fructose via phosphorylation and isomerization.

$$\text{Mannose} \rightarrow \text{Mannose-6-phosphate} \rightarrow \text{Fructose-6-phosphate} \rightarrow \text{Glycolysis}$$
$$\downarrow$$
$$\text{Glycolysis}$$

To date, no genetic errors that would have effects on health have been described with respect to this sugar. Occasionally, the diet provides other sugars as well. These are the pentoses, xylose, and xylulose, found in plums, cherries, and grapes. Mannose and the sugar alcohols are used to produce reduced-sugar or reduced-energy food products. Many of these sugar alcohols are non-digestible/non-absorbable carbohydrates but, because the gut flora can utilize them and provide short-chain fatty acids for absorption, they have an energy value ranging from 1.8 to 4 kcal/gram (8–17 kJ/g) depending on the constituents of the polyol. Maltitol (4-O-α-d-glucopyranopyl-d-glucitol) for example, contains one glucose and one glucose alcohol. It has an energy value of about 2 kcal/gram (8.4 kJ/g). Lactitol, on the other hand, has a higher energy value of approximately 3.6 kcal/gram (15 kJ/g). Xylose is converted to the sugar alcohol xylitol through the action of the NADP-linked enzyme xylose/xylulose dehydrogenase, and the xylitol is excreted in the urine. However, a mutation in the gene for this enzyme has been detected and characterized by the presence of xylose or xylulose in the urine instead of xylitol. This has no clinical significance, except if the urine is screened for reducing sugars without discriminating for glucose just after such a person has consumed the fruits containing these sugars. If the person is not studied more carefully, there is a slight chance of the misdiagnosis of diabetes, based on the presence of these reducing sugars in the urine.

GLYCOGENESIS AND GLYCOGENOLYSIS

Glucose is an essential fuel for working muscle as well as for the brain. To ensure a steady supply of this fuel, some glucose is stored in the liver and muscle in the form of glycogen. This is a ready supply of glucose accessed when these tissues are stimulated to release its glucose from its glycogen by the catabolic hormones glucagon, epinephrine, the glucocorticoids, and thyroxine, or by the absence of food in the digestive tract.

Because the glycogen molecule has molecules of water as part of its structure, it is a very large molecule and cumbersome to store in large amounts. In fact, detailed studies of the nature of the body's fuel stores have shown that the average 70-kg man has less than an 18-hour fuel supply stored as glycogen while that same individual might have up to a 2-month supply of fuel stored as fat. Nonetheless, the synthesis of glycogen and its release of glucose in time of need are important aspects of carbohydrate nutrition. Shown in Figure 5.13 is an overview of glycogenesis.

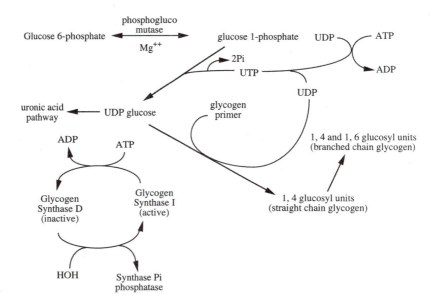

FIGURE 5.13   Glycogen synthesis (glycogenesis).

Figure 5.14 gives details of the glycogenolytic cascade. Muscle and liver glycogen stores have very different functions. Muscle glycogen is used to synthesize ATP for muscle contraction, whereas hepatic glycogen is the glucose reserve for the entire body, particularly the central nervous system. The amount of glycogen in the muscle is dependent on the physical activity of the individual. After bouts of strenuous exercise, the glycogen store will be depleted, only to be rebuilt during the resting period following exercise. One aspect of physical training is concerned with the expansion of the muscle glycogen store. Through repeated depletion–repletion routines, athletes hope to expand the size of this store so as to increase their endurance. Athletes follow an exercise/recovery routine as well as a dietary carbohydrate routine (a normal carbohydrate diet followed by a carbohydrate-rich diet just prior to competition) that they hope will improve their performance through increasing their muscle glycogen store.

The different types of muscle store and use glycogen for glucose and ATP generation differently. Overall, about 8% of muscle glycogen is converted to glucose and some of this is released into the bloodstream. The remainder is oxidized via the glycolytic pathway. Myocytes lack glucose-6-phosphatase, so glucose release from gluconeogenesis is not possible. Exercise or "work" by "red" muscle fibers that are richly endowed with mitochondria can oxidize glucose fully to provide ATP and result in water and carbon dioxide. These fiber types are found in the heart muscle and the long muscles of legs and arms. White muscle, in contrast, has tremendous capacity for glycogenesis, glycogenolysis, and glycolysis, but has far fewer mitochondria the red muscle. Hence, work by white muscle results in an accumulation of lactate released to the bloodstream, since the glucose being used cannot be completely oxidized to CO_2 and water. While red muscle can continue

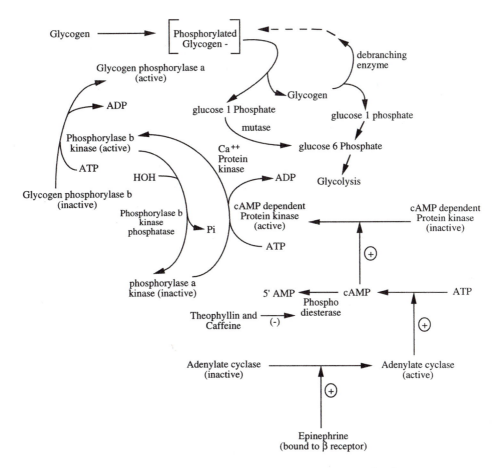

FIGURE 5.14 Stepwise release of glucose molecules from the glycogen molecule.

to work indefinitely, given its generous blood supply and mitochondrial complement, white muscle cannot. It can provide the sudden burst of activity needed for sprinting, for example, but its endurance is limited. Most muscle groups in the human body are mixtures of red and white fibers and, therefore, physical training will capitalize on the fiber type best used for the type of competition (i.e., sprinting vs. marathon running) anticipated.

Hepatic glycogen stores are dependent on nutritional status. They are virtually absent in the 24-hour-starved animal, while being replenished within hours of *ad libitum* feeding. Clusters of glycogen molecules with an average molecular weight of 2×10^7 form quickly when an abundance of glucose is provided to the liver. As noted, the amount of glycogen in the liver is diet dependent. In fact, there is a 24-hour rhythmic change in hepatic glycogen that corresponds to the feeding pattern of the animal. In nocturnal animals such as the rat, the peak hepatic glycogen store will be found in the early morning hours, while the nadir will be found in the evening hours just before nocturnal feeding begins. In humans accustomed to eating during the day, the reverse pattern will be observed.

Glycogen synthesis begins with glucose-1-phosphate formation from glucose-6-phosphate through the action of phosphoglucomutase. Glucose-1-phosphate then is converted to uridine diphosphate glucose (UDP-glucose), which can then be added to the glycogen already in storage (the glycogen primer). UDP-glucose can be added through a 1,6 linkage or a 1,4 linkage. Two high-energy bonds are used to incorporate each molecule of glucose into the glycogen. The straight chain glucose polymer is composed of glucoses joined through the 1,4 linkage and is less compact than the branched chain glycogen, which has both 1,4 and 1,6 linkages, as shown in Figure 5.15. The addition of glucose to the primer glycogen with a 1,4 linkage is catalyzed by the glycogen synthase enzyme, while the 1,6 addition is catalyzed by the so-called glycogen-branching enzyme (Amylo 1→4, 1→6) transglucosidase). Once the liver and muscle cells achieve their full storage capacity, these enzymes are product inhibited and glycogenesis is "turned off." Glycogen synthase is inactivated by a cAMP-dependent kinase and activated by a synthase phosphatase enzyme that is stimulated by changes in the ratio of ATP to ADP. Glycogen synthesis is stimulated by the hormone insulin and suppressed by the catabolic hormones. The process does not fully cease, but operates at a very low level. Glycogen does not accumulate appreciably in cells other than liver and muscle, although all cells contain a small amount of glycogen. Note in Figure 5.13 that a glycogen primer is required for glycogen synthesis to proceed. This primer is carefully guarded so that some is *always* available when glycogen is synthesized. This means that glycogenolysis *never* fully depletes the cell of its glycogen content.

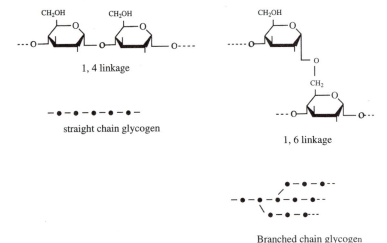

FIGURE 5.15   Glycogen structures.

Glycogenolysis is a carefully controlled series of reactions referred to as the glycogen cascade. It is called a cascade because of the stepwise changes in activation states of the enzymes involved. To release glucose for oxidation by the glycogenolytic pathway, the glycogen must be phosphorylated. This is accomplished by the enzyme glycogen phosphorylase, which exists in the cell in an inactive form (glycogen phosphorylase b) and is activated to its active form (glycogen phosphorylase a) by the enzyme phosphorylase b kinase. In turn, this kinase also exists in an inactive form, which is activated by the calcium-dependent enzyme protein kinase, and active cAMP-dependent protein kinase. These activations each require a molecule of ATP. Finally, the cAMP-dependent protein kinase must have cAMP for its activation. This cAMP is generated from ATP by the enzyme adenylate cyclase which, in itself, is inactive unless stimulated by a hormone such as epinephrine, thyroxine, or glucagon. As can be seen, this cascade of activation is energy dependent, with three molecules of ATP required to get the process started. Once started, the glycolytic pathway will replenish the ATP needed initially as well as provide a further supply of ATP to provide the necessary energy. As mentioned, the liver and muscle differ in the use of glycogen. This also affects how ATP is generated within the glycogen-containing cell and how much is generated by cells that do not store glycogen.

In part, our understanding of how glycogen is used or how glycogenolysis occurs has come about because of some spontaneous mutations in the genes coding for the enzymes involved. While these mutations in several instances are devastating to the affected person, they have shed light on the control of the overall balance of glycogenesis and glycogenolysis.

One very rare autosomal recessive disease is due to a mutation in the gene for the branching enzyme. This results in an accumulation of straight chain glycogen which, because it is less compact than the normally branched chain glycogen, results in an enlarged liver. This disorder is called amylopectinosis and is usually grouped with the other disorders characterized by enlarged glycogen stores. However, this disorder affects synthesis rather than degradation (which is normal) and there is not an excess of glycogen. Infants with this disorder die from cardiac or liver failure, rarely surviving their first year.

Five mutations in the genes that code for the enzymes of glycogenolysis have been described. These include a mutation in the lysomal α-1,4-glucosidase (also called acid maltase), which results in a generalized excess of glycogen not only in the liver and muscle but also in the viscera and central nervous system. This disorder is called Pompe's disease, and is characterized by an enlarged liver and heart and extreme muscular weakness. Death due to heart failure is common.

A mutation in the gene for the debranching enzyme (amylo-1,6-glucosidase) results in the accumulation of highly branched short chain glycogen in the muscles and liver. The usual glycogen has a branch point at every fourth glucosyl residue in the interior of the molecule and farther apart on the outer regions. The glycogen stored in people lacking the debranching enzyme have their branch points very close together. This occurs when glucose is mobilized from glycogen and only the outer limbs of the molecule are used. Without a functioning debranching enzyme, the remaining inner core is untouched. These cores accumulate and are responsible for the enlarged liver and heart. Because the glycogen gives up only a small amount of its glucose, the muscle that needs it for ATP synthesis is very weak. This condition is called Forbes disease.

McArdle's disease affects only the muscle, and the enzyme lacking is the muscle phosphorylase. Patients with this disorder are intolerant to exercise and accumulate glycogen in the muscle but not the liver. This disorder was discovered in military recruits during World War II, when, in a few isolated instances, young men were found who could not endure the rigorous physical training of boot camp. Unfortunately, the first few were thought to be malingerers and were forced to exercise to death by their drill instructors. When their deaths were investigated, the reason for their exercise intolerance was understood. The mutation in the muscle phosphorylase gene might not have been discovered otherwise.

In the liver, a mutation in phosphorylase is far more serious. This disorder, known as Her's disease, results in growth retardation, an enlarged liver due to glycogen accumulation, and elevated serum lipids. In both McArdle's disease and Her's disease, glycogen is not phosphorylated because of a mutation in the enzyme that catalyzes the initial step in glycogenolysis. This is also the case for another glycogen-storage disease, but, instead of a mutation in the gene for phosphorylase, the mutation is in the gene for the phosphorylase kinase, the enzyme that is responsible for the activation of glycogen phosphorylase b to glycogen phosphorylase a. Without the addition of energy through the hydrolysis of ATP, the glycogen phosphorylase cannot transfer this phosphate to the glycogen molecule and produce a molecule of glucose-1-phosphate. People with this disorder have the same symptoms as those with Her's disease and, in addition, have increased rates of gluconeogenesis and hypoglycemia when without food for long periods of time. They also have decreased phosphorylase activity in hepatocytes and leukocytes.

All of these disorders in glycogen synthesis and degradation are rare and all appear as autosomal recessive traits. They are listed in Table 5.7. Their long-term outlook is not very good. Some nutritional manipulations have been tried to reduce the hypoglycemic episodes that characterize some of these disorders. These include a continual nasogastric drip of a starch suspension. Whether this therapy is effective over the long term has not been established. Because the hypoglycemia is due to an inability to normally mobilize the glycogen-glucose, care must be given to avoid prolonged

TABLE 5.7
Amino Acids that Contribute a
Carbon Chain for the Synthesis
of Glucose

Amino Acid	Enters As:
Alanine	Pyruvate
Tryptophane → Alanine	Pyruvate
Hydroxyproline	Pyruvate
Serine	Pyruvate
Cysteine	Pyruvate
Threonine	Pyruvate
Glycine	Pyruvate
Tyrosine	Fumarate
Isoleucine	Succinyl CoA
Methionine	Succinyl CoA
Valine	Succinyl CoA
Histidine → Glutamate	α-ketoglutarate
Proline → Glutamate	α-ketoglutarate
Glutamine → Glutamate	α-ketoglutarate
Arginine → Glutamate	α-ketoglutarate

periods without food. The glucose that is needed by all the body's cells must be provided either by the diet or through an active gluconeogenic process.

GLUCONEOGENESIS

The provision and maintenance of normal blood-glucose levels in the absence of food involves not only glycogenolysis but the synthesis of glucose from noncarbohydrate precursors. This process, called gluconeogenesis, is shown in Figure 5.16. Gluconeogenesis occurs primarily in the liver and kidney. Most tissues lack the full complement of enzymes needed to run this pathway. In particular, the enzyme phosphoenolpyruvate carboxykinase is not found. Shown in Figure 5.16 are the enzymes that are unique to gluconeogenesis. The other reactions shown use the same enzymes as glycolysis (see Figure 5.9) and do not have control properties with respect to gluconeogenesis. The rate-limiting enzymes of interest are glucose-6-phosphatase, fructose-1,6-biphosphatase, and phosphoenolpyruvate carboxykinase (PEPCK). Pyruvate kinase and pyruvate carboxylase are also of interest because their control is a coordinated one with respect to the regulation of PEPCK.

The capacity to synthesize glucose in times of need is absolutely essential to survival. Blood glucose must be maintained so that those tissues, i.e., brain, that have an absolute requirement for this fuel can continue to function. While gluconeogenesis is essential, it must be carefully controlled so that excess glucose is not produced. The process is energetically very expensive. If it were not closely regulated, undue protein catabolism with its associated ammonia load could be devastating because it uses as substrates the carbon chains of deaminated amino acids. Fortunately, a number of fail-safe controls that do not allow this to occur are in place.

Cori and Alanine Cycles

The pathway shown in Figure 5.16 provides glucose to all cells in the body. Under normal dietary conditions, the glucose synthesized in the kidney is used by it as fuel to run its metabolism. Only under conditions of prolonged starvation (more than 48 hours) will the kidney contribute significant amounts of glucose to the circulation. Thus, circulating glucose produced by gluconeogenesis comes

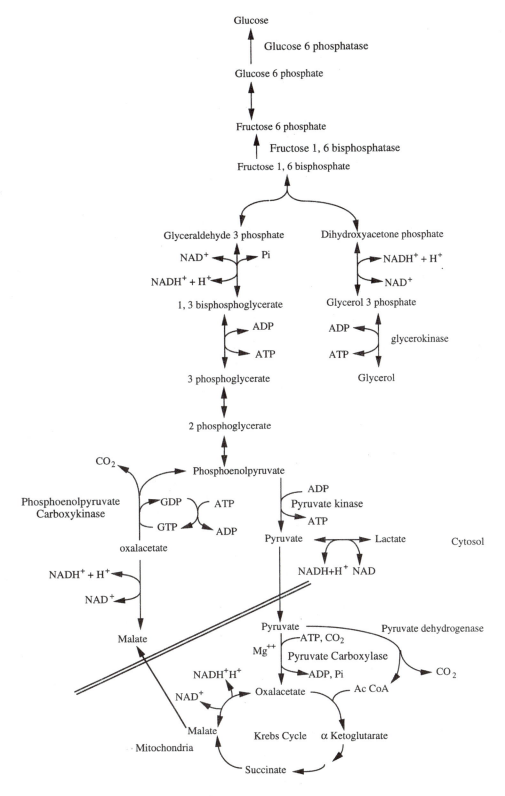

FIGURE 5.16 Pathway for gluconeogenesis.

from the liver. There are two important metabolite or substrate cycles that are crucial to the effective regulation of blood-glucose levels. One is the Cori cycle, shown in Figure 5.17, and the other is the alanine cycle, shown in Figure 5.18. The Cori cycle involves the use of glucose by the red blood cell. Glucose is oxidized via glycolysis to two molecules of lactate. The lactate is delivered to the liver, which converts it back to glucose via gluconeogenesis. The red cell produces 2 ATPs through the glycolytic process while the liver uses six ATPs to resynthesize the glucose.

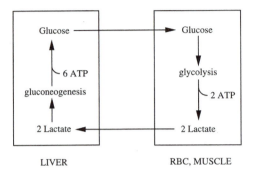

FIGURE 5.17   The Cori cycle.

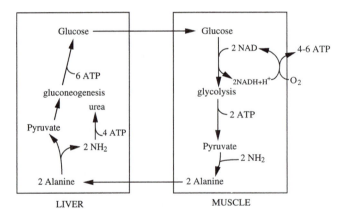

FIGURE 5.18   The alanine cycle. Both the Cori cycle and the alanine cycle serve to ensure a supply of glucose to cells that require it.

The alanine cycle differs in that the exchange is between muscle and the liver. Since the muscle cell has mitochondria, it can use the reducing equivalents generated by the glycolytic sequence to generate 4–6 moles of ATP. Rather than lactate, the muscle cell transaminates the surplus glycolytic product, pyruvate, to alanine and sends this alanine to the liver. Once in the hepatocyte, this alanine is deaminated (the amino group used for urea synthesis) and the resultant pyruvate used to resynthesize glucose via gluconeogenesis. These cycles are important in glucose homeostasis because they provide the means for supplying glucose to tissues that need it and which cannot *complete* its oxidation.

To participate in these cycles, the peripheral cells must release lactate, pyruvate, or alanine as their metabolic end product of glycolysis. Further, the use of the $NADH^+H^+$ generated by the glycolytic sequence differentiates whether the Cori cycle or the alanine cycle is used. If the former, the $NADH^+H^+$ is used to reduce pyruvate to lactate. In the latter, the $NADH^+H^+$ is used as part of a shuttle system for the entry of reducing equivalents into the mitochondrial respiratory chain. This $NADH^+H^+$ is *not* available for pyruvate reduction. Pyruvate is thus available for transamination and is converted to alanine, which, in turn, is used by the liver for glucose synthesis. Although the alanine cycle is an important mechanism in the regulation of blood-glucose level, other amino acids can also serve as glucose precursors. Listed in Table 5.7 are amino acids that can be used in this way. People who consume high-protein, high-fat diets frequently use their excess protein intake to provide the carbon skeletons for glucose synthesis. In addition, when people have been without food for several days, the body proteins are catabolized for energy and to provide glucose precursors. As can be seen in the gluconeogenic pathway shown in Figure 5.16, as well as in the Cori and alanine cycles (Figure 5.18), gluconeogenesis uses more ATP than glycolysis produces. This is a costly process but one that is essential to survival.

The difference in ATPs used and produced implies that the mitochondria are important to the regulation of the pathway. Indeed, one shuttle, the malate-aspartate shuttle shown in Figure 5.19, has rate-controlling properties. The malate-aspartate shuttle works to transport reducing equivalents into the mitochondria. Malate is transported into the mitochondria, whereupon it gives up two reducing equivalents and is transformed into oxalacetate. Oxalacetate cannot traverse the mitochondrial membrane, so it is converted to α-ketoglutarate in a coupled reaction that also converts glutamate to aspartate. Aspartate travels out of the mitochondria (along with ATP) in exchange for glutamate. Once out in the cytosol, the reactions are reversed. Aspartate is reconverted to glutamate, and α-ketoglutarate reconverted to oxalacetate. The oxalacetate, in turn, can be reduced to malate or decarboxylated to form phosphoenolpyruvate. Measurement of the activity of this shuttle has revealed that the more active the shuttle, the more active the gluconeogenesis. This is because the shuttle provides a steady supply of oxalacetate via α-ketoglutarate in the cytosol. This oxalacetate cannot get there any other way. As mentioned, it is generated by the Krebs cycle in the mitochondria, but cannot leave this compartment.

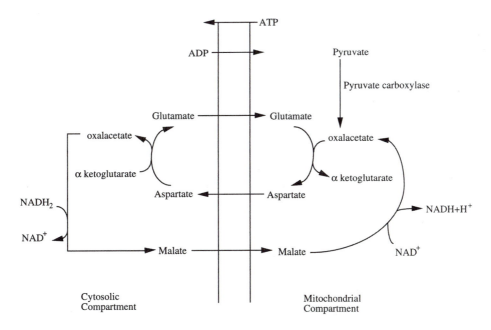

FIGURE 5.19   Malate aspartate shuttle.

Oxalacetate is essential to gluconeogenesis because it is the substrate for PEPCK, which catalyzes its conversion to phosphoenolpyruvate (PEP). This is an energy-dependent conversion that overcomes the irreversible final glycolytic reaction catalyzed by pyruvate kinase. The activity of PEPCK is closely coupled with that of pyruvate carboxylase. Whereas the pyruvate kinase reaction produces 1 ATP, the formation of PEP uses two ATPs: one in the mitochondria for the pyruvate carboxylase reaction and one in the cytosol for the PEPCK reaction. PEPCK requires GTP provided via the nucleoside diphosphate kinase reaction, which uses ATP. ATP transfers one high-energy bond to GDP to form ADP and GTP.

The enzyme PEPCK has been studied extensively as scientists have tried to understand the gluconeogenic process. In starvation or uncontrolled diabetes, PEPCK activity is elevated, as is gluconeogenesis. Starvation elicits a number of catabolic hormones that serve to mobilize tissue energy stores as well as precursors for glucose synthesis. Uncontrolled diabetes elicits similar hormonal responses. In both instances, the synthesis of the PEPCK enzyme protein is increased. Unlike other rate-limiting enzymes, PEPCK is not regulated allosterically or by phosphorylation–dephosphorylation mechanisms. Instead, it is regulated by changes in gene transcription of its single copy gene from a single promoter site. This regulation is unique because all of the known factors (hormones, vitamins, metabolites) act in the same place. They either turn on the synthesis of the messenger RNA for PEPCK or they turn it off. What is also unique is the fact that only liver and kidney cells translate this message into active enzyme protein, which catalyzes PEP formation. Other cells and tissues have the code for PEPCK in their nuclear DNA but do not synthesize the enzyme. Instead, these cell types synthesize the enzyme that catalyzes glycerol synthesis. In effect then, only the kidney and liver have an active gluconeogenic process.

The next few steps in gluconeogenesis are identical to those of glycolysis but are in the reverse direction. When the step for the dephosphorylation of fructose-1,6-bisphosphate occurs, there is another energy barrier and instead of a bidirectional reaction catalyzed by a single enzyme, there are separate forward and reverse reactions. In the synthesis of glucose, this reaction is catalyzed by fructose-1,6-bisphosphatase and yields fructose-6-phosphate. No ATP is involved but a molecule of water and an inorganic phosphate are produced. Rising levels of fructose-2,6-bisphosphatase allosterically inhibit gluconeogenesis while stimulating glycolysis. AMP likewise inhibits gluconeogenesis at this step.

Finally, the removal of the phosphate from glucose-6-phosphate via the enzyme complex glucose-6-phosphatase completes the pathway to yield free glucose. Again, this is an irreversible reaction that does not involve ATP. The glucose-6-phosphate moves to the endoplasmic reticulum, where the phosphatase is located. Should there be a mutation in the gene for the translocation of glucose-6-phosphate to the endoplasmic reticulum or in its phosphatase, glucose cannot be released and hypoglycemia will result. This reaction is also used when glycogenolysis provides the phosphorylated glucose. In either instance, free glucose is not released to the circulation. The resultant disease is called Von Gierke's disease. In addition to hypoglycemia, this rare, autosomally recessive disease is characterized by an enlarged liver due to excess glycogen stores, elevated blood lipids, decreased sensitivity to insulin, brain damage, and a shortened lifespan. About 25% of all patients with some form of glycogen-storage disease have Von Gierke's disease. Aside from providing many small meals throughout the day and night in an attempt to prevent the hypoglycemia, dietary maneuvers can achieve little else.

GLUCOSE HOMEOSTASIS

In the foregoing sections, each of the metabolic pathways involved in the use and production of glucose was discussed with the goal of providing a framework for understanding how the blood-glucose level is maintained within very close limits. Soon after food is consumed, digested, and absorbed, the blood-glucose levels rise. Glucose is a hydrophillic compound and can circulate freely in the blood stream without the need for a special carrier. However, as a hydrophillic compound, it cannot penetrate the plasma membrane surrounding the cells of the body without help. The mechanism for glucose entry is dependent on the hormone insulin and on proteins called glucose transporters. As was discussed in the absorption of glucose by the enterocyte, there are at least four of these proteins. GLUT 1 has a Km that ranges from 16.9–26.2 mM. Under the same conditions, GLUT 2 has a low affinity for glucose and a Km between 3.9 and 5.6 mM. GLUT 3 has a Km of

10.6 and GLUT 4 has a Km of 1.8–4.8 mM. The GLUT 2 transporter can also transport fructose. Its activity is regulated by glucose concentration and by triiodothyronine. Some cell types have only one of these proteins, while others have more than one.

The transporters differ slightly in their structure yet have large areas of homology. They also differ in their affinity for glucose. GLUT 3 and 4 have a higher affinity for glucose than does GLUT 1. These higher affinities assure that glucose transport will be maximal in tissues containing these isoforms even when the substrate levels are relatively low. This is particularly important to the CNS since glucose is its main energy source. GLUT 2 has the lowest affinity for glucose and the rate of transport of glucose through this carrier is directly proportional to the change in glucose concentration. This has importance in the absorption of glucose by the enterocyte, as described in the section on digestion and absorption. It means that the intestinal cell has a fail-safe glucose-uptake system — one that is energy dependent and another that is not. In addition, when the body is in the postprandial state (after a meal has been consumed) and blood glucose levels are high, there is a net flux of glucose into the hepatocytes and islet cells of the pancreas because of the presence of the GLUT 2 transporter. It is not particularly active unless blood-glucose levels are elevated. In contrast, when the body is starving, intracellular glucose levels rise as a result of increased glucose production via gluconeogenesis and glycogenolysis. When the intracellular glucose levels rise, GLUT 2 can work in the opposite direction transporting glucose out of the liver cell for transport to cells lacking significant glucose production capacity. Table 5.8 lists the transporters and their locations. As mentioned in the section on absorption, the glucose transporter is referred to as a mobile transporter because, when it is not in use, it is sequestered in an intracellular pool. When needed, it leaves its storage site, moves to the interior aspect of the plasma membrane, forms a loose bond with the membrane, picks up the glucose molecule and moves it through the membrane into the cytosol, whereupon the glucose can be phosphorylated and metabolized. Figure 5.20 is a cartoon of how these transporters work when the recruitment of the transporter is responsive to insulin signaling.

TABLE 5.8
Location of the Glucose Transporters

Transporter	Location
GLUT 1	Ubiquitous but found mainly in brain, erythrocytes, placenta and cultured cells. Is not particularly responsive to insulin regulation
GLUT 2	Liver, β cells of pancreas, kidney, intestine
GLUT 3	Ubiquitous in human tissue, CNS
GLUT 4	Adipose tissue, heart, skeletal muscle

The action of insulin is initiated when it binds to its plasma membrane receptor. In the binding process, the transport form of insulin, proinsulin, is cleaved with the release of the C-peptide. The insulin receptor extends through the plasma membrane and has an intrinsic protein kinase as part of its structure. When insulin binds to the receptor, almost instantly, autophosphorylation of the receptor occurs with phosphate groups from ATP attached to the exposed tyrosine residues. Phosphorylation of the tyrosine residues requires the movement of the calcium ion from its storage site on the endoplasmic reticulum. This mobilization of calcium occurs when phosphatidyl inositol triphosphate and diacylglycerol are produced from the membrane phospholipid, phosphatidylinositol. In turn, the diacylglycerol stimulates the temporary binding of Ca^{++} to the kinase to facilitate the phosphorylation of the tyrosine residues. All of these reactions result in a change in the phosphorylation state of the transporter in its storage site facilitating its release and migration to

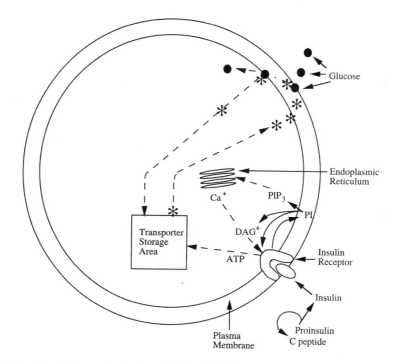

FIGURE 5.20 As blood-glucose levels rise, the β cell of the pancreas releases insulin, which binds to its receptor on the surface of the target cell and signals the release of the mobile glucose transporter from its storage site. The transporter migrates to the plasma membrane, picks up the glucose, transports it to the cytosol, and releases it.

the cell surface. This, then, accomplishes the goal of moving the glucose from the blood stream into the cell for its appropriate disposal.

Not all cells mobilize their glucose transporters under the influence of insulin. Some use a different mechanism. Brain cells are an example, as are the β cells in the islets of Langerhans in the pancreas. These cell types have stringent requirements for glucose as their principal metabolic fuel, yet their use and transport of glucose is independent of insulin bound to a plasma membrane receptor. The presence of glucose transporters in a wide variety of tissues has been ascertained by a number of scientists, yet the details of their recruitment and the signals necessary for this recruitment are not fully known.

As mentioned, insulin bound to its receptor on the plasma membrane is essential to the entry of glucose into insulin-dependent cells. When a person (or animal) consumes a glucose-rich food the blood glucose rises. This glucose stimulates the pancreatic β cells in the islets of Langerhans to release insulin. How the glucose transporter is recruited is not specifically, known but nonetheless, glucose enters the cytosol of the β cell via GLUT 2 and is phosphorylated to glucose-6-phosphate by the enzyme glucokinase. It is thought that this phosphorylation step provides the signal to the β cell to release insulin from its insulin store. Aberrations in pancreatic glucokinase result in impaired insulin release and subsequent impairment in the use of glucose. Again, exactly how this signal is generated is not known. The PIP cycle is involved, as is the tyrosine kinase and the calcium ion, but information is lacking on the specifics of the mechanism. The transport of glucose and subsequent release of insulin via the Golgi complex also involve the calcium, sodium, and potassium ions and ATP.

As the blood-glucose levels fall because of the insulin-stimulated use of this glucose, less glucose is transported into the β cell and thus less insulin is released. In turn, all of the various cells that use glucose will have less glucose to use as well as less insulin bound to receptor signaling glucose use. In the fully fed state, insulin is the key to normal glucose oxidation or conversion to glycogen or fatty acids. However, in the absence of continuous feeding, the body must adjust its metabolism to ensure a continuous fuel supply. Other hormones now play key roles as the blood glucose falls. These hormones switch metabolism from glucose disposal to blood-glucose maintenance. First, they exert an anti-insulin action at insulin target cells by interfering with insulin-stimulated glucose uptake. In so doing, they promote insulin resistance. That is, the cells are resisting the positive effects of insulin on glucose uptake and oxidation via glycolysis. Second, these hormones provide signals that enhance glycogenolysis and gluconeogenesis to provide glucose to those cells that need it. The enhancement of glycogenolysis in the liver precedes that of gluconeogenesis, since glycogen is more readily available than are the substrates for gluconeogenesis. In addition, glycogenolysis is energetically less expensive than is gluconeogenesis. Third, lipolysis and fatty acid oxidation are enhanced to provide energy and glycerol for glucose synthesis. All of these inhibitions and enhancements are coordinated so that the blood-glucose level remains within the normal range of 80–110 mg/dl (4–6 mmol/L). Excursions above and below might occur briefly, but, as soon as they occur, mechanisms are activated that restore overall normoglycemia.

ABNORMALITIES IN THE REGULATION OF GLUCOSE HOMEOSTASIS: DIABETES MELLITUS

Just as we have learned about the details of the synthesis and use of gluconeogenesis, pentose shunt, glycolysis, and glycogen through the study of genetic anomalies in these pathways, so too have we learned about the regulation of glucose homeostasis through the study of a large number of genetic errors that result in the disease diabetes mellitus. Currently, the number of genetic mutations thought to be responsible for the development of this disease are in excess of 200, depending on the definitions used for the disease. According to the American Diabetes Association (ADA), one person in 14 in the U.S. either has diabetes mellitus or will develop it during his or her lifetime. Of this population, 90% will develop the Type 2 or the non-insulin-dependent diabetes mellitus form, and the rest will develop the Type 1 or insulin-dependent form. The risk of developing the secondary complications varies with the particular genetic mutation that has caused the disease. Some of these are listed in Table 5.9. Not all of the genetic mutations that cause the diabetic state have been found. Furthermore, there are twice as many people with mutations that associate with diabetes than there are people with the disease.

Quite a bit of information suggests that the phenotypic expression of these mutations can be modified by environmental factors. These environmental influences may explain the discrepancy between the frequencies of the genotypes and phenotypes. That is, far more people have these genetic aberrations than the number who actually develop diabetic symptoms. Clearly, lifestyle choices (exercise, food choices, etc.) influence the phenotypic expression of the genotype. Of concern is the report of the CDC that, over the last 20 years, the number of people with diabetes has risen. Between 1980 and 1994 there was a 39% increase in this number. The CDC estimates that 5.9% of the population now have this disease.

Of the total population with diabetes mellitus, about 10% have the disease as a result of pancreatic insulin production failure, while 90% develop the disease as a response to one or more failures in the target tissues: liver, muscle, or adipose tissue. This population difference is the basis for the division of the diseases into two broad types. Type 1 takes in the group of diseases that relate to the failure of the pancreas to produce sufficient insulin. Type 2 refers to that group of diseases that develop in response to abnormalities in the target tissues.

People with Type 1 are in the minority with respect to diabetes, yet they have the most severe form of this disorder. People with this form are far more likely to develop the secondary consequences of the disease, are likely to develop the disease quickly, and at an early age. Children are the most frequent victims. The age of onset is often younger than 15 years. The incidence of this

TABLE 5.9
Mutations that Associate with Type 1 and Type 2 Diabetes Mellitus

Gene	Comments
Nuclear DNA	
Hepatic nuclear transcription factor 4α (MODY 1)	Subjects have impaired insulin secretion. 44 different mutations in this gene have been reported
Glucokinase (MODY 2)	Subjects are generally nonobese
Hepatic transcription factor 1α (MODY 3)	Hypertension and Type 2 are found in this genotype, which is polymorphic
Glycogen synthase	Activation of the enzyme is impaired
Glucagon receptor	Susceptibility to Type 2 is variable among different population groups
Insulin receptor	Associated with peripheral insulin resistance in some Type 2 subjects
Insulin receptor substrate (IRS-1)	Results in a signal transmission defect associated with insulin resistance
Mitochondrial α glycerol 3 phosphate dehydrogenase	Associated with Type 2 and with impaired mitochondrial function
Glucose transporters (GLUT 1-4)	Associated with both obesity and Type 2 diabetes
Mitochondrial DNA*	
tRNA^{leu}	7 mutations have been found that associate with diabetes
ND 1	11 mutations have been reported
ND 2, ND 3, ND 4	1 mutation in each of these genes has been reported
tRNA$^{Cys, Ser, Lys}$	1 mutation in each of these genes has been reported
tRNA^{thr}	4 mutations have been found
D-Loop[†]	3 mutations have been reported
COX II	2 mutations have been reported
ATPase 6,8	4 mutations have been reported

* Mutations in the mitochondrial genome that associate with diabetes are heteroplasmic, i.e., there is mixture of normal and abnormal DNA in each cell. The percentage of the abnormal determines the degree to which the function of that cell is impaired.

[†] Promoter regions for the 13 structural genes found in the mitochondrial genome are found here.

form of diabetes varies throughout the world. Table 5.10 shows some incidence rates in several countries for children younger than 15 years of age.

The term *incidence* refers to the number of new cases reported in a given year. In Table 5.10, several years were averaged to provide overall incidence rates for each country. Incidence data for adults have been difficult to acquire, because adults who are insulin dependent may have started out as noninsulin dependent. Nonetheless, Libman et al, in a 1993 *Diabetes Care* article, reported that adults (older than age 20 years) newly diagnosed with Type 1 have an incidence rate of 9.2/100,000. Altogether, the prevalence of Type 1 appears to be approximately 0.12% of the U.S. population. This prevalence is a far smaller number than that for Type 2.

There are year-to-year, seasonal, and regional variations in the incidence of Type 1 diabetes mellitus. Dietary ingredients, viral infections, and exposure to toxins together with genetic factors are the factors that influence disease development. Studies of identical twins have shown a concordance rate that varies from 30–60%, depending on the genotype. Concordance means that if one twin develops the disease, the other has a 30–60% chance of developing that same disease. Where the concordance rate is closer to 30%, the disease development is probably more responsive to environmental influences than when the concordance rate is close to 60%.

TABLE 5.10
Age-Specific Incidence Rates
of Type 1 in Children Younger
than 15 Years

Country	Rate*
Finland	35.3/100,000
Denmark	21.5/100,000
U.S.A.	14.3/100,000
Malta	13.6/100,000
United Kingdom	13.5/100,000
Australia	13.2/100,000
Netherlands	11.0/100,000
New Zealand	10.1/100,000
Algeria	8.1/100,000
Japan	1.8/100,000

* These rates were reported by Karvonen et al. in *Diabetologia* 36:888–892, (1993) and come from an international group (WHO) dedicated to acquiring such data.

Diabetes mellitus is characterized by defective glucose utilization. In its most severe form, the symptoms of excessive thirst, excessive urination, rapid weight loss, and perhaps coma and death are observed. It is a disease that has been known for centuries, having been described in the medical writings of the ancient Greeks and Egyptians. Even then, it was recognized that diet and obesity were important factors in its development.

Although diabetes is a collection of diseases arising for a variety of reasons, its diagnosis is based on the results of a glucose tolerance test. Examples of the results of this test are shown in Figure 5.21. Glucose tolerance in persons suspected of having diabetes mellitus is tested by giving the person a large dose (usually 1 gram/kilogram body weight) of glucose and monitoring the blood-glucose level before and at 30-minute intervals after the glucose.

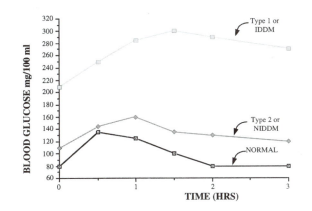

FIGURE 5.21 Typical glucose-tolerance values for normal people and for people with either Type 1 or Type 2 diabetes. Note that the normal response to a glucose challenge includes a rise followed by a fall in the blood glucose. The Type 2 patient may have a normal fasting blood glucose, but the rise following the challenge is greater than normal, and the fall is barely perceptible. The patient with Type 1 may have higher values at all time points. Within each group of subjects, there may be considerable variation.

Variations on the procedure have been developed for screening purposes. A single fasting blood sample may be examined for its glucose content, or a fasting plus a 2-hour post-meal blood sample may be examined, or the test may be 5 hours in duration rather than the usual 2 hours. The type of test used is determined by the patient's symptoms and family history. In normal, nondiabetic, fasted individuals, administration of a bolus of glucose elicits a typical rise then fall in blood glucose levels as shown in Figure 5.21. In contrast, diabetic individuals may have an elevated fasting blood glucose level and may have a failure to appropriately reduce the glucose level after the test dose. Abnormal glucose tolerance is defined in several ways: there may be a departure from the normal fasting blood glucose level (80–110 mg/dl, 4–6 mmol/L) or post-challenge values may be excessively high (exceeding 250 mg/dl) or fail to return to the pre-challenge blood-glucose level by 120 minutes after the challenge. Blood insulin values may exceed normal in some individuals and this is interpreted as a sign of target tissue insulin resistance. These individuals are referred to as hyperinsulinemic. They may be hyperinsulinemic yet have normal blood glucose levels and normal glucose tolerance. There are several variations in response to a glucose challenge and these will be discussed subsequently. However, because the use of glucose is critical to almost every cell in the body, any deviation in any of the many metabolic steps involved in its use must be included in the definition for diabetes mellitus. Table 5.11 lists the abnormalities in cells and tissues that are associated with diabetes mellitus.

TABLE 5.11.
Abnormalities in Cells, Tissues, or Systems that are Associated with Diabetes Mellitus

Abnormality[*]	Result
T cell Receptor (Recognizes self antigen)	Autoimmune destruction of β cells
Inability to repel certain viruses	Viral destruction of β cells
Amino acid substitution in A or B chains of insulin	Major, minor, or no effect on insulin activity
Amino acid substitution at the cleavage site in C chain of proinsulin	No C chain cleavage to produce insulin
β cell glucokinase	Inability to recognize the glucose signal for insulin release
Obesity	Adipose tissue resistance to insulin
Insulin receptor protein	Defective structure fails to fully bind insulin to the target cell membrane or fails to send signal to mobilize glucose transporters; tissue insensitivity to insulin
Glucose transporters	Failure to move glucose into target cell
Intracellular enzymes	Failure to process glucose or produce sufficient ATP

[*] Within each of these disorders, several different mutations causing the same clinical state have been found.

CONSEQUENCES OF INSULIN DEFICIENCY

Much of what has been learned about the consequences of insulin deficiency has been due to the use in experimental animals of β cell cytotoxic agents such as alloxan or streptozotocin. These agents destroy the insulin-producing islet cells, making it possible to study the acute and chronic responses to insulin deficiency. The literature on this aspect of diabetes research is voluminous. From it we have learned how insulin functions in the body.

Insulin release by the β cells of the pancreas involves a number of interrelated metabolic reactions in both the cytosol and the mitochondria, as shown in Figure 5.22. The islet must sense that blood-glucose levels are rising. This is a critical step in insulin release. The glucose phosphorylating enzyme, glucokinase, serves this function. GLUT 2 transports glucose through the plasma membrane, making this glucose available to glucokinase. The glucose is then processed through glycolysis. Once glucose

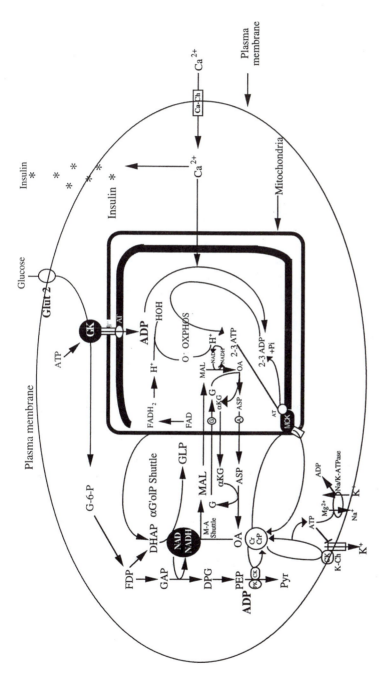

FIGURE 5.22 Proposed mechanism for insulin release by the β cell of the pancreas. Incoming glucose transported by GLUT 2 is phosphorylated by glucokinase (GK) and metabolized via glycolysis. Glucose stimulates binding of GK to the mitochondrial pore protein. Because this binding activates GK increased amounts of G-6-P and ADP are formed. The ADP is transferred across the two boundary membranes through the outer membrane port (P) and the adenylate translocator (AT) in the inner membrane into the mitochondrial matrix, enhancing OXPHOS. Increased phosphorylation of glucose provides substrate for the glycolytic pathway, resulting in elevated production of substrate (NADH) and phosphoenolpyruvate (PEP). Reducing equivalents from external NADH are transported into mitochondria through the glycerol phosphate shuttle or malate–aspartate shuttle. Pyruvate kinase (PK) forms a complex with creatine kinase (CK), and phosphate is directly transferred from PEP to creatine (Cr) yielding CrP. The increase in CrP may change the local concentration of ATP at the K$_{ATP}^+$ channel (K-Ch) through CK activity bound to the cell membrane. This results in a depolarization of the membrane and opens the CA^{2+} channel allowing calcium to flow into the cell. The increase in calcium flux is then followed by insulin (*) release. Mutation of mtDNA results in a reduction in ATP production by OXPHOS, thus affecting the insulin-release mechanism. A shortfall of ATP would also result in reduced insulin synthesis.

is made available to the glucokinase, this enzyme migrates to the mitochondrial membrane pore protein. The ATP produced by the mitochondrial OXPHOS system is needed by glucokinase, as well as by the sodium potassium pump.

Insulin secretion also involves some ion shifts. The Na^+ K^+ pump becomes active as is the K^+ channel allowing these ions to move in and out of the cell. The calcium ion moves in. This ion serves two functions: it stimulates OXPHOS and insulin exocytosis.

As can be seen in Figure 5.22, the flux of substrates through glycolysis and the Krebs cycle contribute reducing equivalents to the mitochondrial respiratory chain. When coupled with ATP synthesis, ATP production is enhanced. This ATP is essential not only for the glucokinase reaction and the sodium potassium pump, but also to support the synthesis of new insulin to replace that which was released. Altogether then, islet function is dependent on optimal mitochondrial function and, in turn, appropriate islet function assures appropriate glucose disposal.

Insulin deficiency characterized by high blood-glucose levels (hyperglycemia) results in the excessive thirst (polydipsia), excessive urine production (polyuria), and rapid weight loss so typical of severe diabetes. The body fat stores are raided, but fatty acid oxidation is incomplete. As a result, acetone, β hydroxybutyrate, and acetoacetate, products of incomplete fatty acid oxidation accumulate. These are the ketone bodies.

Elevated blood levels of these ketones (ketonemia) are observed, as is an elevated urinary excretion (ketonuria). Rising levels of ketones increase the need for buffering power, since they tend to lower pH. Acidosis is a characteristic feature of diabetes. Not only are the fat stores raided, but so is the body protein. Proteolysis (body-protein breakdown) is enhanced and the amino acids thus liberated are used for energy or as substrates for intracellular glucose synthesis. The ammonia released as a product of the deamination of these amino acids assists in the buffering of the accumulating ketones. However, this ammonia is in itself cytotoxic, so the body must increase its capacity to convert it to urea. Humans with uncontrolled diabetes thus are characterized by a loss in body protein, an increase in blood and urine levels of ammonia, an increase in urea synthesis, a negative nitrogen balance, a loss in fat store, elevated blood and urine levels of glucose, and elevated levels of fatty acid oxidation products. Some of these metabolic products are also excreted via the lungs in the expired air. The breath of an uncontrolled diabetic has the aroma of the ketones — somewhat like the aroma of fingernail-polish remover.

Pancreatic β Islet Cell Failure

Several explanations for pancreatic insulin-production failure have been offered. The two most generally accepted are: 1) failure due to autoimmune disease and 2) failure due to viral destruction of the islet β cells. In each of these instances, the genetic heritage of the individual plays a role. In both, the immune system is involved. In autoimmune disease, the insulin-producing pancreatic islet cell is destroyed because the immune system has sensed the presence of an antigen that it recognizes, not as a self-made protein, but as a foreign protein. It then destroys this protein. The interleukins are involved in the autoimmune process and so too is apoptosis.

Autoimmune Disease

Autoimmune diabetes can be accompanied by a number of other diseases; multiple endocrine failure is not uncommon. This means that autoimmune diabetes can be found in a person who also develops psoriasis, rheumatoid arthritis, or thyroiditis (inflammation of the thyroid gland). In autoimmune diabetes, there may be an immune tolerance that is particularly difficult to break. This is because the body may lack antibody specificity. Antibodies can be raised that will react to a group of closely related compounds in an instance of "mistaken identity." Usually, an antibody reacts to a single antigen rather than to a group of closely related antigens. In autoimmune disease, the body tolerates a range of exposures to these antigens before it reacts. Thus, the term, *immune tolerance* means that the individual will tolerate a wide range of exposures to an antigen or group of antigens before a systemic immunologic reaction is elicited. This is not the same thing as food allergies or skin allergies or localized reactions to allergens. Neither should this term, *immune tolerance*, be confused with diseases of the immune system per se.

Autoimmunity is characterized by an increase in the number of T cells. The T cell originates in the thymus, and is a type of cell that is an essential component of the immune system. It recognizes antigens and produces antibodies to them. In some instances, the recognition is non-specific. That is, antibodies are produced that react to a group of related antigens. In autoimmune disease, this is what happens. There is a loss in specificity resulting in a progressive autoimmuno-logically mediated destruction of the islet cells. Immunosuppression can interfere with this destruc-tion, but the use of such drugs has its own set of problems, such as kidney disease or increased susceptibility to infectious disease. The immunologic response is initiated when the T cell receptor recognizes an antigen on the correct histocompatability complex on the surface of the antigen-presenting cell. Transmission of this signal to the nucleus of the cell involves the calcium ion, a complex of related proteins, and the phosphatidylinositol cycle, which is responsible for the movement of the calcium ion from the intracellular store to where it is needed. Antigens are then produced.

Autoimmune disease can result when mutations in the genes that encode the various components of the immune system occur and the body's own protein is recognized as foreign. The body then develops antibodies that effectively destroy that protein. Several cell-surface proteins have been found to stimulate antibody production in susceptible individuals. Several of these are listed in Table 5.12. In autoimmune diabetes, the destruction of the β cell in the islets of Langerhans appears to be associated with one or more mutations in the genes that encode the major histocompatibility complex (MHC). More than 100 genes are involved. These genes have been mapped to the short arm of chromosome 6 and comprise approximately 2×10^6 nucleotides. Mutations in these genes have been divided into two classes (I and II) and are further identified by letter designations. There are so many genes that it would be impossible to list them all in this text. Suffice it to say that the class II HLA genes are more closely linked to autoimmune diabetes than are the class I HLA genes. In rodents (NOD mice and BB rats), several mutations in the MHC region have also been identified that express themselves as autoimmune diabetes mellitus. These rodents have been studied exten-sively and have helped scientists understand the process of the disease.

The development of autoimmune diabetes is associated with an inflammation of the pancreatic islet cells (insulitis). In insulitis, CD4 and CD8 T cells, B cells, macrophages, and killer T cells have all been found. The presence of these marker cells indicates that an immunologic reaction is taking place.

In humans with autoimmune diabetes, islet-cell antibodies to cytoplasmic antigens were reported in 1974. Following this initial report, hundreds of antibodies have been reported in tissues from humans. Glutamic acid decarboxylase (GAD), an enzyme found in β cells that catalyzes the synthesis of the neurotransmitter gammaaminobutyric acid (GABA), has been shown to be an antigen. Islet β cells, like neuronal cells, possess a mechanism for hormone release that depends on a specific trophic stimulus. GABA and GAD are components of this secretion signaling system, as is the glucose transporter, the enzyme, glucokinase, and the mitochondrial oxidative phospho-rylation system that produces ATP. ATP and the calcium ion are major players in the insulin-release mechanism. Autoantibodies to GAD have been observed prior to the development of the clinical state and the presence of these antibodies has been suggested as an early indication of the disease. The gene for GAD has been cloned, characterized, and mapped to chromosome 10. Two isoforms (a 65 kDa and a 67 kDa form) have been isolated and a single gene encodes each. While antibodies to GAD have been found in patients with autoimmune diabetes, the GAD itself is not abnormal nor has its gene been found to be abnormal. Thus, the GAD genes are not candidate genes in this disease.

TABLE 5.12.

Autoantigens that Elicit Islet Cell Reactive Antibodies in Humans with Autoimmune Type 1 Diabetes Mellitus

Autoantigen	Comments
Glutamic acid decarboxylase (GAD)	Antibodies present before clinical state develops
Insulin (58,000 kDa, 51 amino acids)	Antibodies found after diagnosis
Insulin receptor	Antibodies found after diagnosis
38,000 M_r	Antibodies develop in patients with insulinoma
RIN polar	Antibodies are related to those formed in response to certain gangliosides
52,000 M_r	Antibodies present before clinical state develops. Likely the same as GAD
Carboxypeptidase H	Cell surface autoantigen and a major protein in insulin secretory granules
ICA 12/ICA 512	Putative islet cell antigens
PM-1 60,000 M_r	A 24-amino acid peptide that may be a polyclonal activator of autoreactive T cells
IAAb (antiαlgAb)	Anti-immoglobulin antibodies that appear prior to IDDM*
C-peptide	Antibodies found after IDDM diagnosis
ICA 69	Antibodies found prior to IDDM development

*IDDM = insulin-dependent diabetes mellitus

Although GAD antibodies can indicate incipient type 1 diabetes, these antibodies are also elevated in other autoimmune diseases in the absence of diabetic symptoms; yet, in each disease, there are distinct differences in epitope recognition. This suggests that the autoantigen is being presented to the T cells and the B cells by different mechanisms. However, so many have been reported that it is difficult to assign causality to many of them. For example, islet-cell antibodies to plasma insulin C-peptide have been reported in adults having diabetes for at least 10 years. Antibodies to insulin have been found in newly diagnosed children but not in their high-risk relatives. This suggests that these antibodies are a result, not a cause, of the disease. As mentioned, GAD antibodies have been reported to occur prior to the development of diabetic symptoms, so it is possible that they may serve as an early marker of autoimmune disease.

Diabetes Secondary to Viral Infections

Epidemiologists have noted that, following epidemics of diseases such as flu (influenza), there are upsurges in the numbers of people with newly diagnosed Type 1 diabetes. Not all people who develop flu develop diabetes, nor have all people who develop Type 1 diabetes had their disease preceded by flu. Other infections (mumps, rubella) can also precede diabetes. Infections due to cytomegalo virus, the Epstein-Barr virus, the picornaviruses, (which include several strains of encephalomyocarditis virus — the foot-and-mouth disease virus), and a number of the Coxsackie B viruses, can precede diabetes in susceptible individuals. These persistent infections can cause damage in addition to the typical lytic effect that occurs during the acute phase. Damage can take the form of producing (or inducing) small changes in cell proteins that change the function of the protein or change the recognition of this protein as a normal cell constituent. These slightly modified self proteins then are recognized as foreign, and an antibody is produced to destroy it. One such protein is the islet-cell surface protein (ICS). Antibodies to ICS have been found in virally infected humans. Viruses also induce the production of cytokines such as interferon, the interleukins, and tumor necrosis factor. These substances alter the immune response by regulating the expression of β-cell antigens and thus contribute to the development of insulitis. The mechanisms whereby viruses induce diabetes have been the subject of considerable speculation.

There appears to be a genetic determination of susceptibility to these infections that probably involves genes that encode the various components of the immune system. This explains why some humans may develop diabetes secondary to a viral infection while others do not. Notkins and co-workers have demonstrated that susceptibility is compatible with a single gene acting in an auto-somal recessive manner. The mode of action of such a gene would be to control specific virus receptors on the β cell membrane, or perhaps to control the membrane permeability to such viruses, thus facilitating the incorporation of the viral DNA into the β cell DNA and altering its function. Fluorescein labeling of viral antibody has confirmed the entry of the coxsackie B virus into β cells, as well as changes in β cell mRNA. Here is another example of an interaction between the environment and genetics. If the genetic material is such that the immune system is somewhat incompetent in its response to a particular virus, then the viruses will inflict serious damage on the β cell. In persons with a fully competent immune system, such damage does not occur. Evidence of virus-induced diabetes in man has been gathered through post mortem studies of pancreatic tissue excised from children with fatal viral infections. Of the 250 children studied, seven had a coxsackie B infection, and of these, four had significant β cell destruction and evidence of acute or chronic inflammation in the islet tissue. Whether immunization against these viruses is possible and will prevent this disorder is a significant research problem.

Genetic Errors in Insulin Structure

In addition to islet-cell failure, the possibility exists that the islet cell may not be producing insulin in the appropriate amino acid sequence to have full biological activity. Insulin gene mutations have been documented in both man and mouse. These mutations result in a variety of amino acid substitutions and have a variety of effects on insulin action. These mutations are very rare. Steiner et al., for example, studied a number of families with aberrant insulin genes. Ten families were studied that had single point mutations that resulted in amino acid substitutions in the proinsulin molecule. Six of these substitutions resulted in the secretion of defective insulin molecules due to changes within the A or B chains. These changes resulted in molecules that were immunoreactive but did not bind adequately to the plasma membrane insulin receptor on the adipocyte. Four additional families were found to have insulin gene mutations that prevented the recognition of the C-peptide-A chain dibasic cleavage site and its removal. These families had high levels of proinsulin in the blood because the C-peptide was not removed upon binding of the insulin to the receptor site. Proinsulin is the large insulin molecule released by the pancreas. When insulin reaches its target tissue, a fraction of this large molecule is split off. This fraction is called the C-chain or C-peptide. Proinsulin is 1/40th to 1/60th as active as insulin. The aberrant proinsulin molecule may have the appropriate β cell processing protease but not the appropriate C-peptide recognition site.

The variability of the insulin gene in a group of phenotypically normal individuals has been studied. Although several variants have been found, none were considered mutants. That is, the base pair substitutions that coded for specific amino acids in the insulin molecules were in places that did not affect the conformation of the molecule or active site in the insulin molecule, nor did they affect the cleavage of proinsulin to active insulin. The variety of base pair substitutions and subsequent amino acid substitutions in the insulin molecule appears to be large, yet the impact of these aberrations (if they can be called aberrations) is very small or nonexistent. However, should substitutions occur that affect proinsulin cleavage, or reactive sites in the insulin molecule described above, then diabetes would develop. Whether the diabetes is Type 1 or Type 2, would, as mentioned, depend on the nature of the defect.

Also rare are persons with mutations in the gene for the pancreatic glucose-sensing enzyme, glucokinase. The β cell glucokinase plays a pivotal role in the cascade of events leading to the release of the insulin molecule by the β cell. There are several important players: the glucose transporter (GLUT 2), the glucokinase (GK) enzyme and the mitochondrial system (OXPHOS) that produces the energy (ATP) needed for both insulin synthesis and release, the sodium (Na^+), potassium (K$^+$), and calcium (Ca^{++}) ions, and the Na$^+$K$^+$ATPase. Shown in Figure 5.22 is a proposed mechanism whereby the islet cell is stimulated to release insulin. Rising levels of glucose in the blood promote the uptake of this glucose by the β cell. The glucose transporter (GLUT 2) facilitates its entry and the ATP-dependent glucokinase facilitates the phosphorylation of this glucose. If either the glucose transporter or the glucokinase is abnormal due to a mutation in the genes that encode either of the proteins, then the glucose-sensing system that is part of the insulin-release process will not work appropriately and the β cell will not respond appropriately to the glucose signal. Actually, numerous mutations have been reported for the glucokinase gene, yet altogether, these many mutations are thought to account for less than 0.1% of the population with diabetes mellitus. Indeed, there is some argument as to whether these people should be included in the Type 1 category. Usually they are thought to have Type 2 because, although abnormal, the islets do respond to some secretogogues such as amino acids and do produce and release insulin. Again, lifestyle choice determines whether hormone supplements are required for the successful management of the disease. People with these defects are usually referred to as having MODY, maturity onset diabetes of the young. MODY patients are further subdivided into MODY 1, MODY 2, and MODY 3, based on the gene that has mutated.

In MODY 1, the mutated gene is on chromosome 20 and encodes the hepatocyte nuclear transcription factor 4α. Several different mutations in this gene have been found. An aberration in the glucokinase gene on chromosome 7 is responsible for MODY 2. In this gene alone, 44 different mutations have been reported. Finally, MODY 3 is due to a mutation in the hepatocyte nuclear factor 1α on chromosome 12, a transcription factor essential to the expression of several specific hepatic genes as well as several pancreatic β cell genes. All of these mutations are inherited as an autosomal dominant trait. While MODY patients have an islet-cell secretory defect, MODY 1 and MODY 3 patients also manifest a defective responsiveness to the glucose-lowering effect of insulin. Thus, they are classed as insulin resistant. To them, a dose of insulin is less effective in lowering blood glucose than for a person without these genetic defects. This is because the hepatic transcription factors 1α and 4α affect the transcription of several of the genes that encode the enzymes of intermediary metabolism. These enzymes are critical to the appropriate oxidation of glucose and, if less than optimally active, glucose will not be as easily oxidized, hence the apparent reduction in glucose uptake and use by the liver.

TARGET TISSUE DISEASE

The range of disorders in man and laboratory animals that fit the description for Type 2 diabetes is far greater than that for Type 1. Some of these have already been described. For most of the Type 2 disorders, obesity is a concurrent feature. This obesity either precedes or accompanies the development of abnormal glucose tolerance, and hyperphagia is a common characteristic as well. The prevalence of Type 2 is far greater than that of Type 1, as illustrated in Table 5.13.

Animals that are genetically obese usually overeat and studies of the neuroendocrine influence on food intake have suggested that, in part, the genetic error in these animals may reside in the satiety signaling system in the brain. One feature of obesity that is common to Type 2 diabetes is the resistance of the peripheral fat cell to the effects of insulin.

When the fat cell becomes enlarged, it loses its responsiveness to the action of insulin in facilitating the entry of glucose into that fat cell. For decades, it has been known that overly fat people who are insulin resistant can reverse their condition by restricting their energy intake, thereby reducing their excess fat store. When the adipocyte returns to its normal size, it becomes normally responsive to the action of insulin. For many years, it was thought that this defect was simply due to a distortion of the plasma membrane insulin receptor brought about by the increased fat store. Now, however, it is thought that the resistance of the enlarged fat cell favors its smaller neighbors that bind insulin normally. The possibility of mutations in the insulin-receptor gene has been considered and indeed, such have been found. However, mutations in the downstream

Carbohydrates

243

TABLE 5.13
Prevalence[1,2] of Type 2 diabetes, 30–64 Years of Age, in Different Cultural Groups in the U.S.*

Group	Prevalence (%)
Pima Indians (SW U.S.)	55
Hispanics	14
Blacks	~12 females; 8 males
White, European-Americans	8 females; 6 males

*Data from King, H. and Rewers, M., WHO, Ad hoc Diabetes Reporting Group. Global estimates for prevalence of diabetes mellitus and impaired glucose tolerance in adults. Diabetes Care 1993;16:157.

signaling system also have been found, and these result in impaired signal transduction in the cell and consequently impaired glucose use. Signals generated when insulin binds to its receptor on the plasma membrane are needed for the recruitment of the glucose transporters from their storage sites on the endoplasmic reticulum to the plasma membrane and thus transport glucose into the cell and present it to the various enzymes for metabolism. Aberrations in the genes for the glucose transporters likewise can associate with diabetes — particularly that associated with obesity.

In addition to these primary genetic mutations that result in both diabetes and obesity, there are a number of candidate genes that have been found that influence the regulation of food intake (see Unit 3).

Insulin resistance can be observed in muscle as well as adipose tissue. By definition, insulin resistance means that it takes abnormally large amounts of insulin to regulate or control blood glucose within normal limits. A person with insulin resistance may not develop abnormal glucose tolerance *if* the pancreas is able to sustain an abnormally high insulin output. In this circumstance, the individual may be insulin resistant and hyperinsulinemic but not hyperglycemic or have abnormal glucose tolerance. Eventually, the islet β cells may not be able to sustain this high insulin output and the insulin resistance will then progress to abnormal glucose tolerance and subsequently to the diabetic hyperglycemic state. Insulin resistance may be a feature of the fat cell, the muscle cell, or the liver cell, and in each instance, genetic errors in the DNA that code for this particular plasma membrane structure have been found. Insulin receptors have been isolated and their structures analyzed and sequenced. The part of the DNA that codes for these structures has been cloned. It is generally agreed that the receptor is synthesized as a single polypeptide precursor of 1382 amino acids that contains a signal peptide of 27 amino acids, the α subunit of 735 amino acids (including four basic amino acids of the processing site) and the β subunit of 620 amino acids. After glycosylation, processing, and disulfide bonding, it is expressed as a heterotetramer composed of two α-subunits with a molecular weight of 95,000. The α-subunit is entirely located on the exterior aspect of the plasma membrane while the β subunit extends through the plasma membrane into the cytoplasm. The human insulin receptor gene is located on chromosome 19. It consists of 22 exons. The α subunit is encoded by the first 120 kb and includes a signal peptide, an insulin-binding region, and a cysteine-rich region. The β subunit is encoded by the last 30 kb. As mentioned, this subunit is the portion of the receptor molecule that crosses the plasma membrane. It has a proreceptor processing site and the final portion of the unit of the receptor molecule consists of tyrosine kinase. When insulin binds to the α subunit, autophosphorylation occurs, resulting in activation of tyrosine kinase. If the DNA coding for the receptor protein has mutated so that lysine, an important amino acid for ATP binding and receptor activity, is replaced by arginine, alanine, or methionine, the receptor is no longer able to mediate insulin action. Thus, lysine is a critical component of the ATP binding site. Clusters of tyrosine residues are also critical to the autophosphorylation process. If tyrosine is replaced by phenylalanine, again, receptor activity is compromised. Other mutations in the code for the receptor protein that affect its amino acid sequence have been reported. These mutations (depending on their location) likewise can affect the activity of the receptor and, in turn, can explain insulin resistance.

Glucose Transporters

Insulin resistance can also be attributed to post receptor defects. Errors in the codes for the glucose transporter genes (called GLUT 1, 2, 3, and 4) have received considerable attention, especially as these errors may relate to the development of obesity. These are summarized in Table 5.14. Peripheral glucose uptake may be impaired if GLUT 4 in the adipocyte is aberrant. An aberrant adipocyte transporter would result in less insulin-stimulated glucose uptake by these cells, with the result of increased levels of circulating glucose, which in turn would stimulate pancreatic insulin release. Thus, clinically, one could observe both hyperglycemia and hyperinsulinemia. Note the similarity of clinical features between this genetic error and the error described above that involves the gene for the insulin molecule. In both instances, peripheral fat cell resistance, together with compensatory increases in hepatic glycolysis, pentose shunt, glycogenesis, lipogenesis, hepatic lipid output, and adipocyte lipid uptake and storage are observed. The compensatory increases in hepatic metabolism are probably driven by both the hyperinsulinemia, with its effects on anabolic processes, and the hyperglycemia, which provides a continuous high level of substrate for these anabolic pathways.

TABLE 5.14
Aberrant Glucose Transporters and Their Consequences

Protein	Consequences of an Error
GLUT 1	Minimal changes in glucose uptake by all tissues that use glucose
GLUT 2	Liver — glucose metabolic pathways suppressed; increased gluconeogenic activity
	β cell — pancreas unresponsive to glucose stimulation
	kidney — increased gluconeogenic activity
GLUT 3	Minimal changes in glucose uptake and metabolism
GLUT 4	Adipose tissue — decreased glucose use by fat cell; compensatory increase in hepatic glucose use; increase hepatic lipogenesis and lipid output; increase hepatic glycogen store
	Heart, muscle — decreased glucose use by muscle could be lethal if compensatory use of fatty acids and ketones is insufficient

Studies of obese diabetic Zucker (ZDF/drt) rats and obese diabetic A^{vy}/a mice have suggested that the substrate glucose may have regulatory properties with respect to the expression of the gene for the glucose transporters in liver, muscle, and fat cells. This suggestion was based on the observation that alterations in GLUT 2 or GLUT 4 proteins were not associated with the obesity per se, but were secondary to severe hyperglycemia that was the result of the diabetic state. Incidentally, studies of GLUT 1 and GLUT 4 in adipocytes from normal rats showed that feeding a high-glucose diet increases GLUT 4 activity, while feeding a high-fat diet decreased GLUT 4 activity and increased GLUT 1 activity. These results indicated that the two transporters differed in their response to insulin and diet composition. In normal nondiabetic rats, GLUT 1 activity is probably responsible for basal glucose uptake while GLUT 4 is under the control of insulin. When insulin levels are high, GLUT 4 activity is high, whereas GLUT 1 seems to be independent of the hormone, but responsive to the nutritional state of the body. It also appears, from studies of normal and genetically obese or diabetic animals, that the multiplicity of glucose transporters, while seemingly redundant, compose a "fail-safe" mechanism to ensure glucose disposal. Should one of the isoforms be aberrant because of a genetic error, there would be a backup transporter that could increase in activity to compensate for the genetically determined loss.

The study of dietary factors that affected GLUT 1 and GLUT 4 activity also provides some insight into the nature of nutrient–gene interactions that may explain Type 2 diabetes. As mentioned, economic constraints, food rationing, and lifestyle choices can affect the time course and severity of Type 2 diabetes. Lifestyle choices include decisions about the quantity and composition of the food consumed as well as the level of physical activity. As indicated above, the diet composition can affect the recruitment of GLUT 1 and GLUT 4 transporters. If the Type 2 patient had an error in one or the other of these transporters, clearly the choice of diet would be critical in the disposal of glucose by the adipocyte, and in turn critical to the regulation of glucose homeostasis. In addition, exercise has been shown to affect the regulation of glucose transport in skeletal muscle. With exercise, the number of GLUT 4 transporters increases, independent of insulin status. This explains the decrease in insulin need by diabetic athletes, an observation frequently made but poorly understood in practical terms. With exercise, the muscle uses glucose without the need for insulin bound to the receptor. Insulin is thus not needed for the recruitment and translocation of GLUT 4 transporters. With this in mind, if Type 2 diabetes develops as a result of an error in the insulin receptor, then exercise will promote glucose use and facilitate the reduction in blood glucose. If the person thus includes daily exercise and avoids high-energy or high-carbohydrate diets, then the phenotypic expression of the genotype for either a receptor or transporter error might be postponed or avoided. In turn, it is easy to understand why the incidence of Type 2 diabetes decreases with restricted food supplies and increases in physical activity, as happens during times of economic duress or war.

While all of the above-described mutations can lead to abnormal glucose tolerance and, in some people, many of the secondary problems associated with diabetes, diabetes mellitus itself can be a secondary problem as a result of other diseases. While these diseases have not been discussed in detail, the reader should be aware of their occurrence. Lead toxicity and exposure to certain chemicals (Vacor, for example) results in damage to the pancreas and subsequently glucose intolerance. Other toxicities can have similar effects. Diseases of other endocrine organs, especially those producing counter insulin hormones, likewise will result in characteristic changes in glucose tolerance. In this category are diseases of the adrenal cortex (Cushing's disease or excess cortisol release) or tumors in the brain that result in excess ACTH production, or diseases that result in excess growth-hormone release or excess glucagon release, or diseases of the thyroid gland that impair thyroxin release. All of these diseases result in hormonal imbalance and peripheral insulin resistance, and subsequently affect insulin action. When these diseases are treated successfully, frequently the diabetic characteristic disappears. Sometimes, if the primary disease goes too long without treatment, irreversible changes in the pancreas and target tissues occur. Whether there are genetically determined reasons for these other endocrine diseases is not known. Generally speaking, relative to the incidence of diabetes mellitus, these other endocrine diseases are relatively rare. So too are the instances of heavy-metal intoxication. Nonetheless, no discussion of diabetes mellitus in its many forms would be complete without their mention.

Diabetes Due to a Mitochondrial Genomic Mutation

The maternal inheritance pattern of diabetes has led researchers to look for genetic defects in the mitochondrial genome. As mentioned earlier, mtDNA is maternally inherited because the mitochondria contributed to the embryo by the sperm is much less than that present in the egg at the time of fertilization. The ratio is around 1:1000. Thus, mtDNA mutation(s) are transmitted to the progeny via maternal lineage. Mutations in the mitochondrial genome should have an impact on cellular energy production as genes encoded by the mitochondrial genome are components of oxidative phosphorylation (OXPHOS), or are their supporting tRNAs or rRNAs. Inhibition of cellular energy production has been shown to reduce or abolish both insulin secretion and action and, of course, this is central to the diabetic condition. In addition, losses in OXPHOS efficiency mean that there are losses in the control of glucose homeostasis, as evidenced by elevations in the tissue and blood lactate levels as well as impaired glucose tolerance.

To date, 42 different mitochondrial DNA mutations (point mutations, deletions, and duplications) have been found to associate with the Type 2 diabetes phenotype (Table 5.15). Many are associated with other mitochondrial syndromes and involve disturbances in CNS function as well as disturbed muscle and renal function. In these instances, the diabetes symptoms are less important than those associated with the CNS. Patients with diabetes associated with mtDNA mutations generally are not obese. They exhibit hyperglycemia, which is due to a significantly reduced insulin-secretory capacity that progresses with age. This hyperglycemia is not due to decreased insulin sensitivity, aberrant insulin receptors, or aberrant glucose transporters. These patients develop a fatty liver, which is not an uncommon feature of diabetes mellitus. Beta cell loss is seen as well as defects in glucose-induced signaling of insulin release.

The mitochondrial tRNA$^{Leu(UUR)}$ gene is an etiological hot spot for mtDNA mutations. So far, 11 disease-related mutations in this gene have been described, with six associated with Type 2 diabetes. Mutations in this particular gene make up 60% of all of the mitochondrial tRNA gene mutations. An A/G transition at bp 3252 was found to be associated with mitochondrial encephalomyopathy, pigmentary retinopathy, dementia, hypothyroidism and Type 2 diabetes. Another A/G point mutation at bp 3243 has been associated with maternally inherited myopathy and cardiopathy and with MELAS. A C/T exchange at 3256 in a patient with an MERRF-like syndrome has also been reported. It is interesting to note that the 10 different mutations in the same gene can have different phenotypes. The differences in the phenotypes are due to the degree of heteroplasmy, the position of the mutation, and to environmental influences such as diet.

Type 2 diabetes has been reported as a secondary characteristic in many of the mitochondrial diseases. Patients with chronic progressive external ophthalmoplegia (CEOP), and the complete Kearns-Sayre syndrome carrying large mtDNA deletions and duplications have been reported along with Type 2 diabetes. Patients with Pearsons disease, which involves the bone marrow as well as the pancreas, and patients with renal tubular dysfunction also exhibit diabetic symptoms. Glucose intolerance or frank diabetes mellitus occurs in some subjects with mitochondrial myopathy. Of particular interest is the syndrome MELAS, which shares the point mutation at position 3243 in mtDNA with diabetes. Persons with Type 2 diabetes as a result of the 3243 mutation may have no clinical neurological defects. The severity of the symptoms is directly related to the percentage of the mtDNA that is aberrant. Those with MELAS have a large percent of their tRNA with the mutation while those with diabetes (only) have a much smaller percent mutated tRNA. MELAS, LHON, and MERF also develop as results of mutations with the structural genes composing the respiratory chain. Mutations in the any of these genes result in nonfunctional or partially functional respiratory activity and, as a result, ATP production is impaired. Because the CNS depends so heavily on ATP production, large-scale reductions in synthetic capacity will affect this system before any other. Other organs and tissues that have alternative and compensatory mechanisms available for maintaining, at least in part, a "near normal" phosphorylation state will be less seriously compromised. Yet even these mechanisms will fail as the person ages and, when this failure occurs, clinical symptoms of abnormal glucose homeostasis will be observed.

Actually, any mutation of the mitochondrial DNA should affect the synthesis of ATP and, therefore, the supply of cellular energy. Of interest to the current work on mtDNA mutation and diabetes is the discovery that mutations in the mtATPase 6 and 8 genes associate with NIDDM. To date, five mutations that associate with NIDDM (Table 5.16) have been reported in the genes for ATPase 6 and 8. These two subunits, along with the 10 nuclear-encoded subunits, assemble to form complex V of oxidative phosphorylation, the F_1F_oATPase.

TABLE 5.15
Point Mutations in mtDNA
exclusive of the ATPase genes that
Manifest Primarily as Diabetes
Mellitus

Position	Mutation*	Gene
3243	A→G	tRNA^{Leu}
3252	A→G	tRNA^{Leu}
3256	C→T	tRNA^{Leu}
3271	T→C	tRNA^{Leu}
3290	T→C	tRNA^{Leu}
3291	T→C	tRNA^{Leu}
3316	G→A	ND1
3348	A→G	ND1
3394	T→C	ND1
3396	T→C	ND1
3423	G→T	ND1
3434	A→G	ND1
3438	G→A	ND1
3447	A→G	ND1
3480	A→G	ND1
3483	G→A	ND1
4216	T→C	ND1
4917	A→G	ND2
5780	G→A	tRNA^{Cys}
7476	C→T	tRNA^{Ser}
8245	A→G	COX II
8251	G→A	COX II
8344	A→G	tRNA^{Lys}
10398	C→T	ND3
11778	T→C	ND4
12308	A→G	tRNA$^{Leu(cun)}$
14709	T→C	tRNA^{Glu}
15904	C→T	tRNA^{thr}
15924	A→G	tRNA^{thr}
15927	G→A	tRNA^{thr}
15928	G→A	tRNA^{thr}
16069	C→T	D-loop
16093	T→C	D-loop
16126	C→T	D-loop

*When the mutation is heteroplasmic, Type 2
diabetes, rather than a more serious disease,
develops if the mutation is less than 50%.

This complex captures the energy generated by the respiratory chain as it joins two hydrogens to an oxygen to form water. Some of the energy is released as heat, while the remainder is used to form ATP. ATP synthesis is crucial for the synthesis of protein, especially insulin, and the intracellular concentrations of ATP are very important for insulin release. Of course, ATP synthesis is an important component in the regulation of the phosphorylation state that in itself has control properties with respect to intermediary metabolism. Shown in Table 5.16 are the ATPase mutations that have been found in humans and rats. Note that the human and rat ATPase 6 genes are of different lengths. The

TABLE 5.16
ATPase 6 Mutations in Humans and Rats that Associate with Type 2 Diabetes Mellitus

Position	Mutation	Species	Comments
8993	T→G	Human	Heteroplasmic: Accounts for 0.4-10% of NIDDM populations surveyed
8993	T→C	Human	Not as common as the T→G mutation; heteroplasmic
8860	A→G	Human	Similar in position to the rat mutation at 8204
8894	G→A	Human	Cardiomyopathy is a major feature of this disorder.
8204	G→A	Rat	Homoplasmic; found in BHE/Cdb and CFI:CD(SD)BR rats
8289	C→T	Rat	Homoplasmic; found in the BHE/Cdb rat.

human ATPase 6 gene has 636 bp and the rat has 679 bp. Thus, direct species comparison is not possible. Nonetheless, if one were to compare the approximate locations and effects of these mutations, some benefit could be derived. For example, the mutation at bp 8860 in the human is roughly equivalent to the mutation at bp 8204 in the rat. In each species, the mutation has occurred at about the same place in the gene and, while not identical with respect to base sequence, each has the same net effect of changing the polarity of the amino acids coded by the base substitution and in each, this amino acid substitution occurs in the proton channel that is so important in the capture of the energy of the respiratory chain and its transmittance to the high-energy bond of ATP.

Finally, although the mutations described above for diabetes mellitus are many and of clinical and scientific interest, the management of the disease is one of trial and error. Clinicians face some real challenges in devising appropriate strategies for the management of these disorders. What would be appropriate for one genotype might be inappropriate for another. Unfortunately, there are no easy, reliable, inexpensive gene screens available to help the clinician segregate these different genotypes. The American Diabetes Association (ADA) in its 1999 recommendations for clinical practice, suggests that persons with diabetes consume a low-fat diet, and, if they are overweight and sedentary, these patients should be encouraged to reduce their body-fat stores and increase their daily physical activity. The ADA also suggests individualizing the diet, because there have been a number of reports of patients who are better able to manage their glucose homeostasis when consuming a higher-fat diet or a higher-protein diet.

OTHER HEALTH CONCERNS IN CARBOHYDRATE NUTRITION

Already discussed are the genetic errors in glycolysis, shunt-activity, gluconeogenesis, and glycogen turnover. These are summarized in Table 5.17. Few of these affect large numbers of people and few can be managed successfully to normalize health and lifespan. In addition, the dietary and nondietary aspects of the many forms of diabetes mellitus have been presented. In the present section, attention to other issues of importance to carbohydrate nutrition will be given. These are related to the aging process and to the intake of nondigestible fiber, lactose, and alcohol.

AGE

Insulin resistance may be a feature of aging. With age, the pancreas becomes less responsive to signals for insulin release and the target tissues become less responsive to its action. In part, this may be due to age-related increased plasma membrane phospholipid saturation, but it is also due to age-related increases in fat-cell size. As fat cells accumulate stored fat, they become less sensitive to the action of insulin in promoting glucose uptake and use. Muscle cells likewise may have age-related changes in membrane fluidity that impair their response to insulin. As well, there is an

TABLE 5.17 (Continued)
Inherited Disorders of Carbohydrate Metabolism

Digestion	Lactose intolerance	Lactase	Chronic or intermittent diarrhea, flatulence, nausea, vomiting, growth failure in young children
	Sucrose intolerance	Sucrase	Diarrhea, flatulence, nausea, poor growth in infants
Intestinal transport	Glucose-galactose intolerance	Glucose-galactose carrier	Diarrhea, growth failure in infants, stools contain large quantities of glucose and lactic acid
Interconversion of sugars	Galactosemia	Galactose-1-P-uridyl transferase	Increased cellular content of galactose 1-phosphate, eye cataracts, mental retardation, increased cellular levels of galactitol; three mutations have been reported
		Galactokinase	Cataracts, cellular accumulation of galactose and galactitrol; two mutations have been reported
		Galactoepimerase	No severe symptoms; two mutations have been reported
	Fructosemia	Fructokinase	Fructosuria, fructosemia
		Fructose-1-P-aldolase	Hypoglycemia, vomiting after fructose load, fructosemia, fructosuria; in children: poor growth, jaundice, hyperbilirubinemia, albuminuria, amino-aciduria
		Fructose-1,6-diphosphatase	Hypoglycemia, hepatomegaly, poor muscle tone, increased blood lactate levels
	Pentosuria	NADP-lined xylitol dehydrogenase	Elevated levels of xylose in urine
Glucose catabolism	Hemolytic anemia	Glucose-6-phosphate dehydrogenase	Low erythrocyte levels of NADPH, hemolysis of the erythrocyte
		Pyruvate kinase	Nonspherocytic anemia, accumulation of phosphorylated glucose metabolites in the cell, jaundice in newborn
	Type VII glycogenosis	Phosphofructokinase	Intolerance to exercise, elevated muscle glycogen levels, accumulation of hexose monophosphates in muscle
Gluconeogenesis	Von Gierke's disease (Type I glycogenosis)	Glucose-6-phosphatase	Hypoglycemia, hyperlipemia, brain damage in some patients, excess liver glycogen levels, shortened lifespan, increased glycerol utilization
Glycogen synthesis	Amylopectinosis (Type IV glycogenosis)	Branching enzyme Liver amylo (1,4→1,6)-transglucosidase	Tissue accumulation of long-chain glycogen that is poorly branched, intolerance to exercise
Glycogenolysis	Pompe's disease (Type II glycogenosis)	Lysosomal a-1,4-glucosidase (acid matase) Amylo-1,6-gluco-sidase (debranching enzyme)	Generalized glycogen excess in viscera, muscles, and nervous system, extreme muscular weakness, hepatomegaly, enlarged heart
	Forbe's disease (Type III glycogenosis)	Muscle phosphorylase	Tissue accumulation of highly branched, short-chain glycogen, hypglycemia, acidosis, muscular weakness, enlarged heart

TABLE 5.17 (CONTINUED)
Inherited Disorders of Carbohydrate Metabolism

McArdle's disease (Type V glycogenosis)	Liver phosphorylase	Intolerance to exercise
Her's disease (Type VI glycogenosis) Phosphorylase kinase		Hepatomegaly, increased liver glycogen content, elevated serum lipids, growth retardation
(Type IX glycogenosis)		Hepatomegaly, increased liver glycogen levels, decreasd phosphorylase activity in hepatocytes and leukocytes, elevated blood lipids, hypoglycemia after prolonged fasting, increased gluconeogenesis

age-related decrease in muscle use. Working muscles have little need for insulin bound to its receptor to facilitate glucose use.

Altogether then, this decrease in muscle activity plus the increase in fat-cell size has a negative effect on the insulin–glucose relationship. Glucose levels rise and the β cells of the pancreatic islets of Langerhans increase their output of insulin to meet the glucose challenge. However, this excess output does little good in reducing the blood glucose in the aging, overly fat, inactive individual, and it is not uncommon to have Type 2 diabetes develop as a consequence. Age-related impaired glucose tolerance can be mitigated by food restriction and increased activity, which reverses the above physiological state. Because insulin is one of the main regulators of intermediary metabolism and because its action is counterbalanced by the glucocorticoids, the catecholamines, the thyroid hormones, glucagon, and several other hormones, it should be no surprise that age changes in these hormones occur as well. Again, some of these changes can be attributed to age changes in membrane lipids but some can be attributed to changes in hormone production and in the synthesis and activity of the receptors that mediate their action.

TABLE 5.18
Hormone Changes with Age

Hormone	Age - Effects
Serum Thyroxine (T4)	↓
Serum Triiodothyronine (T3)	↓
Thyroid binding globulin	No change or ↑
Thyroid stimulating hormone (TSH)	↓
Insulin	↑ followed by ↓
ACTH	↓
Epinephrine	↓
Glucagon	↓
Growth Hormone	↓
Estrogen	↓
Testosterone	↓
Cortisol (Glucocorticoids)	↓
Pancreatic polypeptide	↓

↑ increase; ↓ decrease

Table 5.18 lists some hormones affected by age. The blood levels of most of these hormones decrease in the aging human and laboratory animal. A few pass through a phase where they are elevated above normal then fall below normal as aging continues. All of these hormones serve to regulate the metabolism of carbohydrate, lipid, and protein. Age has unique effects on each of these tissues and their respective metabolic processes. The pathways of intermediary metabolism are outlined in Table 5.19. Each of these pathways has specific control points that are affected by age. Although various studies have shown age-related declines in enzyme activities, it should be remembered that these are *in vitro* measurements in conditions where substrates and coenzymes are in optimal amounts to assure saturation. This rarely occurs *in vivo*. Hence, a decline in activity may not mean a decline in *in vivo* function. In a number of instances, the age-related decline in activity of a pathway or reaction can be inhibited by chronic food restriction. This inhibition of aging effects on metabolism probably has to do with the decreased fat stores that are the result of food restriction. A decrease in fat store reduces the supply of fatty acid precursors to free radicals and this may lead to a reduction in error rates in the genetic material as well as a reduction in protein damage with resultant loss of function. In addition, a reduced fat store has effects on peripheral cell responsivity to insulin vis à vis glucose use and, of course, in the absence of hyperinsulinemia, there is a decreased release of the anti-insulin hormones. As described above, age-related alterations in hormone balance do occur and these alterations have an impact on carbohydrate oxidation, glycogen storage and mobilization, hexose monophosphate shunt, and gluconeogenesis.

As aging proceeds, there is a rise in blood lipids coupled with a decrease in adipose tissue lipoprotein lipase. With age, adipocytes have a less competent lipid-uptake system due to this decline in lipase activity. In normal aging animals, the rates of cholesterol synthesis do not change; however, the uptake of this cholesterol as well as its oxidation and excretion decline. This has the result of an age-related increase in serum cholesterol levels. Genetics plays an important role in these age-related changes in serum lipids (see Unit 6). Some genotypes are characterized by a sharper decline with age in lipid-uptake processes than other genotypes. For example, those whose lipoprotein receptors are genetically aberrant will, as a result, show a far earlier rise in serum lipids than those whose receptors are fully functional. Some may have a decline in only cholesterol uptake or triacylglyceride uptake, while others will have a decline in the uptake of both. Age-related declines in thyroid hormone production, thyroxine conversion to triiodothyronine, glucocorticoid release, and the insulin:glucagon ratio will have effects on fatty acid mobilization and oxidation and the results of this decline in hormone-stimulated lipolysis are observed as an age-related expansion of the fat stores. While age has effects on fatty acid synthesis in rats and mice, these effects are minimal in humans consuming the typical Western diet. This is because this diet is relatively rich in fat, so the need for its synthesis is almost nonexistent. Humans tend to use the dietary carbohydrate as their primary fuel and the surplus dietary fat is transported to the adipose tissue for storage. Hence, *de novo* fatty acid synthesis is negligible. In rats and mice, this is not the usual situation. The typical rodent diet is low in fat. Most of the energy comes from carbohydrate and deaminated amino acids (those in excess of need for protein synthesis). In the young animal there is considerable protein synthesis and with age there is a decline in this synthetic activity. With an age-related decline in protein synthesis, there is an increased need to rid the body of amino groups as the surplus amino acids are deaminated for use in gluconeogenesis and lipogenesis. This means that if the protein intake is not reduced to accommodate the decreased need for protein, there will be an increase in the activity of the urea cycle. Studies in aging rats have shown that dietary intake excess of energy and protein are associated with an age-related increase in urinary protein and renal disease that is preceded by first an increase, then a fall, in ureogenesis. Food restriction or protein intake restriction ameliorates these age-related changes in renal function and urea synthesis.

All of these age-related changes in intermediary metabolism are linked together by age changes in mitochondrial oxidative phosphorylation. As discussed in Units 2, 3, and 6, age carries with it a progressive change (increase) in mitochondrial membrane saturation, a progressive loss in ATP

TABLE 5.19
Effects of Age on Intermediary Metabolism and its Control

Pathway		Control Points	Effects of Age
Glycolysis	a)	Transport of glucose into the cell (mobile glucose transporter)	↓
	b)	Glucokinase	↓
	c)	Phosphofructokinase	↓
	d)	α-Glycerophosphate shuttle	
	e)	Redox state, phosphorylation state	
Pentose phosphate shunt	a)	Glucose-6-phosphate dehydrogenase	↓
	b)	6-Phosphogluconate dehydrogenase	↓
Glycogenesis	a)	Stimulated by insulin and glucose	ND
	b)	High-phosphorylation state (ratio of ATP:ADP)	ND
Glycogenolysis	a)	Low-phosphorylation state	ND
	b)	Stimulated by catecholamines	ND
Lipogenesis	a)	Stimulated by insulin	
	b)	Acetyl-CoA carboxylase	
	c)	High-phosphorylation state	
	d)	Malate citrate shuttle	↓
Gluconeogenesis	a)	Stimulated by epinephrine	
	b)	Malate aspartate shuttle	↓
	c)	Redox state	↑
	d)	Phosphoenopyruvate carboxykinase	↓
	e)	Pyruvate kinase	
Cholesterogenesis	a)	HMG CoA reductase	
Ureogenesis	a)	Carbamyl phosphate synthesis	↑, ↓
	b)	ATP	ND
Citric acid cycle	a)	All three shuttles	ND
	b)	Phosphorylation state	↓
Lipolysis	a)	Lipoprotein lipase	↓
Respiration	a)	ADP influx into the mitochondria	↓
	b)	Ca²⁺ flux	
	c)	Shuttle activities	↓
	d)	Substrate transporters	↓
Oxidative phosphorylation	a)	ADP:ATP exchange	↓
	b)	Ca²⁺ ion	
Protein Synthesis	a)	Accuracy of gene transcription	↓
	b)	Availability of amino acids	↓
	c)	ATP	↓

↑ - Increased as the animal ages

↓ - Decreased as the animal ages

ND - No data

NC - No change

synthetic efficiency, and an increase in free radical damage to mitochondrial DNA and its translation products. These progressive changes mean a progressive loss in the tight control of intermediary metabolism exerted by the concentration and flux of the adenine nucleotides. In turn then, one might expect to find progressive changes as described above in carbohydrate, lipid, and protein metabolism in addition to, and in response to, the progressive changes with age in the endocrine system and those changes associated with the central nervous system.

FIBER

A number of years ago, several scientists noticed that populations whose traditional diets were rich in fibrous food had low incidences of colon cancer as well as heart disease and diabetes mellitus. They compared these diets to those typically consumed by people in the U.S. and Europe and suggested that the health status of these populations was related to their high-fiber diets. With the consumption of high-fiber diets, the feces were bulkier, moister, and more frequent than when low-fiber diets were consumed. These reports attracted a lot of attention and a plethora of high-fiber foods appeared in the market place. People began to consume these products in the hope of having similar benefits conferred. It is not clear that such benefits have been collected.

Dietary fiber refers to those carbohydrates that are indigestible and unabsorbed. The component glucose moieties are joined by β linkages rather than α linkages. They may also contain additional substituents, but their chief characteristic is that of nondigestibility by the α amylases of the mammalian gastrointestinal system. These nondigestible carbohydrates are plant products and fall into five major categories: celluloses, hemicelluloses, lignins, pectins, and gums. The first three provide bulk to the gastrointestinal contents due to their property of absorbing water. The increased bulkiness of the gut contents stimulates peristalsis and results in shorter passage time and more frequent defecation. In addition to the water-holding property, fibers of the lignin type adsorb cholesterol, aiding in its excretion in the feces. Pectins and gums also influence gastric emptying but in the opposite direction. These fiber types form gels that slow gastric emptying and interfere with the absorption of sugars, starches, and also fats. The fibers, collectively, help to lower the level of serum cholesterol while increasing its excretion. It is for these reasons that nutritionists encourage the consumption of fiber-rich plant foods. Fruits are good sources of pectin, while cereal grains and the woody parts of vegetables are good sources of the celluloses, hemicelluloses, and lignins. Dried beans and oats are good sources of gums. The inclusion of foods containing all of these fiber types will no doubt be of benefit with respect to intestinal transit time and may also result in a small decrease in cholesterol absorption. This may have some impact on cholesterol balance. If fiber increases cholesterol excretion and reduces cholesterol recirculation, a small decrease in serum cholesterol level may occur. However, since cholesterol synthesis may rise to compensate for decreased absorption and reabsorption, the net effect with respect to cardiovascular-disease development may be minor indeed.

The increased transit speed of high-fiber diets may be of benefit to those people susceptible to colon cancer. The fiber not only adsorbs cholesterol and hastens its excretion, but also adsorbs potentially noxious components of the ingesta, hastening their excretion as well. Thus, carcinogenic compounds have less time for exposure to colon cells and thus less opportunity to convert a normal cell to a cancer cell.

Finally, as with all comparisons of population groups, one must be careful in the interpretation of the data. Yes, a certain primitive group has less degenerative disease than we do in the U.S. and yes, the diet contains more fiber. Is this a cause-and-effect scenario? No, it is not. The picture is incomplete without observations on the incidence of other diseases, the average lifespan, the availability of clean water, immunizations, medical care, and observations on other aspects of lifestyle that can affect disease development.

ETHANOL

Alcoholic beverages have been consumed by humans since the dawn of history. They have been used to ease anxiety, to promote social interaction, and as a vehicle to dominate others. Ethanol, the alcohol in beverages, is the quantitative end product of yeast glycolysis. Small amounts can be synthesized in mammalian cells. Thus, ethanol is a drug, a food, and a metabolite. It has been estimated that upward of 90 million Americans consume alcoholic beverages every day and that about 10% of these people are addicted to its consumption. This affliction is called alcoholism.

Alcoholism is truly a disease that is a result of a diet–gene interaction. The dietary ingredient in this instance is alcohol; the gene is as yet unidentified. However, there is ample evidence in the literature that supports the concept that the tendency toward alcoholism is inherited. Studies of twins reared by adoptive parents as well as multigeneration studies of families give support to this idea. An alcoholic is more likely than a nonalcoholic to have an alcoholic relative. At least 33% of alcoholics have an alcoholic parent. This has been observed in adopted individuals where the biological parent was unknown to the alcoholic and so the parent's proclivities were not taught. Studies of monozygotic (identical) and dizygotic (fraternal) twins indicated a high degree of concordance for alcoholism. If one twin became an alcoholic, the other twin also became one if that twin chose to consume alcohol. The concordance was greater in the identical twins than in the fraternal twins. While scientists agree on the heritable nature of alcoholism, no one gene or group of genes has been identified and found culpable for the disorder.

Ethanol, once consumed, is rapidly absorbed by simple diffusion. The diffusion is affected by the amount of alcohol consumed, the regional blood flow, the surface area, and the presence of other foods. The different segments of the gastrointestinal tract absorb ethanol at different rates. Absorption is fastest in the duodenum and jejunum, slower in the stomach, ileum, and colon, and slowest in the mouth and esophagus. The rate of absorption by the duodenum depends on gastric emptying time, which, in turn, depends on the kinds and amounts of foods consumed with the ethanol. Certain drugs may also influence gastric-emptying time and thus influence absorption. Complete absorption may vary from 2 to 6 hours. The type of beverage can influence ethanol absorption. Ethanol from beer is absorbed slower than that found in whisky, which is slower than gin, and red wine. Of course, pure ethanol is absorbed the fastest of all.

Once absorbed, ethanol is rapidly distributed between the intracellular and extracellular compartments. This is because ethanol is completely miscible in water and thus freely travels any place water travels. The uptake of ethanol by the fat depots is minimal. Ethanol crosses the plasma membranes but, in so doing, changes them. When ethanol is in contact with a protein, it denatures it. Thus, large and frequent ethanol exposures results in damage to proteins both within and around the cells. The most damaged tissue is the liver, since ethanol is carried directly to this tissue via the portal blood. While gut cells are also damaged, these cells have such a rapid turnover time (less than 7 days) that such damage due to intermittent ethanol consumption is not as long lasting as the damage that happens in the liver. Liver cells, in contrast, have a longer half-life and, once damaged, do not repair as readily. Alcoholic liver disease is a major cause of death among those who drink heavily.

Ethanol diffuses from the blood to the alveolar air so the ethanol content of expired air bears a constant relationship to pulmonary arterial blood ethanol levels. The partition coefficient is 2100:1. This means that 2100 ml of expired air contains the same amount of ethanol as 1 ml of blood. If the blood contains 100 mg of ethanol, the expired air will contain 232 ppm. This is the basis for the "breathalyzer" tests for intoxication. Intoxication occurs at 150 mg/100 ml of blood but most states prosecute drivers having blood levels exceeding 100 mg/dl.

Of the ethanol consumed, 90–98% is oxidized to carbon dioxide and water. The rest is excreted as ethanol in the breath or in the urine. The metabolism of ethanol is shown in Figure 5.23. The rate of oxidation is fairly constant at about 10–20 mg/ml. This indicates that the first rate limiting reaction catalyzed by alcohol dehydrogenase is saturated at this level. This is a zero-order reaction. The average rate at which alcohol can be metabolized is about 10 ml/hr (or 7 g/hr). The ethanol in 4 oz of whisky requires 5–6 hr to metabolize completely to CO_2 and water. One mole of ethanol requires 16 moles of ATP for its conversion to CO_2 and HOH.

While ethanol is distributed throughout the body, the liver is the chief site for its oxidation. As mentioned, the first rate-limiting reaction is catalyzed by alcohol dehydrogenase and converts ethanol to acetaldehyde. Acetaldehyde is quite damaging to cellular proteins and part of the hepatic injury found in alcoholics is due to this metabolite. It binds covalently to protein, impairs the microtubular assembly and the mitochondrial respiratory chain, it depletes pyridoxine supplies,

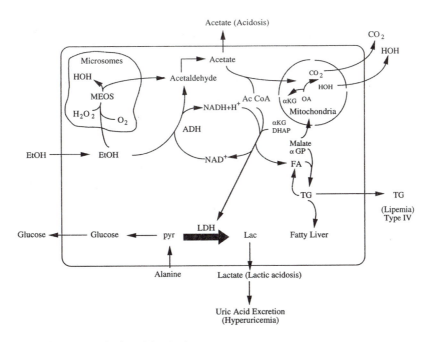

FIGURE 5.23   Metabolism of ethanol by the hepatocyte.

stimulates inappropriate collagen synthesis, and inhibits DNA repair. Acetaldehyde is also produced when ethanol is metabolized by the microsomal ethanol oxidizing system (MEOS). This system uses peroxide (H_2O_2) and produces a molecule of water as well as the acetaldehyde. The acetaldehyde is converted to acetate, which can either be joined with a CoA or released to the circulation. If too much acetate is released, acidosis develops.

Acetyl CoA can either be used for fatty acid synthesis or be shuttled into the mitochondria via carnitine to be oxidized as through the citric acid cycle. A fatty liver typifies the alcoholic. The fatty liver may progress to alcoholic hepatitis, to cirrhosis, liver failure, and death. The fatty liver is due to accelerated hepatic fatty acid synthesis as well as due to an ethanol-induced impairment in hepatic lipid output. If the hepatocyte accumulates too much lipid, the cell will burst and die. Areas of dead tissue within the liver is known as cirrhosis. When too much tissue dies, the liver may cease to function and the alcoholic dies.

In addition to the direct effects of ethanol on cell function, there are a number of auxiliary health concerns related to ethanol consumption. People who consume large quantities of ethanol find that their needs for thiamin, niacin, pyridoxine, and pantothenic acid increase dramatically. The alcoholic frequently manifests symptoms of beriberi, pellegra, and other deficiency diseases. In part, this is due to the increased need for these vitamins when ethanol is metabolized and in part because alcoholics may choose to consume alcoholic beverages in preference to nourishing food. Those alcoholics who continue to eat nourishing food in addition to consuming ethanol do not develop overt deficiency diseases as frequently. Nonetheless, the nutritionist should be aware of ethanol-induced increases in the needs for the B vitamins.

Finally, there is another concern with respect to ethanol consumption. That is the development of fetal malformations in women who drink ethanol during pregnancy. In 1973, eight cases of unrelated children were described having similar congenital defects. Particularly noticeable were the facial malformations involving eye placement, and nose and mouth development. All of these children had mothers who were alcoholic. In a subsequent report, it was noted that alcoholism in mothers was associated with an increased incidence of spontaneous abortions, premature delivery of fetuses who were poorly developed for their gestational age, and infants born with respiratory distress syndrome. Many of these children failed to grow and develop normally with full intellectual capacity. Various learning disabilities (partial hearing or visual loss) also characterized these children. How the ethanol affects fetal development, particularly the development of the central nervous system, is not known. Yet awareness of the potential damage of ethanol to the developing embryo and fetus should dictate abstinence prior to and during the gestational period.

CARBOHYDRATE REQUIREMENTS

Carbohydrates are not considered essential nutrients aside from their use as providers of energy. As discussed in the section on gluconeogenesis, the body can usually synthesize sufficient glucose to sustain its absolute need for this fuel. Those cells that require other monosaccharides likewise can synthesize them. The mammary gland, for example, can convert glucose to galactose (see Figure 5.12) and use it (joined to glucose) to make the milk sugar lactose. The seminal vesicles likewise can isomerize glucose to fructose (see Figure 5.11) to meet the need for this particular monosaccharide. Thus, the traditional definition of nutrient essentiality is not met. Neither the normal human nor members of other animal species need to consume glucose in any set amount if synthesis is sufficiently active to meet need and if the diet provides sufficient gluconeogenic precursors. It has been estimated that the average human uses about 125 g of glucose per day to sustain neural activity. If this glucose is supplied by gluconeogenesis, 40% will come from lipid precursors and 60% will come from protein components (see Table 5.7). As mentioned, this synthesis is very expensive with respect to the energy needed and, more important, with respect to the amount of dietary protein that must be consumed in order to support glucose synthesis. If no dietary carbohydrate is consumed, more than 155 g of protein (2–3 times the usual protein need) must be consumed to provide the 75 g of the 125 g glucose per day that is needed.

Are there circumstances where this is not true? Are there times when glucose serves a vital function that is in addition to its role as an energy provider? The answer to these questions is yes. Just as the growing child needs dietary arginine, while the adult does not, the traumatized or septic patient needs glucose, when otherwise this need could be met by gluconeogenesis.

In trauma or sepsis, the energy requirement is greatly increased (see Unit 3) because these conditions elicit a stress response. This response means an increase in levels of the catabolic hormones, which are anti-insulin hormones as well as anti-inflammatory hormones. The stress hormones mobilize body protein and fat stores to provide the means for repair of injured tissues. When this catabolic response is prolonged (days to weeks), it must be reversed or patients could die if their protein and energy stores are insufficient to sustain the prolonged mobilization. If sufficient glucose is provided in a hypertonic solution via a central vein such as the subclavian, it can reverse this catabolic response. This treatment is called parenteral nutrition. This will minimize the loss in body muscle mass. The effect of this hypertonic solution of glucose is to overcome (through mass action) the anti-insulin effects of the catabolic hormones and thereby stimulate glycolysis, glycogenesis and inhibit proteolysis and lipolysis.

The questions are, how much carbohydrate (glucose) is needed to have the above effect and how long should glucose be provided at this high level? The estimates vary. If the liver is functioning normally, 50–80% of the energy intake should have the desired anticatabolic effect. This would mean a 5–30% increase over the usual carbohydrate intake of 45–55% of the total energy intake, presuming that the patient can and will eat. This is not always possible. The patient may be in a coma, have a broken jaw, or the injury or sepsis may involve the gastrointestinal tract. In such instances, all needed nutrients, including glucose, must be supplied by the parenteral route. This creates other kinds of problems with respect to our knowledge about micronutrient needs in the absence of the protective role of the gastrointestinal system. Micromineral needs are especially difficult to manage under these circumstances. Humans need small amounts of most of these nutrients. If supplied in excess, a toxic state can develop.

With respect to the absolute amount of glucose that must be provided to the traumatized or septic patient, the estimates vary from 4 g/kg body weight (280 g/day/70 kg man) to 7 g/kg body weight (490 g/day/70 kg man). This would provide between 1120 to 1960 kcal (4686-8200 kJ) from glucose per day. The period of administration of this high a level of glucose to achieve anticatabolism has been estimated to be from 4 days to 2 weeks. After this period, a more normal distribution of macronutrients may be more appropriate.

SUPPLEMENTARY READINGS

Baily, D.L. and Horuk, R. (1988) The biology and biochemistry of the glucose transporter. *Biochem. Biophys. Acta* 947:541-590.

Barnard, R.J. and Youngren, J.F. (1992) Regulation of glucose transport in skeletal muscle. *FASEB J.* 6:3238-3244.

Beale, E.G., Clouthier, D.E., and Hammer, R.E. (1992) Cell-specific expression of cytosolic phosphoenolpyruvate carboxykinase in transgenic mice. *FASEB J.* 6:3330-3337.

Bowman, B.A., Forbes, A.L., White, J.S., and Glinsman, W.H., Eds. (1993) Health effects of dietary fructose. *Am. J. Clin. Nutr.* 58:721S-823S (Special issue).

Cherrington, A.D. (1999) Control of glucose uptake and release by the liver *in vivo*. *Diabetes* 48:1198-1214.

Chiu, K.C., Tanizawa, Y., and Permutt, M.A. (1993) Glucokinase gene variants in the common form of NIDDM. *Diabetes* 42:579-582.

Devor, E.J. and Cloninger, C.R. (1989) Genetics of alcoholism. *Ann. Rev. Genet.* 23:19-39.

Elwyn, D.H. and Bureztein, S. (1993) Carbohydrate metabolism and requirements for nutritional support. *Nutrition* 9:50-66; 164-175; 255-267.

Gerbitz, K-D., Gempel, K., and Brdiczka, D. (1996) Mitochondria and Diabetes. *Diabetes* 45:113-126.

Goering, H.K. and van Soest, J.P. (1970) Forage fiber analysis. *Agriculture Handbook No. 379*, Agriculture Research Service, U. S. Department of Agriculture, (Washington, D.C.: U.S. Government Printing Office).

Gould, G.W. and Bell, G.I. (1990) Facilitative glucose transporters: An expanding family. *TIBS* 15:18-23.

Hoek, J.B., Thomas, A.P., Rooney, T.A., Higashi, K., and Rubin, E. (1992) Ethanol and signal transduction. *FASEB J.* 6:2386-2396.

Jensen, B.A., Rosenberg, H.S., and Notkins, A.L. (1980) Postmortem tissue changes in children with fatal viral infections. *Lancet* 2:354-358.

Joost, H.G. and Weber, T.M. (1989) The regulation of glucose transport in insulin sensitive cells. *Diabetologia* 32:831-838.

Kahn, B.B. and Pedersen, O. (1992) Tissue specific regulation of glucose transporters in different forms of obesity. *Proc. Soc. Exp. Biol. & Med.* 200:214-217.

Lieber, C.S. (1993) Herman Award Lecture, 1993: A personal perspective on alcohol, nutrition and the liver. *Am. J. Clin. Nutr.* 58:430-442.

Makino, H., Taire, M., Shimada, F., Hasimoto, N., Suzuki, Y., Nozaki, O., Hatanaka, Y., and Yoshida, S. (1992) Insulin receptor gene mutation: A molecular and functional analysis. *Cellular Signaling* 4:351-363.

McCrane, R.A., Widdowson, E.M., and Shackelton, L.B. (1936) The nutritive value of fruits, vegetables, and nuts. Medical Research Council Special Report Series No. 213, London.

Nandan, S.D. and Beale, E.G. (1992) Regulation of phosphoenolpyruvate carboxykinase mRNA in mouse liver, kidney, and fat tissues by fasting, diabetes and insulin. *Lab. An. Sci.* 42:473-477.

Nordlie, R.C., Bode, A.M., and Foster, J.D. (1993) Recent advances in hepatic glucose-6 phosphatase regulation and function. *Proc. Soc. Exp. Biol. & Med.* 203:274-285.

Olansky, L., Janssen, R., Welling, C., and Permutt, M.A. (1992) Variability of the insulin gene in American Blacks with NIDDM. *Diabetes* 41:742-749.

Olson, A.L. and Pessin, J.E. (1996) Structure, function and regulation of the mammalian facilitative glucose transporter gene family. *Ann. Rev. Nutr.* 16:235-256.

Petry, K.G. and Reichardt, J.K.V. (1998) The fundamental importance of human galactose metabolism: Lessons from genetics and metabolism. *Trends in Genetics* 14:98-102.

Rondinone, C.M., Wang, L-M., Lonnroth, P., Wesslau, C., Pierce, J.H., and Smith, U. (1997) Insulin receptor substrate (IRS) 1 is reduced and IRS 2 is the main docking protein for phosphatidyl inositol 3-kinase in adipocytes from subjects with NIDDM. *Proc. Natl. Acad. Sci.* 94:4171-4175.

Sharp, S.C. and Diamond, M.P. (1993) Sex steroids and diabetes. *Diabetes Rev.* 1:318-342.

Short, M.K., Clouthier, D.E., Schaefer, I.M., Hammer, R.E., Magnuson, M.A., and Beale, E.G. (1992) Tissue specific, developmental, hormonal and dietary regulation of rat phosphoenolpyruvate carboxykinase-human growth hormone fusion genes in transgenic mice. *Mol. Cell. Biol.* 12:1007-1020.

Smith, G.N., Patrick, J., and Sinervo, K.R. (1991) Effects of ethanol exposure on the embryo-fetus: Experimental considerations, mechanisms, and the role of prostaglandins. Can. *J. Physiol. Pharmacol.* 69:550-569.

Southgate, D.A.T. (1969) Determination of carbohydrates in food. II. Unavailable carbohydrates, *J. Sci. Food & Ag.* 20:331.

Steiner, D.F., Tager, H.S., Chan, S.J., Nanjo, K., Sanke, T., and Rubenstein, A.H. (1990) Lessons learned from molecular biology of insulin gene mutations. *Diabetes Care* 13:600-609.

Stoffel, M., Froguel, P.H., Takeda, J., Zouali, H., Vionnet, N., Nishi, S., Weber, I.T., Harrison, R.W., Pilkis, S.J., Lesage, S., Vaxillaire, M., Velho, G., Sun F, Iris, F., Passa, P.H., Cohen, D., and Bell, G.I. (1992) Human glucokinase gene: Isolation, characterization, and identification of two missense mutations linked to early onset-non insulin-dependent (type 2) diabetes mellitus. *Proc. Natl. Acad. Sci. USA* 89:7689-7702.

Thacker, S.B., Veech, R.L., Vernon, A.A., and Rutstein, D.D. (1984) Genetic and biochemical factors relevant to alcoholism. *Alcoholism: Clinical and Experimental Res.* 8:375-383.

van Soest, P.J. and McQueen, R.W. (1973) The chemistry and estimation of fibre, *Proc. Nutr. Soc.* 32(1936):123.

Yoon, J-W., Austin, M., Onodera, T., and Notkins, A.L. (1979) Virus induced diabetes mellitus. Isolation of a virus from the pancreas of a child with diabetic ketoacidosis. *N. Eng. J. Med.* 300:1173-1179.

Yoon, J-W. (1995) A new look at viruses in Type 1 diabetes. *Diabetes/Metabolism Reviews* 11:83-107.

Books

Bjorntorp, P. and Brodoff, B.N. (Eds.). (1992) *Obesity.* J. B. Lippincott Co., Philadelphia, PA, 805 pages.

Dickens, F., Randle and P.J., and Whelan (Eds.) (1968) *Carbohydrate Metabolism and its Disorders.* 2 volumes. Academic Press, New York.

Ellenberg, M. and Rifkin, H. (1985) *Diabetes Mellitus, Theory and Practice.* 3rd Edition, Medical Examination Publishing Co., New Hyde Park, NY, 1105 pages.

Leiter, E.H. and Wilson, G.L. (1988) Viral interactions in pancreatic β cells. In: *Pathology of the Endocrine Pancreas* (Ripeleers, D., Lefebore, P., Eds.). Springer Verlag, pp 8-105.

Magnuson, M.A. and Jetton, T.L. (1993) Tissue specific regulation of glucokinase. In: *Nutrition and Gene Expression* (C.D. Berdanier and J.L. Hargrove, Eds.), CRC Press, Boca Raton, FL, pp. 143-167.

Marble, A., Krall, L.P., Bradley, R.F., Christlieb, A.R., and Soeldner, J.S. (1985) *Joslin's Diabetes Mellitus.* Lea & Febiger, Philadelphia, 1007 pages.

Notkins, A.L., Yoon, J.W., Onodera, T., Toniolo, A., and Jenson, A.B. (1981) Virus-induced diabetes mellitus. In: *Perspectives in Virology XI* (Pollard, M., Ed.), Alan R. Liss, Inc., NY, pp 141-162.

Shafrir, E. and Renold, A.E. (1991) *Frontiers in Diabetes. Lessons from Animal Diabetes II.* John Libby, London, Vol. III, 682 pages.

Shallenberger, R.S. and Birch, G.G. (1975) *Sugar Chemistry.* Avi Publishing Co., Westport, CT.

Sipple, H.L. and McNutt, K.W. (1974) *Sugars in Nutrition.* Academic Press, NY.

6 Lipids

CONTENTS

The third macronutrient group comprises the lipids. They are energetically more dense, having more than twice the energy value of carbohydrate per gram. Americans consume approximately 32–42% of their total energy as lipid. The lipids make up a group of compounds which are, in general, insoluble in water and soluble in such solvents as diethyl ether, carbon tetrachloride, hot alcohol, chloroform, and benzene. They are present in various amounts in all living mammalian cells. Nerve cells and adipose cells are rich in lipid; muscle cells and epithelial cells have considerably less.

In addition to being a very important source of energy, lipids serve a variety of other needs. They perform a basic role in the structure and function of biological membranes. In the body, they are the precursors of a variety of hormones and important cellular signals. They help to regulate the uptake and excretion of nutrients by the cell. Each cell has a characteristic lipid content.

CLASSIFICATION

Lipids, as has been mentioned, have the property of being relatively insoluble in water and relatively soluble in such solvents as ether, chloroform, benzene, and some alcohols. Additionally, some lipids are saponifiable; others are not. Saponifiable lipids, when treated with alkali, undergo hydrolysis at the ester linkage, resulting in the formation of an alcohol and a soap. Triacylglycerol (triglyceride), for example, when treated with sodium hydroxide, is hydrolyzed yielding a mixture of soaps and free glycerol. Traditionally, saponifiable lipids have been classified into three groups, each with subgroups.

A. Simple lipids: esters of fatty acids with various alcohols
   1. Fats: esters of fatty acids with glycerol (acylglycerols)
   2. Waxes: esters of fatty acids with long chain alcohols
   3. Cholesterol esters
B. Compound lipids: esters of fatty acids that contain substituent groups in addition to fatty acids and alcohol
   1. Phospholipids: esters of fatty acids, alcohol, a phosphoric acid residue, and usually an amino alcohol, sugar, or other substituent
   2. Glycolipids: esters of fatty acids that contain carbohydrates and nitrogen (but not phosphoric acid). in addition to fatty acids and alcohol
   3. Lipoproteins: loose combinations of lipids and proteins
C. Derived lipids: substances derived from the above groups by hydrolysis. They are the results of saponification

Two other terms that are frequently used in the classification of lipids (but are not a division of the system just described). are neutral and polar lipids. Neutral lipids are uncharged lipids and include triacylglycerols (also called triglycerides), cholesterol, and cholesterol esters. Polar lipids have positive and negative charges on certain atoms of the molecule. Examples of these are the phospholipids that compose the cell membrane. Phosphatidyl inositol, phosphatidyl choline, and phosphatidyl ethanolamine are membrane phospholipids and are polar.

STRUCTURE AND NOMENCLATURE

SIMPLE LIPIDS

Fatty Acids

Fatty acids are carboxylic acids. They have a polar group (the carboxyl group) at one end and a methyl group at the other. A hydrocarbon chain is in the middle. Fatty acids can have few carbon atoms or more than 20; however, chain lengths of 16 and 18 carbons are the most prevalent. There is usually an even number of carbon atoms (with no branching) in the chain. The chain may be saturated (containing no double bonds) or unsaturated (containing one or more double bonds). Monounsaturated acids have one double bond; polyunsaturated acids have two or more.

The nomenclature of fatty acids is frequently confusing because the same fatty acid can have more than one name: its common (or trivial) name and its systematic name. The common name is rarely, if ever, related to the structure of the molecule. It is sometimes derived from the plant or animal source from which the acid was first isolated. The student has no choice but to memorize these names. Common names for nutritionally important fatty acids are given in Table 6.1

TABLE 6.1
Structure and Names of Fatty Acids Found in Food

Structure	# Carbons: Double Bonds	Systematic Name	Trivial Name	Source
Saturated Fatty Acids				
$CH_3(CH_2)_2COOH$	4:0	n-Butanoic	Butyric	Butter
$CH_3(CH_2)_4COOH$	6:0	n-Hexanoic	Caproic	Butter
$CH_3(CH_2)_6COOH$	8:0	n-Octanoic	Caprylic	Coconut oil
$CH_3(CH_2)_8COOH$	10:0	n-Decanoic	Capric	Palm oil
$CH_3(CH_2)_{10}COOH$	12:0	n-Dodecanoic	Lauric	Coconut oil, nutmeg, butter
$CH_3(CH_2)_{12}COOH$	14:0	n-Tetradecanoic	Myristic	Coconut oil
$CH_3(CH_2)_{14}COOH$	16:0	n-Hexadecanoic	Palmitic	Most fats and oils
$CH_3(CH_2)_{16}COOH$	18:0	n-Octadecanoic	Stearic	Most fats and oils
$CH_3(CH_2)_{18}COOH$	20:0	n-Eicosanoic	Arachidic	Peanut oil, lard
Unsaturated Fatty Acids				
$CH_3(CH_2)_5CH=CH(CH_2)_7COOH$	16:1	9-Hexadecenoic	Palmitoleic	Butter and seed oils
$CH_3(CH_2)_7CH=CH(CH_2)_7COOH$	18:1	9-Octadecenoic	Oleic	Most fats and oils
$CH_3(CH_2)_5CH=CH(CH_2)_9COOH$	20:1	11-Octadecenoic	trans-Vaccenic	Hydrogenated vegetable oils
$CH_3(CH_2)_4CH=CHCH_2CH=CH(CH_2)_7COOH$	18:2	9,12-Octadecadienoic	Linoleic	Linseed oil, corn oil, cottonseed oil
$CH_3CH_2(CH=CHCH_2)_3(CH_2)_7COOH$	18:3	9,12,15-Octadecatrienoic	Linolenic	Soybean oil, marine oils
$CH_3(CH_2)_4(CH=CHCH2)_4(CH_2)_2COOH$	20:4	5,8,11,14-Eicosatetraenoic	Arachidonic	Cottonseed oil

The systematic method of naming fatty acids is based on a modification of the name of the straight chain hydrocarbon having the same number of carbon atoms. The final -e from the hydrocarbon name is removed and -oic added, followed by the word acid. To name the salt of the acid, the -e from the hydrocarbon base is replaced with -ate. For example, the saturated, 18-carbon hydrocarbon, $C_{18}H_{38}$, has as its systematic name n-octadecane (the n means normal or no branching); its saturated fatty acid counterpart is n-octadecan*oic acid* (its common name is stearic acid); the salt is n-octadecan*ate*. The monounsaturated, 18-carbon is 9-octadecen*e*; one form of the unsaturated acid is cis-9-octadecen*oic acid* (common name, oleic acid) The salt is cis-9-octadecen*ate*.

In the systematic name it is possible to address each carbon atom as was done in the last example just cited. There are two ways of doing this: with lower-case Greek letters or with Arabic numerals. With Greek letters, the carbon adjacent to the carboxyl group is α (alpha); the next one is β (beta); the last in the molecule is ω (omega). The carboxyl carbon is not given a designation.

With Arabic numerals, the carboxyl carbon is 1; the next carbon, 2; the next, 3; and so on. The number 9 in the above example means that a double bond exists between carbons 9 and 10.

Other conventions are also used to indicate the position of the double bond. In one of them, Δ 9 indicates a double bond between carbons 9 and 10. In another, the number of carbon atoms, the number of double bonds, and the position of each double bond are all clearly shown. For example, oleic acid is 18:1 Δ 9 or 18 carbons with one double bond between the ninth and tenth carbons. Similarly, the 18-carbon acid with two double bonds is linoleic acid; in this system it would be referred to as 18:2 Δ 9, 12. In yet another convention, the position of the double bond from the terminal carbon (the methyl group) is indicated. The number of carbon atoms and the number of double bonds are shown as in the previous convention. The position of the double bond from the terminal carbon is then shown. For instance, oleic acid is 18:1ω9; linoleic acid is 18:2ω6. This convention is particularly useful in discussions about the interconversion of fatty acids; since carbon atoms are added between this double bond and the carboxyl group, it remains the terminal carbon.

As mentioned, fatty acids are either saturated or unsaturated. These two forms of fatty acids differ significantly in their structural considerations. In the saturated fatty acid, the hydrocarbon tail can exist in an infinite number of conformations because each carbon atom can rotate freely.

Unsaturated fatty acids, on the other hand, have a rigid feature to their structure because the carbons in the double bonds are not free to rotate; they exist as the *cis* or *trans* geometrical isomers. The *cis* configuration produces a bond in the hydrocarbon chain so that it resembles the shape of the letter U. Each *cis* configuration in the tail will add another bend. The *trans* configuration has nearly the same shape as the extended conformation of the saturated fatty acid. These structural features of the unsaturated fatty acids have a biological significance, as will be discussed in later sections.

In polyunsaturated fatty acids, the double bonds are not conjugated; that is, the double bonds will be separated by more than one single bond as in: $-CH_2-CH=CH-CH_2-CH=CH-CH_2-$, The unsaturated fatty acids of higher plants and animals are usually palmitoleic, oleic, linoleic, and linolenic acids, the first double bond will be between atoms 9 and 10; others, if present, will be at carbon 12 or greater. Most of these unsaturated fatty acids will exist in the *cis* configuration. When vegetable oils are solidified to make margarine, some of the double bonds will be converted to single bonds through the addition of hydrogen. The process is called dehydrogenation and the oils must be heated before hydrogenation will take place. When this occurs, some of the residual unsaturated fatty acids will change from the *cis* to the *trans* residual form. Margarine and vegetable shortening are thus sources of the *trans* fatty acids in the human diet. Some fatty acids exist naturally in the *trans* configuration. Eight percent of the unsaturated fatty acids in cows' milk is in the *trans* form. In this instance, the presence of *trans* fatty acids is due to their production by the rumen flora.

Fatty acids with an odd number of carbon atoms are found in limited amounts in natural products. Less than 0.4% of the total fatty acids in olive oil and 0.8% of those in lard contain an odd number of carbon atoms. In contrast, 60% of olive oil and 40% of lard consists of the even-numbered monounsaturated fatty acid, oleic acid. Few oils or waxes contain significant amounts of odd-numbered fatty acids. Odd-numbered fatty acids can be found in vitamin B_{12}-deficient individuals because B_{12} is an essential coenzyme in the conversion of methylmalonyl CoA to succinyl CoA. When this conversion is impaired, methylmalonic acid accumulates and some of this is used to synthesize odd-numbered fatty acids.

Of the polyunsaturated fatty acids, linoleic and linolenic are designated as the *essential fatty acids* (EFA). Linoleic is an 18-carbon fatty acid with two double bonds (ω6,18:2, $\Delta^{9,12}$). Linolenic acid is also an 18-carbon fatty acid but with three double bonds (ω3, 18:3, $\Delta^{9,12,15}$). Both are in the *cis* configuration. Food oils of plant origin are good sources of linoleic acid, while the marine oils are good sources of linolenic acid. A few oils of plant origin contain linolenic acid (i.e., primrose oil). Most mammals require these fatty acids and cannot synthesize them. Felines, in addition, cannot convert linoleic acid to arachidonic acid (ω6, 20:4, $\Delta^{5,8,11,14}$). Hence, for these animals, arachidonic acid is an esential fatty acid.

Fats

Fats are formed when one or more fatty acids react with the hydroxyl group(s) of glycerol to make an ester. They are called neutral fats, glycerides, or acylglycerols. The fat most frequently found in nature has all three hydroxyl positions esterified; it is known as triacylglycerol. Triacylglycerols that contain the same fatty acid residue on all three carbons are simple triacylglycerols. An example would be tripalmitin. In nature, the triacylglycerols usually contain more than one fatty acid and thus are called mixed triacylglycerols or triglycerides.

Most fats in nature are complex mixtures of simple and mixed triacylglycerols. As yet, no general rule has been devised to determine the manner in which the fatty acids attach to glycerol. Many oils and fats contain between six and ten different saturated and unsaturated fatty acids. The number of possible combinations with this many fatty acid residues is very large.

The ratio of unsaturated to saturated fatty acids is defined as the P/S ratio. A high ratio of 3:1 means that there are three molecules of unsaturated fatty acids to every saturated fatty acid present. Animal fats and the foods rich in these fats usually have a low P/S ratio. Most vegetable oils have a high P/S ratio. However, there are some exceptions to this. The tropical plants (palm and coconut) provide a solid fat with a low P/S ratio. These fats, although called "oils" are rich in medium chain (chain lengths of 8–14 carbons) saturated fatty acids. By convention, these lipids are called oils because they are fluid at much lower temperatures (the ambient temperature of the tropics) than are the fats of animal origin. Thus, we have coconut oil, palm oil, and palm kernel oil as solids at temperatures of 18–22°C but liquid at 26–30°C. The P/S ratio of the fat in the adipose tissue of humans reflects the P/S ratio of the food these humans consumed. In order to assess the P/S ratio of the fat intake of populations, only a small sample of adipose tissue would need to be obtained and analyzed for its P/S ratio. Because the body metabolizes the fat it consumes, both lengthening and shortening the food fatty acids, an exact copy of the food lipid fatty acids will not be obtained, but some general trends will be observed.

SOURCES OF LIPIDS

When discussing food sources of lipids, the food sources of triacylglycerols are primarily meant, because they are the lipids that occur in foods in large quantities. Lipids are found in almost every natural food. Fruits and vegetables have small amounts of lipids while meat, milk, cheese, eggs, and table spreads have larger amounts. A few plant foods — olives and avocados — contain as much as 20% (by weight) fat. Nuts are rich sources of fat: pecans are 71% fat and walnuts are 60% fat. Table 6.2 shows the total fat content of several foods and also gives some values for the saturated fatty acid content and the amount of two common unsaturated fatty acids, oleic and linoleic.

More than one-half of dietary fat is contributed from invisible sources: from the fat in milk and eggs, whole grain cereals, baked products, and convenience foods. The other fraction of dietary fat is visible. The marbling in meat, butter on bread or vegetables, and salad oil on lettuce are examples of the latter.

The fatty acid composition of several fats and oils is given in Table 6.2. Of the saturated fatty acids, palmitic (16:0) and stearic (18:0) are the most prevalent in nature. Of the unsaturated fatty acids, oleic (18:1) and linoleic (18:2) are the most abundant. Together, these two fatty acids make up 90% of the unsaturated fatty acids in the American diet.

As mentioned earlier, fats of plant origin tend to be less saturated than animal fats. Beef fat contains a lot of stearic acid. Mutton fat and cocoa butter contain a similar array of fatty acids but not in the same amounts. Mutton fat has as much as 27% saturated fatty acids by weight whereas cocoa butter has 2.5%. This accounts for the marked difference in the physical properties of these two fats. Milk fat is similar to lard (pig fat) because it contains large amounts of palmitic and oleic acid. Fish, on the other hand, tends to have much more polyunsaturated fatty acid in its glycerides.

TABLE 6.2
Percent Fat in 100 g Portions of Common Food

Item	Total Fat (% by weight)	Total Sat'd Fatty Acids (% of the Total Fatty Acids in the Fat)	Unsaturated Fatty Acids	
			Oleic	Linoleic
Animal				
Bacon	53	20	27	7
Butter	81	45	27	3
Chicken, broiled	3.5	1	1	1
Egg, whole	12	4	5	Trace
Hamburger	12	6	4.7	Trace
Ice cream, 10% fat	10	6	4	Trace
Lamb, leg, roasted	19	10	7	Trace
Milk, whole	3.5	2	1.2	Trace
Milk, 2%	2	1.2	0.8	Trace
Milk, skim	Trace	Trace	Trace	Trace
Pork chops	21	8	9	2
Salmon, pink	6	1	1	Trace
Vegetable				
Avocados	13	2.3	6	1.8
Bread, whole wheat	2.6	0.4	1.3	0.4
Bread, white enriched	3.3	0.7	1.8	0.4
Broccoli	0.6	Trace	Trace	Trace
Cereal, 40% bran	2.8	Trace	Trace	Trace
Cereal, oatmeal	0.8	Trace	Trace	Trace
Orange juice, fresh	0.4	Trace	Trace	Trace
Peanut butter	50	12.5	25	12.5
Pecans	71	4.6	44	14
Potato, baked	Trace	Trace	Trace	Trace
Strawberries, raw	0.7	Trace	Trace	Trace
Walnuts	60	3	24	33

Source: Nutritive Values of the Edible Part of Foods, Home and Garden Bulletin No. 72, Washington, D.C., 1970, U.S. Department of Agriculture

Freshwater fish contain more unsaturated C_{18} and less unsaturated C_{20} and C_{22} than do marine fish. Fatty marine fish such as mackerel contain long chain polyunsaturated fatty acids of the omega ω-3 or n-3 type.

Cholesterol, cholesterol esters, free fatty acids, phospholipids, and sphingolipids are also present in the foods humans consume. These compounds represent only a small fraction of the total fat consumed. Because of the population studies linking heart disease to cholesterol levels in the blood, nutritionists are frequently interested in the levels of this lipid in the food. Listed in Table 6.3 are some human foods and their cholesterol content. Greater detail on the composition of the tremendous variety of foods that humans consume may be found in the USDA *Handbook of Food Composition* (U. S. Government Printing Office, Washington, D.C.). These food-composition data are computerized and can be obtained on disk. Other handbooks and computer programs have been developed to assess the nutrient intakes of not only man, but other species as well. The data provided in these sources are averages of several different analyses, but are not absolute. Variation in the source of the food, how it is prepared, and how much fat is removed prior to preparation and consumption contributes to the uncertainty associated with these values.

TABLE 6.3
Total Lipid and Cholesterol Content of 100 g
Portions of Several Common Foods*

Food	% Fat	% Cholesterol
Codfish	0.67	0.043
Halibut	2.94	0.041
Mackerel	6.30	0.076
Salmon	3.45	0.052
Beef steak, cooked	31.8	0.36
Hamburger, cooked	12.8	0.10
Stew meat	18.8	1
Lamb chops, cooked	36.0	1.11
Pork chops, cooked	21.1	1.03
Pork sausage	46.2	1.35
Bologna	28.6	1.04
Chicken, white meat	3.5	0.64
Eggs, whole	12	4.2
Egg white	<3	–
Whole milk	3.3	0.32
Skim milk	Trace	Trace
Cheddar cheese	32	1.0
Cottage cheese (4%)	4.29	0.21
Mozzarella cheese, skim milk	17.9	4.5
Butter	81.4	2.4
Margarine	81.4	–
Fruits, all kinds	<1	–
Avocado	13	–
Leafy vegetables	<1	–
Legumes (except peanuts)	1	–
Root vegetables	<1	–
Cereals and grains	1-2	0
Crackers	1	0
Bread, white, enriched	4	<0.1

*Foods are selected from the vast array of foods presented in Handbooks 8-15, U.S. Department of Agriculture, Human Nutrition Information Service, U.S Government Printing Office, Superintendent of Documents, Washington, D.C. 20402.

Interest in the sphingolipids in food has emerged as reports have appeared suggesting that these lipids might have an anti-cancer or antilipemia function. Sphingolipids are complex lipids having a sphingosin backbone, of which there are more than 60 variants. There are various alkyl chain lengths (4–22 carbons) and varying degrees of saturation as well as varying positions for these double bonds, chain branching, and presence of a hydroxyl group. The amino group of the sphingoid base is usually substituted with a long chain fatty acid to produce a ceramide. There are so many variants of these compounds that this group is the largest group of complex dietary lipids, yet their nutritional significance has not been well studied.

DIGESTION AND ABSORPTION

The digestion and absorption of the various food lipids involves the mouth, stomach, and intestine (Figure 6.1). The digestion of lipid is begun in the mouth with the mastication of food and the mixing with the acid-stable lingual lipase. Digestion can proceed only when the large particles of food are made smaller through chewing. The action of the tongue and teeth mixes the food with the lingual lipase. Later, the churning action of the stomach mixes the food particles with hydrochloric acid. These actions separate the lipid particles, exposing more surface area for enzyme action and emulsion formation. The changes in physical state, illustrated in Figure 6.2, are essential steps that precede absorption. In the stomach, lipid-protein complexes are cleaved, releasing lipid when the proteins of these complexes are denatured by gastric hydrochloric acid and attacked by the proteases (pepsin, parapepsin I, and parapepsin II) of the gastric juice. The remaining lipid components of the diet are mixed with other diet ingredients by the churning action of the stomach. Little degradation of fat occurs in this organ except that catalyzed by lingual lipase, which is thought to originate from glands in the back of the mouth and under the tongue. This lipase is active in the acid environment of the stomach. However, because of the tendency of lipid to coalesce and form a separate phase, lingual lipase has limited opportunity to attack the triacylglycerols. Those that are attacked release a single fatty acid, usually a short or medium chain one. The remaining diacylglycerol is subsequently hydrolyzed in the duodenum. In adults consuming a mixed diet, lingual lipase is relatively unimportant. However, in infants having an immature duodenal lipase, lingual lipase is quite important. In addition, this lipase has its greatest activity on the triacylglycerols commonly present in whole milk. Milk fat has more short and medium chain fatty acids than fats from other food sources.

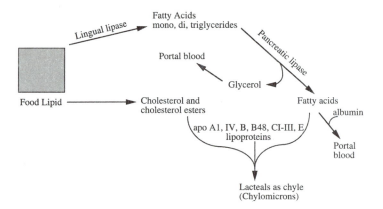

FIGURE 6.1 Overview of digestion and absorption of food lipid.

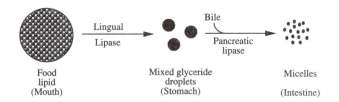

FIGURE 6.2 Changes in the physical state of food lipid as it is prepared for absorption.

Although the action of lingual lipase is slow relative to lipases found in the duodenum, its action to release diacylglycerol and short and medium chain fatty acids serves another function: these fatty acids serve as surfactants. Surfactants spontaneously adsorb to the water–lipid interface, stabilizing emulsions as they form. Other dietary surfactants are the lecithins and the phospholipids. Altogether, these surfactants plus the churning action of the stomach produce an emulsion that is then expelled into the duodenum as chyme.

The chyme's entry into the duodenum stimulates the release of the gut hormones pancreozymin and cholecystokinin into the blood stream. Cholecystokinin stimulates the gall bladder to contract and release bile. Bile salts serve as emulsifying agents and to further disperse the lipid droplets at the lipid–acqueous interface facilitating the hydrolysis of the glycerides by the pancreatic lipases. The bile salts impart a negative charge to the lipids, which in turn attracts the pancreatic enzyme colipase.

Pancreozymin (secretin) stimulates the exocrine pancreas to release pancreatic juice, which contains three lipases (lipase, lipid esterase, and colipase). These lipases act at the water–lipid interface of the emulsion particles. One lipase acts on the fatty acids esterified at positions 1 and 3 of the glycerol backbone, leaving a fatty acid esterified at carbon 2. This 2-monoacylglyceride can isomerize and the remaining fatty acid can move to carbon 1 or 3. The pancreatic juice contains another less specific lipase (called a lipid esterase), which cleaves fatty acids from cholesterol esters, monoglycerides, or esters such as vitamin A ester. Its action requires the presence of the bile salts. The lipase that is specific for the ester linkage at carbons 1 and 3 of the triacylglycerols does not have a requirement for the bile salts and, in fact, is inhibited by them. The inhibition of pancreatic lipase by the bile salts is relieved by the third pancreatic enzyme, colipase. Colipase is a small protein (mol. wt. 12,000 Da) that binds to both the water–lipid interface and to lipase, thereby anchoring and activating the lipase. The products of the lipase-catalyzed reaction, a reaction that favors the release of fatty acids having 10 or more carbons, are these fatty acids and mono-acylglyceride. The products of the lipid esterase-catalyzed reaction are cholesterol, vitamins, fatty acids, and glycerol. Phospholipids present in food are attacked by phospholipases specific to each of the phospholipids. The pancreatic juice contains these lipases as prephospholipases, which are activated by the enzyme trypsin.

As mentioned, the release of bile from the gall bladder is essential to the digestion of dietary fat. Bile contains the bile acids, cholic acid and chenodeoxycholic acid. These are biological detergents or emulsifying agents. At physiological pH, these acids are present as anions, so they are frequently referred to as bile salts. At pH values above the physiological range, they form aggregates with the fats at concentrations above 2–5 mM. These aggregates are called micelles (Figure 6.3). The micelles are much smaller in size than the emulsified lipid droplets. Micelle sizes vary depending on the ratio of lipids to bile acids, but typically range from 40 to 600 Å.

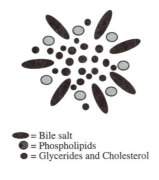

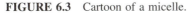 = Bile salt
= Phospholipids
= Glycerides and Cholesterol

FIGURE 6.3   Cartoon of a micelle.

Micelles are structured such that the hydrophobic portions (triglycererols, cholesterol esters, etc.) are toward the center of the structure, while the hydrophilic portions (phospholipids, short chain fatty acids, bile salts) surround this center. The micelles contain many different lipids. Mixed micelles have a disc-like shape whereby the lipids form a bilayer and the bile acids occupy edge positions, rendering the edge of the disc hydrophilic. During the process of lipase and esterase digestion of the lipids in the chyme, the water-insoluble lipids are rendered soluble and transferred from the lipid emulsion of the chyme to the micelle. In turn, these micelles transfer the products of digestion (free fatty acids, glycerol, cholesterol, etc.) from the intestinal lumen to the surface of the epithelial cells, where absorption takes place. The micellar fluid layer next to this cell surface is homogenous, yet the products of lipid digestion are presented to the cell surface and, by passive diffusion, these products are transported into the absorptive cell. Thus, the degree to which dietary lipid, once digested, is absorbed, depends largely on the amount of lipid to be absorbed relative to the amount of bile acid available to make the micelle. This, in turn, is dependent on the rate of bile acid synthesis by the liver and bile release by the gall bladder. People who have had their gall bladder removed still have their bile acids. Instead of stockpiling them in the gall bladder to be released upon the cholecystokinin signal, surgeons simply remove the gall bladder and make a direct connection between the liver and the duodenum. Once the fat has been absorbed, the bile acids pass on through the intestine, where they are either reabsorbed or conjugated and excreted in the feces.

The primarily bile acids, cholic and chenodeoxycholic acids, are produced from cholesterol by the liver. They are secreted into the intestine, where the intestinal flora convert these acids to their conjugated forms by dehydroxylating carbon 7 (see Figure 6.4). Further metabolism occurs at the far end of the intestinal tract where lithocholate is sulfated. While the dehydroxylated acids can be reabsorbed and sent back to the liver via the portal blood, the sulfated lithocholate is not. It appears in the feces. All four of the bile acids, the primary and dehydroxylated forms, are recirculated via the entero-hepatic system so that very little of the bile acid is lost. It has been estimated that the bile acid lost in the feces (~ 0.8 g/day) equals that newly synthesized by the liver so that the total pool remains between 3–5 g. The amount secreted per day is on the order of 16–70 g. Since the pool size is only 3–5 g, this means that these acids are recirculated as often as 14 times a day.

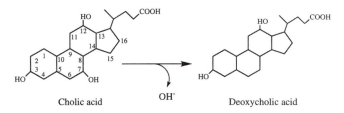

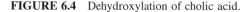

Cholic acid   OH⁻   Deoxycholic acid

FIGURE 6.4 Dehydroxylation of cholic acid.

The function of the bile acids is thus quite similar to that of enzymes. Neither are "used up" by the processes they participate in and facilitate. In the instance of fat absorption, the bile acids facilitate the formation of micelles, which, in turn, facilitate the uptake of the dietary fatty acids, monoglycerides, sterols, phospholipids, and other fat-soluble nutrients by the enterocyte of the small intestine. Not only do these bile acids recirculate, so too does cholesterol. Gallstones develop when the resecreted material is supersaturated with cholesterol, and this cholesterol-laden bile is stored in the gall bladder. With time, the cholesterol precipitates out, providing a crystalline structure for the stone. Since the bile also contains a variety of minerals, these minerals form salts with the bile acids and are deposited within and around the cholesterol matrix. Eventually, these stones irritate the lining of the gall bladder or may lodge themselves in the duct connecting the bladder to the duodenum. When this happens, the bladder becomes inflamed, the duct may be blocked, and the patient becomes unable to tolerate food. In some cases, treatment consists of reducing the irritation and inflammation through drugs, but often the patient has the gall bladder and its offending stones removed. This surgery is called a cholesystectomy.

Virtually all of the fatty acids, monoacylglyceride, and glycerol are absorbed by the enterocyte. Only 30–40% of the dietary cholesterol is absorbed. The percent cholesterol absorbed depends on a number of factors, including the fiber content of the diet, the gut passage time, and the total amount of cholesterol present for absorption. At higher intake levels, less is absorbed and vice versa at lower intake levels. Compared with fatty acids and the acylglycerides, the rate of cholesterol absorption is very slow. It is estimated that the half-life of cholesterol in the enterocyte is 12 hours. With high fiber intakes, less cholesterol is absorbed because the fiber acts as an adsorbent, reducing cholesterol availability. Unit 5 discusses the different fibers and their biological activity. Cellulose and lignens are good adsorbants of cholesterol, while transit through the intestine can be hastened by cellulose and hemicellulose. Pectins and gums increase transit time, yet they lower serum cholesterol levels by creating a gel-like consistency of the chyme, rendering the cholesterol in the chyme less available for absorption. High-fiber diets reduce gut passage time, which, in turn, results in less time for cholesterol absorption.

The fate of the absorbed fatty acids depends on chain length. Those fatty acids having 10 or fewer carbons are quickly passed into the portal blood stream without further modification. They are carried to the liver bound to albumin in concentrations varying between 0.1 to 2.0 μeq/ml. Those fatty acids remaining are bound to a fatty acid-binding protein and transported through the cytosol to the endoplasmic reticulum, whereupon they are converted to their CoA derivatives and reesterified to glycerol or residual monoacylglycerides to reform triacylglycerides. These reformed triacylglycerides adhere to phospholipids and fat-transporting proteins that are members of the lipoprotein family of proteins. This relatively large lipid–protein complex migrates to the Golgi complex in the basolateral basement membrane of the enterocyte. The lipid-rich vesicles fuse with the Golgi surface membrane, whereupon the lipid–protein complex is exocytosed or secreted into the intercellular space which, in turn, drains into the lymphatic system. The lymphatic system contributes these lipids to the circulation as the thoracic duct enters the jugular vein prior to its entry into the heart.

TRANSPORT

Blood lipid values vary depending on the age, sex, lifestyle, genetics, and diet of the population. Typical values for the different lipids are shown in Table 6.4. After a meal, the blood lipids rise. The time it takes for the peak value to appear depends on a variety of factors but, most notably, on the proximate composition of the meal. A high-fat meal leaves the stomach at a slower rate than does a low-fat meal. A high-fat meal will result in more total lipid entering the blood than a low-fat meal, but this lipid will enter the blood at a slower rate.

As fat digestion and absorption proceed, TG and cholesterol are processed in the intestinal epithelial cells into lipid-rich particles containing about 1% protein. The lipid associates with amphipathic protein known as lipoprotein. Lipoproteins carry not only the absorbed food lipids, but also the lipids synthesized or mobilized from organs and fat depots. Nine different lipid-carrying proteins have been identified, and each plays a specific role in the lipid-transport process. In addition, there are several minor proteins that may be involved in some aspects of lipid cycling and uptake. The proteins involved in lipid transport are listed in Table 6.5. Mutations in the genes that encode these proteins can lead to aberrant lipid transport and the individual may have either abnormally high or low blood lipid values. The hepatic and intestinal apolipoproteins can be distinguished using electrophoresis, a technique of separating proteins based on their electrophoretic mobility. Typically, these lipid-carrying proteins contain protein, triacylglycerols, phospholipids, and cholesterol. When separated, they have distinct characteristic lipid content, as shown in Table 6.6.

The intestinal cell has three apolipoproteins, called A-1, A-IV, and B-48. Apolipoprotein B-48 is unique to the enterocyte and is essential for chylomicron release by the intestinal cell. A-1 is

TABLE 6.4
Blood Lipid Levels for Normal Fasting Humans

Fraction	Range of Values[*]
Total	450–1000 mg/dl
Triacyglycerides	40–150 mg/dl
Phospholipids	9–16 mg/dl as lipid P
Cholesterol	120–220 mg/dl
Free Fatty Acids	6–16 mg/dl

[*]Selected from a table published in *N. Eng. J. Med.* 314:39, 1986.

TABLE 6.5
Proteins Involved in Lipid Transport

Protein	Function
apo A-II	Transport protein in HDL
apo B-48	Transport protein for chylomicrons; synthesized in the enterocyte in the human
High density lipoprotein binding protein (HDLBP)	Binds HDL and functions in the removal of excess cellular cholesterol
apo D	Transport protein similar to retinol-binding protein
apo (a)	Abnormal transport protein for LDL
apo A-I	Transport protein for chylomicrons and HDL; synthesized in the liver and its synthesis is induced by retinoic acid
apo C-III	Transport protein for VLDL
apo A-IV	Transport protein for chylomicrons
CETP	Participates in the transport of cholesterol from peripheral tissue to liver; reduces HDL size
LCAT	Synthesized in the liver and is secreted into the plasma where it resides on the HDL. Participates in the reverse transport of cholesterol from peripheral tissues to the liver; esterifies the HDL cholesterol.
apo E	Mediates high-affinity binding of LDLs to LDL receptor and the putative chylomicron receptor. Required for clearance of chylomicron remnant. Synthesized primarily in the liver.
apo C-I	Transport protein for VLDL
apo C-II	Chylomicron transport protein required cofactor for LPL activity
Apo B-100	Synthesized in the liver and is secreted into the circulation as part of the VLDL. Also serves as the ligand for the LDL receptor mediated hepatic endocytosis.
Lipoprotein lipase	Catalyzes the hydrolysis of plasma triglycerides into free fatty acids
Hepatic lipase	Catalyzes the hydrolysis of triglycerides and phospholipids of the LDL and HDL. It is bound to the surfaces of both hepatic and nonhepatic tissues.

synthesized in the liver. Apo B-48 is actually an edited version of the hepatic apo B-100. It is the result of an apo B mRNA editing process that converts codon 2153 to a translational stop codon. Apo B-48 is, thus, an edited form of apo B-100 and this editing is unique to the intestinal cell. Failure to appropriately edit the apo B gene in the intestinal cell will result in a disorder called

TABLE 6.6
Characteristics of the Various Lipoproteins

Fraction	% Protein	Density	% Lipid as		
			Triacylglycerol	Phospholipid	Cholesterol
Chylomicrons	1.5–2.5	<0.95	84–89	7–9	1–5
VLDL	5–10	0.95–1.006	50–65	15–20	5–15
LDL*	20–25	1.006–1.019	7–10	15–20	35–401
LDL**	20–25	1.019–1.063	7–10	15–20	7–102
HDL	40–55	1.068–1.210	5	20–35	4–12

*Primarily esterified cholesterol
**Primarily unesterified cholesterol

familial hypobetalipoproteinemia. In this disorder, there will be a total or partial (depending on the genetic mutation) absence of lipoproteins in the blood. Hypobetalipoproteinemia can also develop should there be base substitutions in the gene for the apo b protein. In addition to very low blood lipids, patients with this disorder also have fat malabsorption (steatorrhea). The feces contain an abnormally large amount of fat and have a characteristic peculiar odor. In this disorder, not only is the triacylglyceride absorption affected, but so too are the fat-soluble vitamins. Without the ability to absorb these energy-rich food components and the vital fat-soluble vitamins, the patient does not thrive and survive. Fortunately, this genetic mutation is not very common. It is inherited as an autosomal recessive trait.

The particles of absorbed lipid and transport proteins are called chylomicrons. They are present in the blood of feeding animals but are usually absent in starving animals. As the chylomicrons circulate, they acquire an additional protein, apo C-II. This additional protein is an essential cofactor for the recognition and hydrolysis of the chylomicron by the capillary endothelial enzyme, lipoprotein lipase (LPL). The LPL hydrolyzes most of the core triglycerides in the chylomicron leaving a remnant that is rich in cholesterol and cholesterol esters. During the LPL catalyzed hydrolytic process, the excess surface compounds, i.e., the phospholipids and apolipoproteins B, A-I, and A-IV are transferred to high density lipoproteins and, in exchange, apo-E is transferred from the HDL to the cholesterol ester-rich chylomicron remnant. These remnants are then cleared from the blood by the liver. On the hepatocyte is a lipoprotein receptor which recognizes Apo-E and this receptor plays an important role in remnant clearance. Figure 6.5 illustrates the process of exogenous lipid absorption, transport, and clearance.

The chylomicron is a relatively stable way of ensuring the movement, in an aqueous medium (blood), of hydrophobic molecules such as cholesterol and triacylglycerols from their point of origin, the intestine, to their point of use or storage. As mentioned, there are several unique proteins that facilitate this movement. These lipid-transporting proteins determine which cells of the body receive which lipids. At the target cell, the particles lose their lipid through hydrolysis facilitated by an interstitial lipoprotein, lipase, which is found in the capillary beds of muscle, fat cells, and other tissues using lipid as a fuel. Lipoprotein lipase is synthesized by these target cells but is anchored on the outside of the cells by a polysaccharide chain on the endothelial wall of the surrounding capillaries. Should this lipoprotein lipase be missing or genetically aberrant (Type I lipemia or chylomicronemia) so that the chylomicrons cannot be hydrolyzed, these chylomicrons accumulate and the individual develops a lipemia characterized by elevated levels of triacylglyceride and cholesterol-containing chylomicons. Also characteristic of this condition is considerable abdominal discomfort, the presence of an enlarged liver and spleen, and of subcutaneous xanthomas (clusters of hard, saturated fatty acid and cholesterol-rich nodules). Like familial hypolipoproteinemia, this condition is rare. Of interest is the observation that, despite the very high blood lipid

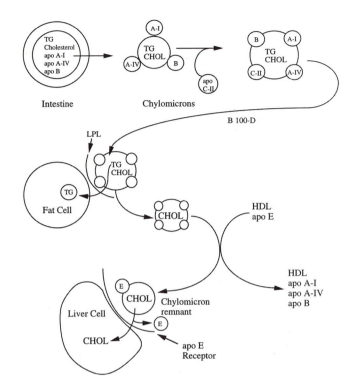

FIGURE 6.5   Schematic representation of the uptake, transport, and disposal of dietary lipids. TG: triacylg-lycerides; CHOL: cholesterol and cholesterol esters; apo A-I, apo B, Apo E: polypeptide lipid carriers; HDL: high-density lipoprotein.

levels of these people, few die of coronary-vessel disease. Their shortened life span is due to an inappropriate lipid deposition in all of the vital organs which, in turn, has a negative effect on organ function and life span.

ENDOGENOUS LIPID TRANSPORT

Fatty acids, TG, cholesterol, cholesterol esters, and phospholipids are synthesized in the body and are transported from sites of synthesis to sites of use and storage. While the transport of these lipids is, in many instances, similar to that of the dietary lipids, there are differences in the processing and in some of the proteins involved. Endogenous fat transport (Figure 6.6) involves the production and secretion of very-low-density lipoproteins (VLDL) by the liver. These lipid–protein complexes are rich in TG but also contain cholesterol. The polypeptides that transport these lipids make up approximately 10% of the weight of the VLDL. They include the polypeptides apo-B, B-100, apo C-I, apo C-II, apo C-III, and apo E. As mentioned, several of these polypeptides are also involved in exogenous lipid transport. Once the VLDLs are released by the hepatocyte, they are hydrolyzed by the interstitial lipoprotein lipase, and intermediate-density lipoproteins (IDL) are formed. These are cleared from the circulation as they are recognized and bound to hepatic IDL receptors. The hepatic receptors recognize the apo E that is part of the IDL. Any of the IDL that escapes hydrolysis at this step is available for hydrolysis by the hepatic lipoprotein lipase. This hydrolysis leaves a cholesterol-rich particle of low density (LDL). The LDL has apo B-100 as its polypeptide carrier and both hepatic and extrahepatic cells have receptors that recognize this polypeptide. Normally, about 70% of LDL is cleared by the LDL receptors and most of this is cleared by the liver. The endogenous fat transport and disposal system is diagrammed in Figure 6.6. From the foregoing, it is apparent that considerable lipid recycling occurs in the liver. The VLDLs originate in the liver,

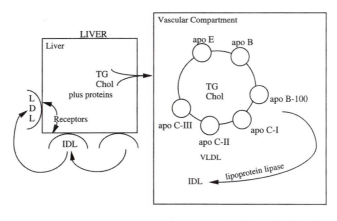

FIGURE 6.6 Lipid recycling: endogenous lipid transport and disposal. Very-low-density lipoproteins (VLDL) are secreted by the liver and circulated back to it, where various receptors (shown as a half-moon on the cell surface) bind and removes the lipid in a stepwise sequence. TG: triacylglycerides; CHOL: cholesterol and cholesterol esters; apo A E, apo B, apo B-100, apo C-III, apo C-II, apo C-I: polypeptide lipid carriers; IDL: intermediate-density lipoproteins; LDL: low-density lipoproteins.

which is the primary site for LDL disposal. Other organs and tissues also participate in disposal, but their participation is minor compared with that of the liver.

GENETIC BASIS FOR LIPOPROTEINEMIA

As mentioned, there are a number of proteins involved in the uptake, synthesis, and disposal of lipid. The genes for the transport proteins, apo A-I, apo A-II, apo A-IV, apo (a), apo B, apo D, apo C-I, apo C-II, apo C-III, apo D, and apo E have been identified, as have mutations that result in lipid transport abnormalities (Table 6.7). In addition to these transport proteins, we have the proteins that are the important rate-limiting enzymes and receptors that are involved in lipoprotein processing; the peripheral lipoprotein lipase and the hepatic lipoprotein lipase; the lipoprotein receptors on the plasma membrane of the cells that receive and oxidize or store the transported lipids; and the rate-limiting enzymes of lipid synthesis and use. Included in this last category are the fatty acid synthase complex, acetyl CoA carboxylase, HMG CoA reductase, HMG CoA synthase, cholesterol ester transfer protein (CETP), fatty acid-binding protein (FABP), lecithin-cholesterol acyltransferase (LCAT), cholesterol 7-hydroxylase, and the high-density lipoprotein-binding protein (HDLBP). Many of these proteins have been isolated and studied in detail. Several of their cognate genes have been identified and mapped. Listed in Table 6.7 are the chromosomal locations of these genes and shown in Figure 6.7 are the gene structures of seven of the apolipoproteins. With this many genes involved in the uptake, synthesis, transport, and degradation of the circulating lipids, it is not surprising to find mutations that phenotype as either lipemia or fat malabsorption. Not all of these diseases of lipid transport are associated with atherosclerosis. Table 6.7 lists the known defects as well as estimates of their frequency.

Defects in exogenous fat transport are manifested in several ways. As described above, defective chylomicron formation due to mutations in either the apo B gene or its editing leads to and is characterized by fat malabsorption. This includes the malabsorption of fat-soluble vitamins as well. Twenty different mutations have been identified in the gene for the apo B protein. These mutations are inherited via an autosomal recessive mode and are characterized not only by fat malabsorption, but also by acanthocytes, retinitis pigmentosa, and muscular neuropathies. To a large extent, these symptoms can be attributed to a relative deficiency of the fat-soluble vitamins due to malabsorption. While a defect in the apo B gene can account for defective fat absorption, Wetterau and Shoulders et al. have suggested the presence of another mutation (in the microsomal triglyceride transfer protein)

TABLE 6.7
Location of Genes Involved in Lipoprotein Metabolism

Gene	Chromosome Location	Characteristics of Mutation	Frequency of Mutation
apo A-II	1	Transport protein in HDL	?
apo B 48	2 p 23-24	Hypobetalipoproteinemia	1:1,000,000
High density lipoprotein binding protein (HDLBP)	2 q 37		?
apo D	3	Transport protein similar to retinol-binding protein	?
apo (a)	6	Abnormal transport protein for LDL	?
LPL	8 p 22	Defective chylomicron clearance	1:1,000,000
apo A-I	11	Defective HDL production (Tangier's disease)	1:1,000,000
apo C-III	11		?
apo A-IV	11		?
Hepatic LPL (HTGL)	15 q 21	Defective IDL clearance	?
CETP	16 q 22.1		?
LCAT	16 q 22.1	Familial lecithin:cholesterol transferase deficiency. 2 types.	Rare
LDL receptor	19	Familial hypercholesterolemia	1:500
apo B 100	2	Familial defective apo B 100	1:500-1:1000
apo E	19	Type III hyperlipoproteinemia	1:5000
apo C-I	19	Transport protein for VLDL	?
apo C-II	19	Defective chylomicron clearance	1:1,000,000

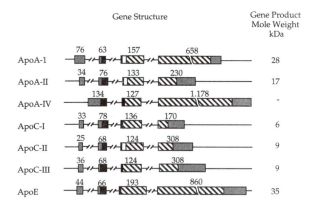

FIGURE 6.7 Gene structures and molecular weights of several of the lipid transport proteins. The 5,3' untranslated region is shown shaded, the leader sequence is shown black, the prosequence is white, the region coding for the mature protein is striped. From Rosseneu and Lebeur, *FASEB J*, 1995.

that also might result in fat malabsorption. This transfer protein is essential for apo B translocation and subsequent synthesis of chylomicrons. Defects in this transfer protein would impair apo B availability and chylomicron formation. In these defects, very low levels of chylomicrons are found in the blood. Persons with this disorder are rare (one in a million). In this circumstance, the severity of the disease is related to the size of the mutated gene product and whether it can associate with the lipids it must carry. The size of the truncated apo B can vary from apo B-9 (41 residues) to apo B-89

(4487 residues). Except in the case of the apo B-25, the result of a deletion of the entire exon 21, all the truncated forms reported to date are C-T transitions or base deletions. These deletions can involve misaligned pairing deletion mechanisms. Frameshift mutation can be compensated by a reading frame restoration of the apo B gene.

Familial hyperchylomicronemia is characterized by elevations in chylomicrons having both triglycerides and cholesterol. Hyperchylomicronemia was found to be due to mutations in the genes that encode the enzyme lipoprotein lipase needed for the hydrolysis of chylomicrons. This enzyme is a glycoprotein having an apparent monomeric molecular weight of about 60,000 daltons on SDS gel electrophoresis and 48,300 daltons by sedimentation-equilibrium ultracentrifugation. The enzyme is linked to the endothelial cells of the capillary system. Lipoprotein lipase is quite similar to hepatic triglyceride lipase, an enzyme found in the hepatic sinusoids. The main difference between the two lipases is that the interstitial lipase has a requirement for the lipid-carrying protein, apo C-II, for full activity whereas hepatic LPL does not. Mutations in the gene for apo C-II can result in aberrant lipase activity because apo C-II serves as a cofactor in the lipoprotein lipase-catalyzed reaction. Hepatic triglyceride lipase has no such requirement. Aberrations in the hepatic triglyceride lipase result in an accumulation of VLDL rather than accumulations of chylomicrons. Mutations in the genes for LPL and apo C-II are very rare, occurring at a frequency of one in a million. The gene for LPL has been mapped to chromosome 8, while that for apo C-II has been mapped to chromosome 19, and the hepatic LPL to chromosome 15. Other features of these disorders include an inflammation of the exocrine pancreas and eruptive xanthomas. Chylomicronemia does not appear to be atherogenic. The mutations in the LPL gene appear to be insertions or deletions or due to aberrant splicing, while those in the apo C-II gene seem to be due to splice site mutations or small deletions. Twenty-two mutations in the apo C-II gene have been reported. With respect to the aberrant splicing of the LPL gene in three unrelated humans, Holzl et al. reported a C→A mutation in position 3 of the acceptor splice site of intron 6, which caused aberrant splicing. The major transcript showed a deletion of exons 6 through 9 and amounted to about 3% of normal. Trace amounts of both a normally spliced LPL mRNA and a second aberrant transcript devoid of exon 7 were found. In one of these patients, Holzl et al. found a 3' splice mutation on one allele while on the other allele they found a missense mutation resulting in Gly 188→Glu substitution. All three subjects were classed as hyperchylomicronemic due to LPL deficiency.

The absence of LPL activity in certain tissues or in certain individuals can be attributed to mutations in lipoprotein lipase promoter region. Studies of tissue-specific expression of LPL in a variety of murine tissues by Gimble et al. showed that cis acting elements located within the − 1824-bp of the 5' flanking region were required for the expression of LPL. These include nuclear factors recognizing both the CCAAT box and the octamer sequence immediately flanking the transcriptional start site. Those tissues that have no LPL activity lack this promoter region. Since humans and mice have identical CCAAT and octamer sequences, one could suppose that humans having an intact LPL gene of normal sequence but lacking LPL activity might have a deficient or mutated promoter region. Although such has been suggested by Sparkes et al., proof that this might occur is presently lacking.

Mutations in the gene for hepatic lipoprotein lipase result in elevated blood levels of triglycerides and cholesterol and these elevations are related to an increased risk for atherosclerosis. Hepatic LPL must be secreted by the hepatocyte into the sinusoids to function as a catalyst for the hydrolysis of core TG and surface phospholipids of chylomicron remnants, HDL, and IDL. Through its activity, it augments the uptake of HDL cholesterol by the liver (reverse cholesterol transport) and is involved in the reduction of HDL size from HDL_2 to HDL_3. Hepatic LPL aids in the clearance of chylomicron remnants by exposing the apo E epitopes for enzymatic action. Missense mutations in the hepatic LPL gene include substitutions of serine for phenylalanine at amino acid position 267, threonine for methionine at position 383, and asparagine for serine at position 291. These mutations result in poorly secreted enzyme and thus the phenotypic expression of the mutation is low hepatic lipase activity. The frequency of the Asn 291 Ser mutation in a population having premature CVD has been reported as 5.2%.

Defects in chylomicron remnant clearance are much more common than any of the above mutations. Defective clearance due to mutations in the apo E gene result in a lipemia known as Type III hyperlipoproteinemia. It is associated with premature atherosclerosis and patients with these defects have high serum triglyceride levels as well as high serum cholesterol levels. Xanthomas are found in nearly three-quarters of the population with these defects. The lipemia is responsive to energy restriction using diets that have 40% of energy from carbohydrate, 40% from fat, and 20% from protein. Weight loss is efficacious for most people with this defect. The apo E gene codes for the protein on the surface of the chylomicron remnant that is the ligand for receptor-mediated clearance of this particle.

A number of mutations in the apo E gene have been reported, and the phenotypes of these mutations are grouped into three general groups labeled E_2, E_3, and E_4. Those of the E_2 groups fail to bind the particles to the cell surface receptor for the chylomicron remnant. Those of the E_3 and E_4 groups have generally low remnant clearance rates. The apo E allele and phenotype frequency varies. The E_2 frequency is about 8%, the E_3 about 77%, and the E_4 about 15% of the total population with an apo E mutation. The incidence of apo E gene mutations is about 1% of the population. Since apo E is involved in both endogenous and exogenous lipid transport and clearance, a faulty apo E gene is devastating. Mature human apo E is a 299 amino acid polypeptide. Apo E as well as other apolipoproteins contain 11 or 22 amino acid repeated sequences as one of their key features. These appear to encode largely amphipathic helices, which are needed for lipid binding. There is a high degree of conservation among species of nucleotide sequences in the gene fragment that encodes the amino acid repeats. The gene for apo E has been mapped to chromosome 19, as have the genes for apo C-I, apo C-II, and LDLR. There appears to be a tight linkage among these genes that coordinates their expression. Among the common mutations are amino acid substitutions at positions 112 and 158, while less-frequent substitutions occur at other positions in the polypeptide chain. Several of these involve the exchange of neutral amino acids for acidic amino acids with the net result of alterations in polypeptide charge and subsequent inadequate binding to the appropriate cell surface receptors.

In a rare form of the disorder, the mutation is such that no useful apo E is formed. Transgenic mice have been constructed with an apo E mutation that mimics apo E deficiency. These mice, like humans, develop hypercholesterolemia and increased susceptibility to atherosclerosis. When these mice were fed low- (5%) or high-fat (16%) diets, a differential serum cholesterol pattern was observed: those fed the high-fat diet had significantly higher levels of cholesterol and VLDL and LDL than those fed a low-fat or stock diet. The transgenic mice, even when fed the stock diet, had significantly higher levels of cholesterol and VLDL and LDL than the normal control mice. There was a gender difference as well. Male transgenic mice were less diet responsive in terms of their cholesterol levels than female transgenic mice. As mentioned, there is some sequence homology between humans and mice in the apo E DNA and it could be inferred that these responses to dietary fat intake in mice could be observed in humans as well.

While the above transgenic approach used the gene-knockout paradigm (an extreme in the variants of apo E mutants) it nonetheless suggests that variation in the apo E genes could determine the responsiveness of humans with apo E defects to dietary manipulation. Indeed, such nutrient–gene interactions have been reported. The dietary fat clearance in normal subjects appears to be regulated by the genetic variance in apo E sequence and this, in turn, is related to fat intake. Not only is triacylglycerol clearance affected, but so too is cholesterol clearance. One study reported that the apo E genotype declares the response to cholesterol intake with respect to blood cholesterol levels and that this genotype influences cholesterol synthesis. Those subjects who respond poorly to an oral cholesterol challenge vis à vis blood cholesterol clearance had higher rates of cholesterol synthesis than those who could rapidly clear their blood of cholesterol after an oral challenge. One of the more interesting variants of the apo E is called the Milano variant. In this variant, blood lipid levels are elevated, but these elevations are not associated with an increased risk of athero-sclerosis.

Cholesterol traffic is also controlled by the LDL receptor and the transport protein apo B-100. Mutations in the gene for the LDL receptor or in the gene for apo B-100, the ligand for the LDL receptor results in high serum levels of cholesterol. The former results in the disorder called familial hypercholesterolemia and occurs with a frequency of about one in 500. Familial hypercholester-olemia is associated with early death from atherosclerosis in man and related primates. Dietary-fat saturation affects transcription of LDL receptor mRNA, in that feeding a diet containing saturated fat results in decreased LDL receptor mRNA, compared with feeding an unsaturated-fat diet. These results suggest that unsaturated fatty acids may interact with proteins that in turn serve as either cis or trans acting elements for this gene in much the same way as polyunsaturated fatty acids affect fatty acid synthetase gene expression.

Familial defective apo B-100 hypercholesterolemia is due to a mutation in the coding sequence of the apo B gene at bp 3500 that changes the base sequence such that glutamine is substituted for arginine. This is in the LDL receptor-binding region of the apo B protein and results in a binding affinity of less than 4% of normal. Polymorphic variation in the genes for both the LDL receptor and the apo B-100 have been reported for mice, and this variation has provided the opportunity to identify the genetic and molecular constraints of lipoprotein gene expression.

Both apo B and apo E serve as ligands for the LDL receptor. In contrast to apo E, apo B has little homology with the other apolipoproteins. Apo B in mice is quite variable, and this variation imparts or confers a diet-responsive characteristic in inbred mouse strains vis à vis polypeptide sequence and activity. That is, some mouse strains have reduced levels of plasma apo B when fed a high-fat diet compared with controls fed a stock diet, while other mouse strains are unresponsive to diet vis à vis their plasma apo B-100 levels. Such polymorphism also exists in humans. Apo B has been mapped to chromosome 2 and produces two gene products, apo B-100 and B-48. In the intestine, the apo B primary transcript is co- or post-transcriptionally modified. This modification converts codon 2153 from a glutamine (CAA) to an in-frame, premature termination codon (UAA), thereby causing translation to terminate after amino acid 2152. This mRNA editing thus explains the difference in size of these two proteins. If more of the apo B gene is deleted, hypocholesterolemia is observed. This is because apo B-48 is required for the transport of the chylomicrons from the intestine. If lacking, chylomicron formation is impaired and low serum cholesterol levels are observed. Both familial defective apo B-100 and familial hypercholesterolemia are characterized by high levels of LDL. Both are associated with CVD, but only the familial hypercholesterolemia is characterized by tendon xanthomas. Both are inherited as autosomal dominant disorders. Col-lectively, these mutations have a cumulative frequency of 1 in 250. However, because polymorphism in the apo B gene can and does occur, there is the possibility that, collectively, the frequency is much greater, perhaps as high as one in five. If this is the case, then the population variation in plasma cholesterol levels could be explained on the basis of these genetic differences alone, apart from those mutations that are associated with the rest of the genes that encode components of the lipid transport system.

Genetically determined abnormalities in LDL metabolism may also be due to mutation in the large glycoprotein, apo (a). Apo (a) is a highly variable disulfide protein bonded to the apo B-100. It is thought to resemble plasminogen. In fact, the genes that encode Lp(a) and plasminogen are very close to each other on the long arm of chromosome 6. In general, LDLs containing apo (a) do not bind well to the LPL receptor, and people having significant amounts of apo (a) have a two- to threefold increase in CVD risk. Many individuals have little or no apo (a) and it has been suggested that those who have it are abnormal with respect to LPL activity.

Several mutations in the genes that encode the endogenous lipid transport have been reported. The reverse cholesterol transport pathway is part of this endogenous lipid-transport system. It involves the movement of cholesterol from peripheral tissues to the liver. The peripheral tissues cannot oxidize cholesterol and so must send it to the liver, where it is prepared for excretion, via cholesterol 7 α

hydroxylase, as bile acids. This pathway uses the HDL to shuttle the cholesterol in this direction. HDL consists primarily of apo A-1 and cholesterol, which is esterified by the enzyme lecithin:cholesterol acyl transferase (LCAT). Mutations in the LCAT gene have been reported and result in one of two diseases: familial LCAT deficiency and fish eye disease. Thirteen different mutations have been identified and in one, a single T→A transversion in codon 252 in exon 6, converting met (ATG) to Lys (AAG), was observed. Three unrelated families were found to have this mutation; however, the severity of their disease varied. In these families, no other mutation in LCAT was observed. Of the remaining 12 LCAT mutations, 10 were point mutations, three were frameshifts and one consisted of a three-base insertion that maintained its reading frame. For fish eye disease, three mutations have been reported. This disorder is less serious than familial LCAT deficiency and is characterized by dyslipoproteinemia and corneal opacity. LCAT activity is 15% of normal and there is a reduced level of HDL in the plasma. In contrast, familial LCAT deficiency is characterized by a variety of symptoms, including lipoprotein abnormalities, renal failure, premature atherosclerosis, reduced levels of plasma cholesterol esters, and high plasma levels of cholesterol and lecithin.

The LCAT enzyme requires apo A-I as a cofactor. If there is a mutation in the gene for apo A-I, defective HDL production results. This is a rare mutation and its frequency is estimated as one in a million. Individuals with this defect have premature CVD, corneal clouding, and very low HDL levels. Plasma apo A-I has a variety of charge isoforms with similar antigenicity and amino acid composition. Humans, baboons, African green monkeys, and cynomolgus monkeys have been studied, and there are species differences in hepatic and intestinal apo A-I production. In all instances, the differences in apo A-I were reported between intestine and liver. In the liver, there was a twofold higher level of apo A-I mRNA than in the intestine, and the abundance of this mRNA was species specific. The apo A-I gene is regulated at the level of transcription and a portion of the species-specific difference in apo A-I gene expression is due to a sequence divergence in the 5' regulatory region, including the exon/intron 1 of the apo A-I gene. The capacity to produce HDLs is both genetically controlled and tissue specific, and probably explains why some genotypes respond normally to a high-fat diet by producing more HDL while other genotypes become hypercholesterolemic under these same conditions. Attempts to create a transgenic mouse expressing a human apo A-I gene have not been fully successful, but have provided additional information about the relationship of apo A-I to HDL size. The human apo A-I gene was inserted into the mouse, and in these mice, both the mouse and the human genes were expressed. This dual expression suggests a species difference in the control of this expression. In other words, the control points differed and this resulted in a broader spectrum of HDL particles.

Defective HDL metabolism due to a mutation in the apo A-I gene results in a rare autosomal-dominant disorder described in a small group of villagers in Italy. Affected individuals have reduced levels of HDL cholesterol and apo A-I levels, but have no increased risk of CVD. The disorder, named Apo A-I Milano is due to a point mutation in the apo A-I gene, changing codon 173 so that cysteine is used instead of arginine. Normal apo A-I has no cysteine, so this change has an effect on the apo A-I structure.

Defective lipoprotein processing has already been discussed with respect to LDP, LCAP, and apo C-II deficiencies. A deficient cholesterol ester transport protein (CETP) has been reported due to a mutation of the gene for this protein located on chromosome 16. A mutation in this gene has been used to explain the atherogenicity of high-fat diets in primates, but, to date, no evidence of such a mutation in humans has been put forward.

NUTRIENT–GENE INTERACTIONS IN LIPID TRANSPORT

The above-described observations of diet and genetic factors suggest that CVD could develop as a result of a nutrient–gene interaction. There are a number of genes involved in the regulation of blood lipid levels. Further, the diet influence involves not only the amount of fat consumed but also the type of fat and the amount and type of carbohydrate. For example, the editing of the apo

B gene is enhanced by dietary carbohydrate. A number of genes have carbohydrate-response elements and it is possible that this gene has this element in its promoter region. A carbohydrate response element has been identified in the apo E gene. Carbohydrate influences mRNA stability and RNA processing of this gene. Similarly, the gene that encodes the seven-enzyme complex of mammalian fatty acid synthetase has a fatty acid response unit in its promoter. The expression of this gene is down regulated by dietary polyunsaturated fatty acids. The lipid transport genes might also have a lipid-response element.

Over transcription of the fatty acid synthase gene (which has a lipid response element) has been shown to occur in genetically obese Zucker rats. Mouse apo A-IV gene expression in C57BL/6 mice, which were shown by Paigen et al. to develop atherosclerosis, is induced by high-fat feeding. In normal mice, this does not occur. The apo A-IV gene consists of three exons and two introns. The introns separate the evolutionarily conserved and functional polypeptide domains. Intron 1 divides most of the apo A-IV signal peptide from the amino terminus of the mature plasma protein. The second intron separates a highly conserved variant amphipathic peptide repeat from the remainder of the mature apo A-IV protein. The 5' flanking region has several features: variant TATA- and CAT-box sequences (TTTAAA and CCAACG); five G rich direct repeats of 10 nucleotides and a short inverted repeat. The variants found in this region may determine whether dietary fat can induce apo A-IV gene expression. Some may constitute a lipid-response element, while other sequence variants may not be lipid responsive. Further studies showed that the genetic control of apo A-IV mRNA levels involves both cis acting elements and genetically distinct trans acting factors. The cis acting elements (nucleic acid sequences) and the trans acting factors (specific proteins) determine both the rate of mRNA transcription and its turnover. Transcription requires the recognition of promoter sequences by protein transcription factors. These factors may bind lipid and be part of the lipid response unit or the lipid response unit may be entirely separate. This has not been determined, merely speculated.

Dietary lipids, even in the absence of direct effects on transcription and translation, influence the phenotypic expression of specific genotypes either because of overconsumption or because they have effects on certain of the hormones, i.e., insulin or the steroid hormones, or the catabolic hormones that regulate or influence lipid synthesis, oxidation, and storage. For example, Chen et al. showed that, in diabetic mice, insulin regulated the transcription of the apo C-III gene and that this regulation in turn affected serum triglyceride levels. Triglyceride levels fell in the insulin-treated diabetic mice subsequent to an insulin-induced increase in apo C-III mRNA level. In turn, Chen et al. were able to show that this mRNA increase was due to a specific effect of insulin on apo C-III gene transcription.

The level of cholesterol in the blood depends on the diet consumed and how much cholesterol is being synthesized. The cholesterol content of the gut LDL of a person on a low-cholesterol diet might run as low as 7–10% of the total lipid in the lipoprotein, while the hepatic LPL of this same individual might be as high as 58% of total lipid. People consuming a low-cholesterol, low-saturated-fat diet may reduce the contribution of the diet to the blood cholesterol while increasing the hepatic *de novo* cholesterol synthesis. Persons having an LPL receptor deficiency are characterized by high serum cholesterol levels and, in some cases, by high serum triacylglycerides. The reason these blood lipids are elevated is that the individuals cannot utilize the lipids carried by the LPL due to the error(s) in the receptor molecule. Further, because these circulating lipids do not enter into the adipose and hepatic cell in normal amounts, the synthesis of triacylglycerides and cholesterol is not appropriately down regulated. Hence, this individual has elevated serum lipids not only because the LPL lipid is not appropriately cleared from the blood, but also because of high rates of endogenous lipid synthesis. Individuals with this disorder have lipid deposits in unusual places such as immediately under the skin, around the eyes, on the tendons, and in the vascular tree. It is this last feature that probably accounts for the shortened life span of these people, with the cause of death being cardiovascular disease. As can be seen from the metabolic characteristics of this disorder, low-cholesterol diets are probably useless in reducing serum cholesterol levels because *de novo* synthesis of cholesterol from non-lipid precursors can and does occur. Treatment with lipid adsorbents (high-fiber diets, the drug cholestyramine) will help reduce the cholesterol (but not triacylglycerides) coming from the intestine, and there are drugs that can safely lower *de novo* cholesterol synthesis as well as increase intracellular lipid oxidation. All of these therapies may help reduce the serum lipid levels, but even doing this only treats the symptoms, not the genetic disorder. Gene therapy is needed to correct the genetic disorder that is the basic underlying cause of the symptoms.

Heart disease in its various forms is also associated with elevated levels of the VLDL. A specific genetic error has not been identified; however, the disorders have been subdivided into three general categories. In one, Type III lipemia, the patients are characterized by elevated serum cholesterol, phospholipid, and triacylglyceride levels, elevated VLDL levels (and sometimes LDL levels), fatty deposits on the tendons and in areas on the arms just under the skin, vascular atheromas, and ischemic heart disease. This type of lipemia is inherited as an autosomal dominant trait in one person in 5,000. Another lipemia (Type IV) having a normal cholesterol level but an elevated triacylglyceride level and elevated VLDL levels is also associated with ischemic heart disease and premature atherosclerosis. It is frequently seen in obese patients with Type 2 diabetes. People with diabetes mellitus have five times the risk of normal people of developing premature atherosclerosis and its associated coronary events. A combination of cardiovascular disease that is followed by renal disease is the leading cause of death for people with diabetes mellitus.

Those people with Type 1 diabetes mellitus are more likely to develop a lipemia (Type V lipemia) that is slightly different from the aforementioned Type 2-related lipemia. While the incidence of both is two in 1000, those with the latter problem inherited their trait in an autosomal recessive manner, while those with the Type 2-related lipemia inherited their trait as an autosomal dominant trait. Elevated chylomicron and VLDL levels and reduced dietary fat tolerance characterize this type of lipemia. Patients with this disorder are usually of normal body weight.

METABOLISM

Once the dietary lipids are transferred to the target tissues, one of several processes occurs. The fatty acids of the triacylglycerols either are oxidized for energy, are stored as resynthesized triacylglycerols, or are incorporated into the membranes within and around the cells. An overview of these processes is shown in Figure 6.8. Certain of the fatty acids, the essential fatty acids, linoleic and linolenic, have a special role as precursors for the 20 carbon compounds called eicosanoids. Diet can affect all of these processes and, as well, stimulate lipid synthesis.

Fatty Acid Synthesis

In humans consuming a typical American diet containing 35 to 45% of its energy as fat, very little fatty acid synthesis occurs. However, in certain circumstances, for example, humans consuming a very low-fat diet that is high in refined sugar, synthesis can and does occur. The magnitude of this synthesis is dependent on a variety of factors, of which diet is one. In laboratory rats accustomed to a very low-fat diet composed mainly of cereal grains, lipid synthesis occurs at a significant rate. Furthermore, in people who are obese, it is suspected that significant fatty synthesis also occurs despite their high fat intake. In humans, primates, and birds, the liver is the primary site for fat synthesis. In rats and mice, lipogenesis occurs in the adipose tissue as well as in the liver. In pigs, lipogenesis occurs primarily in the fat depots. In those humans having a very high synthetic rate, a fatty liver may be observed. Humans sustained by parenteral nutrition (nutrients provided through a catheter placed in the subclavian vein) or those who derive a significant (more than 60%) amount of their energy from carbohydrate, may have high lipogenic rates and a fatty liver if the export of these newly synthesized lipids via the VLDL is impeded.

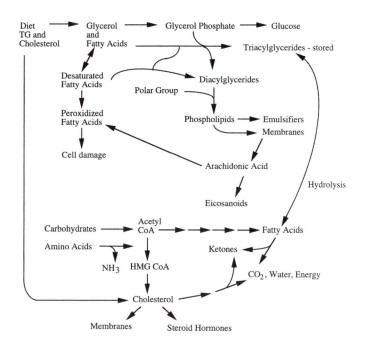

FIGURE 6.8   Overview of lipid metabolism.

If VLDL synthesis keeps pace with the high lipogenic rate, a fatty liver does not develop. In rats fed high-sugar (65% by weight) diets, lipogenesis is quite high. However, normal rats will adapt to this diet so that the initial fatty liver will disappear as the hepatic lipid output increases to match the increased synthesis.

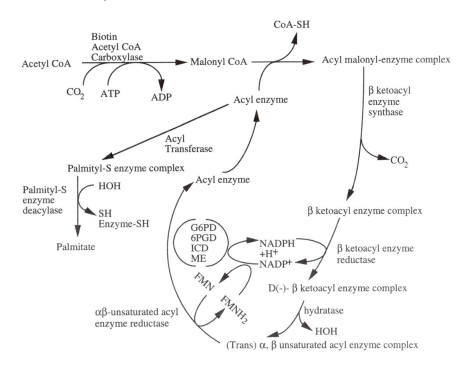

FIGURE 6.9   Fatty acid synthesis.

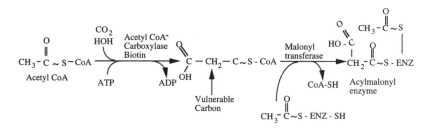

FIGURE 6.10   Details of the initial steps in fatty acid synthesis.

Fatty acid synthesis (Figure 6.9) begins with acetyl CoA, which arises from the oxidation of glucose or the carbon skeletons of deaminated amino acids. Acetyl CoA is converted to malonyl CoA with the addition of 1 carbon (from bicarbonate) in the presence of the enzyme acetyl CoA carboxylase. The reaction uses the energy from 1 molecule of ATP and biotin as a coenzyme. This reaction is the first committed step in the reaction sequence that results in the synthesis of a fatty acid. In many respects, it resembles the carboxylation of pyruvate, the first committed step in gluconeogenesis. In both reactions, activated carbon dioxide attached to the biotin–enzyme complex is transferred to the methyl end of the substrate. Although most fatty acids synthesized in mammalian cells have an even number of carbons, this first committed step yields a 3-carbon product. Figure 6.10 illustrates these initial reactions. This results in an asymmetric molecule that becomes vulnerable to attack (addition) at the center of the molecule with the subsequent loss of the terminal carbon. The

vulnerability is conferred by the fact that the carboxyl group at one end and the $\overset{\overset{0}{\parallel}}{C} \sim$ S-CoA group at the other end are both powerful attractants of electrons from the middle carbon group. This leaves the carbon in a very reactive state, and a second acetyl group carried by a carrier protein with the help of phosphopantethine, which has a sulfur group connection, can be joined to it through the action of the enzyme malonyl transferase. Subsequently, the "extra" carbon is released via the enzyme β–ketoacyl enzyme synthase leaving a 4-carbon chain still connected to an SH group at the carboxyl end. This SH group is the docking end for all the enzymes that the fatty acid synthase complex comprises. These enzymes catalyze the addition of two carbon acetyl groups in sequence to the methyl end of the carbon chain until the final product, palmityl CoA, and then palmitic acid, is produced. Members of this fatty acid synthase complex include the aforementioned malonyl transferase and β–ketoacyl synthase, β–ketoacyl reductase, which catalyzes the addition of reducing equivalents carried by FMN, and an acyl transferase. Upon completion of these six steps, the process is repeated until the chain length is 16 carbons long. At this point, the SH-acyl carrier protein is removed through the action of the enzyme palmityl-S-enzyme deacylase, and the palmitic acid is available for esterification to glycerol to form a mono-, di-, or triacylglyceride.

Fatty acid synthesis does not occur as an uncontrolled sequence of reactions. It has a number of direct and indirect controllers. As mentioned above, the synthesis of malonyl CoA is the first committed step in the pathway. It also is the first rate-limiting reaction. Acetyl CoA carboxylase as a rate-limiting enzyme has been studied in detail. It is synthesized as an inactive protomer which, when citrate levels increase, aggregate to form the active enzyme. Other tricarboxylates can stimulate aggregation but citrate is the preferred anion. Citrate, a citric acid cycle intermediate in the mitochondria, is exchanged for malate or pyruvate. Figure 6.11 illustrates the relationship of the citric acid cycle to fatty acid synthesis. The malate–citrate shuttle is very active in cells also having a very active lipogenic process. This shuttle also has rate-limiting properties. Pyruvate, from the oxidation of glucose via the glycolytic sequence (Unit 5), is also actively exchanged for citrate in the lipogenic cell. These exchanges are described and discussed in Unit 3. Citrate is cleaved through the action of the ATP-citrate lyase (citrate cleavage enzyme) producing oxalacetate and

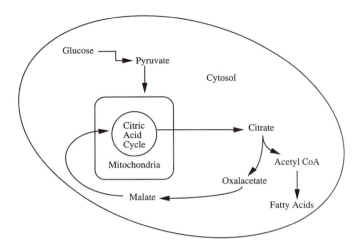

FIGURE 6.11 Citric acid cycle activity is important to active lipogenesis.

acetyl CoA. This acetyl CoA is the beginning substrate for fatty acid synthesis. Feedback inhibition of acetyl CoA carboxylase is exerted when palmitoyl CoA accumulates.

Acetyl CoA carboxylase is sensitive to the phosphorylation state of the cytosol. High levels of ATP are needed for the carboxylation of acetyl CoA to form malonyl CoA. Thus, high phosphorylation states (high concentrations of ATP relative to ADP and inorganic phosphate) are a characteristic of high rates of lipogenesis. Acetyl CoA carboxylase is also controlled by a cAMP-mediated phosphorylation-dephosphorylation mechanism in which the phosphorylated enzyme is less active than the dephosphorylated enzyme. Insulin promotes dephosphorylation while glucagon promotes phosphorylation. Thus, when insulin levels are high, one would anticipate high rates of lipogenesis and the reverse when insulin levels are low and glucagon levels are high. One might also anticipate an increase in lipogenesis in hyperinsulinemic individuals, and, indeed, obese people as well as genetically obese experimental animals are characterized by both. As a corollary, one might also anticipate that the consumption of a high-glucose, low-fat diet that stimulates insulin release and also provides ample glucose for conversion to fatty acids would be characterized by high rates of lipogenesis, particularly in the liver. In rodents, this anticipation is justified. However, in humans, there is some discussion as to whether the human diet is sufficiently high in simple sugar and sufficiently low in fat to have the same sort of lipogenic response. Species differences in habitual diet composition as well as species differences in biological time frame complicate the discussion. A 24-hour day in a rat is roughly equivalent to a 30-day time span in the human, with respect to total life span. The peaks and nadirs in the lipogenic rates in the rat will thus be further apart within a 24-hour period than will lipogenic rates in the human. Thus, one can elicit an increase in acetyl CoA carboxylase activity and in lipogenesis in the rodent with a short interval (1–2 days) of high-glucose diet feeding where that same interval for the human will show little, if any, change.

Genetic factors also influence acetyl CoA carboxylase activity. In the human, the gene for acetyl CoA carboxylase is located on chromosome 17. Should this gene mutate, a nonfunctional enzyme will be produced and *de novo* fatty acid synthesis will not occur. Such an inborn error has been reported in humans. However, since humans consuming a high-fat diet, such as that consumed in the U.S., synthesize very little lipid *de novo*, the absence of a functioning acetyl CoA carboxylase is not as devastating as the absence of an important rate-limiting step in some other pathway. In contrast, such a deficiency in rats, animals that usually consume a low-fat, high-carbohydrate diet, would seriously impair survival unless the rat was fed a human-like diet.

Another control of fatty acid synthesis is exerted by the complex of enzymes known as the fatty acid synthase. All of the dietary and hormonal factors described above for activating or inhibiting acetyl CoA carboxylase have the same effects on the fatty acid synthase complex. Further, phosphorylated sugars have allosteric effects on this enzyme complex. An allosteric effect is one that promotes (or inhibits) the activity of an enzyme or enzyme complex by binding to a site other than the active catalytic site that promotes (or inhibits) the activity of the active catalytic site. An allosteric effector may not be involved in the reaction itself, but, through its binding, causes a change in the conformation of the enzyme. In the case of inhibition, such a conformational change may "hide" the active catalytic portion of the molecule. In promotion, the reverse occurs; the "business end" of the molecule is readily accessible to substrate, cofactors, and coenzymes.

While dietary ingredients affect the activity of fatty acid synthase through effects on the supplies of acetyl CoA, they have other effects as well. These effects occur at the level of the genes for fatty acid synthase. Diets high in simple sugars increase the synthesis of fatty acid synthase. Diets rich in polyunsaturated fatty acids decrease this synthesis. Clarke and Jump (1993) reviewed the literature on this aspect of fatty acid synthesis and concluded that polyunsaturated fatty acids suppress the rapid transcription of genes coding for fatty acid synthesis. They speculate that in liver cells there is a nuclear fatty acid-binding protein that selectively binds 18:2 (ω6 or N6) polyenoic fatty acids and their metabolites. Upon binding, the putative trans acting protein would bind to a cis-acting element linked to the fatty acid synthase (or S14) gene which, in turn, would result in a suppression of gene transcription. This in turn would result in less enzyme activity.

Numerous publications report in detail how the various enzymes in metabolism work *in vitro*. However, one must appreciate the fact that most *in vitro* studies of enzyme activity are conducted with idealized amounts of substrate and cofactors and with little subsequent product removal. Usually the enzyme is studied at saturation, a condition that seldom occurs in the living organism. *In vivo*, enzymes are rarely saturated; they usually are working so rapidly that 10–20% saturation is more likely. This allows for greater control of the flux of metabolites through the system by factors other than the amount and activity of the enzyme per se. Thus, as measured *in vitro*, in cells having 50% less of a given enzyme than normal cells, the flux of substrate through the pathway *in vivo* would not necessarily be slower. In fact, the inheritance of a number of the genetic diseases characterized by an absence of activity of a certain enzyme can be tracked within a given family by the activity of that enzyme in unaffected homozygotes and heterozygotes. Heterozygotes will have reduced enzyme activity yet be normal with respect to their metabolism. This may also be true for the fatty acid synthase complex in animals fed polyunsaturated fatty acids. That is, they may have less enzyme but the flux of acetyl CoA through the fatty acid synthesis pathway as reflected in the total amount of accumulated lipid in the tissue may differ from animals fed a low-polyunsaturated-fatty-acid diet. There are many reasons that this occurs. Suffice it to say that the amount of rate-limiting enzyme does not always predict the activity of the pathway of which it is a part or the amount of product the pathway produces that accumulates.

Despite the gaps in our knowledge about the details of acetyl CoA carboxylase and fatty acid synthase, the reaction sequence shown in Figure 6.8 is well established, as are the effects of certain dietary ingredients and hormones on fatty acid synthesis in living creatures. We know that the fatty acid chain is continually bound to the fatty acid synthase complex and is sequentially transferred between the 4'-phosphopantetheine (pantothenic acid) group of the acyl carrier protein and the sulfhydryl group of a cystein residue on ketoacyl-ACP synthase during the condensation step.

There are other aspects of fatty acid synthesis that should be mentioned. Although the hexose monophosphate shunt NADP-linked enzymes are not rate controlling, it is recognized that the reactions catalyzed by these enzymes provide about 50% of the reducing equivalents needed in the reaction sequence catalyzed by the fatty acid synthase complex. The remaining reducing equivalents are provided by the NADP-linked isocitrate dehydrogenase (~ 10%) and the malic enzyme (~ 40%) Fatty acid synthesis is one of the few synthetic pathways that incorporate reducing equivalents into the product. Most pathways for the synthesis of large molecules release reducing equivalents as part of their condensation reactions. Because fatty acid synthesis incorporates these reducing equivalents, one can measure the rate of incorporation of ^{3}H (from radio-labeled water) into palmitate. This technique was devised by Lowenstein and refined by Fain and Jungas.

The pathway for the synthesis of fatty acids, shown in Figure 6.8, has been well studied. It produces the 16-carbon saturated fatty acid palmitate. This fatty acid is then the substrate for a variety of other reactions to produce the full array of endogenously produced fatty acids found in the body. Palmitate can be elongated, desaturated, oxidized, and esterified. Descriptions of all of these processes follow.

FATTY ACID ELONGATION

Elongation occurs in either the endoplasmic reticulum or the mitochondria. The reaction differs depending on where it occurs and in what species. Mammalian *de novo* fatty acid synthesis from excess dietary carbohydrate results mainly in palmitic, stearic, and oleic acid. Some longer-chain fatty acids are produced by specific tissues. Oleic acid is usually produced by the desaturation of palmitic acid, followed by elongation rather than the desaturation of stearic, although both reactions do occur. Chain elongation following desaturation of stearic acid to oleic acid will produce eicosenoic (20:1ω9), erucic (22:1ω9), and nervonic (24:1ω9) acids. These are of the ω9 series of fatty acids. Fatty acid elongation and desaturation of the ω9 series in the endoplasmic reticulum essentially stops with the formation of 22:3 ω9. In the ω7 series, elongation stops at 18:3ω7. The ω6 series ends with the formation of arachidonate, while the ω3 series continues on up to the formation of 22:6ω3. In the endoplasmic reticulum, the reaction sequence is similar to that just described for the cytosolic fatty acid synthase complex. The source of the 2-carbon unit is malonyl CoA and NADPH provides the reducing power. The intermediates are CoA esters not the acyl carrier protein 4'-phosphopantetheine. The reaction sequence (Figure 6.12) in the brain can proceed producing fatty acids containing up to 24 carbons. In the mitochondria, elongation uses acetyl CoA rather than malonyl CoA as the source of the 2-carbon unit. It uses NADH$^+$H$^+$ as the source of reducing equivalents and uses, as substrate, carbon chains of less than 16 carbons. Mitochondrial elongation is the reversal of fatty acid oxidation, which also occurs in this organelle.

FATTY ACID DESATURATION

Desaturation occurs in the endoplasmic reticulum and microsomes. The enzymes that catalyze this desaturation are the Δ4, or Δ5, or Δ6 desaturases. Again, desaturation is species specific. Mammals for example, lack the ability to desaturate fatty acids in the n6 or n3 position. Only plants can do this, and even among plants there are species differences. Cold-water plants can desaturate at the n3 position while land plants of warmer regions cannot. The cold-water plants are consumed by cold-water creatures in a food chain that includes fish as well as sea mammals. These, in turn, enter the human food supply and become sources of the n3 or omega 3 fatty acids in the marine oils. In animals, desaturation of *de novo* synthesized fatty acids usually stops with the production of a monounsaturated fatty acid with the double bond in the 9–10 position counting from the carboxyl end of the molecule. Hence, palmitic acid (16:0) becomes palmitoleic acid (16:1) and stearic acid (18:0) becomes oleic acid (18:1).

In the absence of dietary EFA, most mammals will desaturate eicosenoic acid to produce eicosatrienoic acid. Increases in this fatty acid with unsaturations at ω7 and ω9 positions characterize the tissue lipids of EFA-deficient animals. They are sometimes called mixed-function oxidases, because two substrates (fatty acid and NADPH) are oxidized simultaneously. These desaturases prefer substrates with a double bond in the ω6 position but will also act on ω3 fatty acid bonds and on saturated fatty acids. Desaturation of *de novo* synthesized stearic acid to form oleic acid results in the formation of a double bond at the ω9 position. This is the first committed step of this desaturation–elongation reaction sequence. Oleic acid can also be formed by the desaturation and elongation of palmitic acid.

Fatty acid desaturation can be followed by elongation and repeated such that a variety of mono- and polyunsaturated fatty acids can be formed. These fatty acids contribute fluidity to membranes

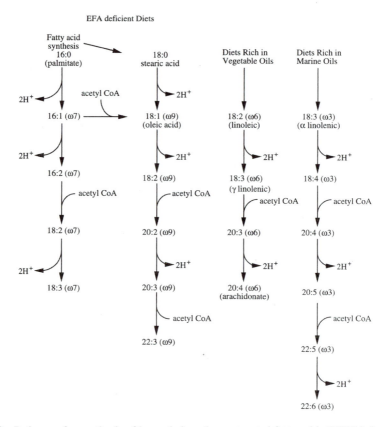

FIGURE 6.12   Pathways for synthesis of long-chain polyunsaturated fatty acids (PUFA) through elongation and desaturation. Not all of these reactions occur in all species. The ω symbol is the same as the n symbol. Thus, 18:2ω6, linoleic acid, could also be written 18:2n6.

because of their lower melting point. An increase in the activity of the desaturation pathway is a characteristic response of rats fed a diet high in saturated fatty acids. The body can convert the dietary saturated fatty acids to unsaturated fatty acids thus maintaining an optimal P:S ratio in the tissues.

There are two unsaturated fatty acids the body cannot make. These are the so-called essential fatty acids, linoleic (18:2, ω6) and linolenic (18:2ω3) acids (Figure 6.13). In addition, felines cannot make arachidonic acid. The consequences of inadequate essential fatty intake are both subtle and various. In the absence of linoleic acid in the diet, microsomal desaturation and elongation activity increases and $\Delta^{5,8,11}$ eicosatrienoic acid (20:3ω9) accumulates. These fatty acids are synthesized in the plant kingdom and, when consumed by animals, find their way into the food chain. Linoleic acid is used to make arachidonic acid (20:4ω6) while linolenic acid is used to make eicosapentanoic acid (20:4ω3) through elongation and desaturation. Figure 6.12 shows the overall pathway for the synthesis of these unsaturated fatty acids including the conversion of linoleic to arachidonic acid.

The activity of the desaturases can be increased through feeding saturated fat or high sugar diets. Both dietary maneuvers increase the need to synthesize unsaturated fatty acids. Desaturase activity is stimulated by insulin, triiodothyronine, and glucocorticoid. Desaturase activity is decreased when high polyunsaturated fats are fed.

FATTY ACID AUTOOXIDATION

Unsaturated fatty acids, particularly the polyunsaturated fatty acids, are more reactive than saturated fatty acids. The double bonds can be attacked by oxygen radicals in a process called autooxidation.

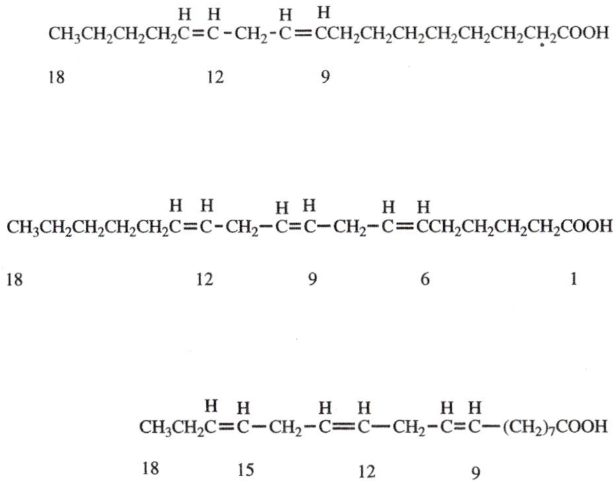

CH₃CH₂CH₂CH₂C=C - CH₂ - C=CCH₂CH₂CH₂CH₂CH₂CH₂COOH   linoleic acid [18:2, (9, 12)]

18   12   9

CH₃CH₂CH₂CH₂CH₂C=C - CH₂ - C=C - CH₂ - C=CCH₂CH₂CH₂CH₂COOH   γ linolenic acid [18:3, (6, 9, 12)]

18   12   9   6   1

CH₃CH₂C=C - CH₂ - C=C - CH₂ - C=C - (CH₂)₇COOH   linolenic acid [18:3 (9, 12, 15)]

18   15   12   9

FIGURE 6.13 Essential fatty acids.

In food, autooxidation is responsible for the deterioration of food quality. The discoloration of red meat upon exposure to air at room temperature is an indication of the autooxidation process. The off odor that accompanies this discoloration is the result of the autooxidation of the fatty acids in the meat fat. In living systems, the process of autooxidation is suppressed to a large extent. This is essential because the products of this oxidation, fatty acid peroxides, can be very damaging. Peroxides denature proteins, rendering them inactive, and attack the DNA in the nucleus and mitochondria, resulting in base-pair deletions or breaks in the DNA which, in turn, result in mutations or errors. In the nucleus, these breaks or deletions can be repaired. In the aging animal, the repair mechanism loses its efficiency and one of the characteristics of aged cells is the loss of its DNA-repair ability. To prevent widespread damage to cellular proteins and DNA by these radicals, there is a potent antioxidation system. This system includes the selenium-containing enzyme, glutathione peroxidase, catalase, and superoxide dismutase. These enzymes are found in the peroxisomes. Superoxide dismutase is also found in the mitochondria. All of these components serve to suppress free radical formation.

The free radical chain reaction is shown in Figure 6.14. Free radicals can form when the oxygen atom is excited by a variety of drugs and contaminants and by ultraviolet light. The excited oxygen atom is called singlet oxygen (O_2^-). Pollutants such as the oxides of nitrogen or carbon tetrachloride can provoke this reaction. *In vivo*, the detoxification reactions catalyzed by the cytochrome P450 enzymes generate free radicals. In the respiratory chain of the mitochondria, the possibility of oxygen radical production exists, and it is for this reason the mitochondria possess a particularly potent peroxide suppressor, superoxide dismutase or SOD. SOD in the mitochondria requires the manganese ion as a cofactor. The cytosol also has SOD but this enzyme requires the copper and zinc ions. Both forms of the enzyme catalyze the reaction $O_2^- + O_2^- + 2H^+ \rightarrow H_2O_2 + O_2$. Two superoxides and two hydrogen ions are joined to form one molecule of hydrogen peroxide and a molecule of oxygen. In turn, the peroxide can be converted to water through the action of the enzyme catalase. Peroxides can also be "neutralized" through the action of glutathione s-transferase. This reaction requires 2 moles of reduced glutathione and produces 2 molecules of oxidized glutathione and 2 molecules of water. Fatty acid radicals can also be neutralized by glutathione peroxidase, producing a molecule of an alcohol with the same chain length as the fatty acid. Glutathione-S-transferase can duplicate the action of glutathione peroxidase. These enzymes and the reactions they catalyze are listed in Table 6.8.

In addition to the reactions that counteract the *in vivo* formation of oxygen radicals or fatty acid peroxides, certain of the vitamins have this role as well. Ascorbic acid has an antioxidant function

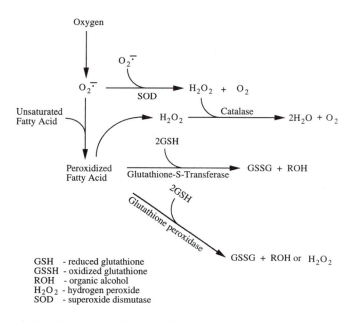

GSH   - reduced glutathione
GSSH - oxidized glutathione
ROH   - organic alcohol
H_2O_2 - hydrogen peroxide
SOD   - superoxide dismutase

FIGURE 6.14   Free radical formation and suppression *in vivo*.

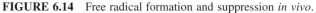

TABLE 6.8
Antioxidant Enzymes Found in Mammalian Cells

Enzyme	Required Mineral Cofactor	Reaction Catalyzed
Superoxide dismutase	CuZn Mn	$2O_{-2} + 2H^+ + H_2O_2$
Glutathione peroxidase	Se	$H_2O_2 + 2GSH \rightarrow GSSG + 2H_2O$
		$ROOH + 2GSH \rightarrow GSSG + ROH + H_2O$
Catalase	Fe	$2H_2O_2 \rightarrow 2H_2O + O_2$
Glutathione-S-transferases	–	$ROOH + 2GSH \; GSSG + ROH + H_2O$

as it can donate reducing equivalents to a peroxide converting it to an alcohol. β carotene can quench singlet oxygen and thus convert it into O_2. Vitamin E is perhaps the best known antioxidant vitamin, and its action is similar to that of ascorbic acid. It donates reducing equivalents to a peroxide, converting it to an alcohol.

Although the foregoing has emphasized the negative aspects of the partial reduction products of oxygen, there is some evidence that peroxide formation has some benefit. For example, leukocytes produce peroxides as a means of killing invading bacteria. Other examples no doubt will emerge as scientists struggle to understand the role of peroxidation (and the peroxisomes) in mammalian metabolism.

AGING AND FREE RADICALS

Aging is characterized by a progressive decline in the biochemical and physiological functions of various organs in an individual. It has been proposed that the process of aging is related, in part, to the accumulated effects of free radical damage to cell membranes and to DNA. Although cells have developed various enzymatic and nonenzymatic systems to protect them from damage by these free radicals, a fraction of these may escape the cellular defense mechanisms and cause permanent or transient damage to proteins, lipids, and nucleic acids. The free-radical attack of mitochondrial DNA (mtDNA) could be involved in these pathological conditions because of the fact that mitochondria are the major source of free radicals in cells. There are several reasons this occurs. The mtDNA is naked (has no protective histone coat), it is compact, and is preferentially attached to the mitochondrial inner membrane, which is the major site of lipid peroxidation in the mitochondria.

Free radical damage can result in large-scale deletions in the mtDNA of various tissues. Shown in Figure 6.15 are the results of one such study of aged humans. Shown are various deletion mutations in this genome. Base substitutions in this genome were found as well. With age, mitochondrial respiratory function declines in a variety of tissues coincident with rising levels of lipid peroxides and evidence of cumulative mtDNA damage. Figure 6.16 illustrates the age-related increase in the proportion of deleted mitochondrial DNA in three tissues. While the amount of mutated DNA is quite small, these data do support the notion that free radical damage could be involved in the aging process. Of course, there are so many mitochondria in each cell (500–25,000 depending on cell type), and each mitochondrion has 8–10 copies of its genome, that the damage reported in this aging study could be rather trivial. In contrast, free radical damage to the nuclear DNA, if unrepaired, could be more serious.

FATTY ACID ESTERIFICATION

Most fats in food, as well as those stored in the adipose tissue depots and those present in small amounts in other tissues, exist as triacylglycerides. Triacylglycerides are hydrolyzed to their component fatty acids and glycerol and reesterified at each of several points in their metabolism. Already described is the process of fat absorption that involves hydrolysis and reesterification prior to entry into the blood stream as either chylomicrons or VLDL. This hydrolysis and reesterification also occurs when lipids arrive at the hepatocyte, the myocyte, or the adipocyte. The triacylglyceride is hydrolyzed by interstitial lipoprotein lipase and the fatty acids are transported into the target cell and reesterified to glycerol-3-phosphate. In the fat cell, this glycerol-3-phosphate usually is a product of glycolysis rather than the glycerol liberated when the triacylglycerol is hydrolyzed. The liberated glycerol usually passes back to the liver, which has a very active glycerokinase to phosphorylate it. In the liver, the phosphorylated glycerol is either used as a substrate for glucose synthesis or recycled into hepatic phospholipids or triacylglycerides or oxidized to CO_2 and water.

The formation of triacylglycerides, regardless of the source for the glycerol-3-phosphate, follows the same pattern in all tissues. With some modification, it is the pathway used for the synthesis of phospholipids. These pathways are shown in Figure 6.17.

Triacylglycerides are formed in a stepwise fashion. First, a fatty acid (usually a saturated fatty acid) is attached at carbon 1 of the glycerophosphate. The phosphate group at carbon 3 is electronegative and, because it pulls electrons toward it, leaves carbon 1 more reactive than carbon 2. The fatty acid (as an acyl CoA) is transferred to carbon 1 through the action of a transferase. The attachment uses the carboxy end of the fatty acid chain and makes an ester linkage releasing the CoA. Now the molecule has electronegative forces at each end: the phosphate group on carbon 3 and the oxygen plus carbon chain at carbon 1. Now carbon 2 is vulnerable and reactive and another carbon chain can be attached. In this instance, the fatty acid is usually an unsaturated fatty acid. At this point, the 1,2-diacylglyceride-phosphate loses its phosphate group so that carbon 3 is now reactive. The 1,2-diacylglyceride can either be esterified with another fatty acid to make triacylglyceride or can be used to make the membrane lipids phosphatidylcholine, phosphatidylethanolamine, phosphatidylinositol, cardiolipin, and phosphatidylserine. These membrane lipids have very special functions, as will be discussed later.

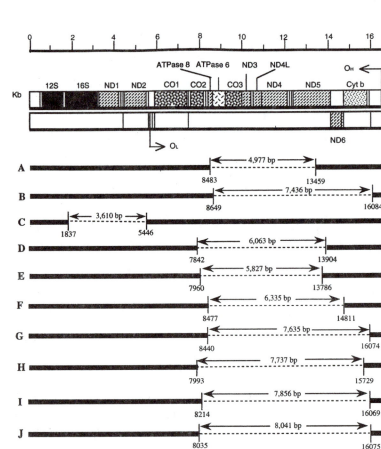

FIGURE 6.15 Mitochondrial DNA deletions that have been identified in various tissues of aged human subjects. The shaded or stippled boxes above represent the coding regions for protein subunits constituting the respiratory enzyme complexes. OH and OL represent the origins of replication of heavy and light strands of mtDNA, respectively. 12S and 16S denote the genes coding for the 12S rRNA and 16S rRNA, respectively. ND indicates NADH dehydrogenase, CO indicates cytochrome oxidase, Cyt *b* indicates cytochrome *b*, and ATPase represents Fo,F1-ATPase. From this figure it is easy to identify the genes that are truncated or removed by each type of deletion. (From Wei and Kao, with permission, CRC Press.)

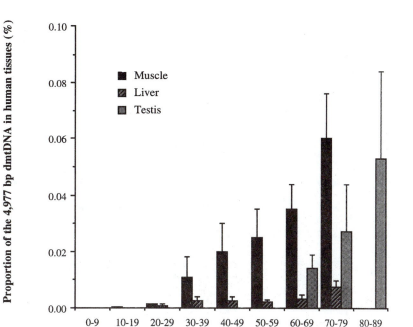

FIGURE 6.16   Age-dependent increase in the proportion of the 4,977 bp-deleted mitochondrial DNA in human tissue. The black bar in each age group represents the average proportion (mean ± S.D.) of the 4,977 bp-deleted mtDNA in the muscle tissue from subjects in the group. (From Wei and Kao, with permission, CRC Press.)

In the stored triacylglycerides, most unsaturated fatty acids are found at carbon 2. In the membrane phospholipids, the unsaturated fatty acid at carbon 2 is usually arachidonic acid. This arachidonic acid, produced by elongation and desaturation of dietary linoleic acid, is preferentially used in the membrane phospholipid. It can either be attached to the glycerol backbone when the phospholipid is made or exchanged for another fatty acid as the lipids in and around the cells remodel themselves. There is constant hydrolysis and reesterification in the cell. Thus, there is a rapid exchange of fatty acids between those in the membranes and those inside the cell. In fact, if the fatty acid composition of the diet were to be changed, it would take less than a week to observe corresponding changes in the fatty acid composition of the stored lipids and even less time to observe changes in membrane phospholipid fatty acids. Scientists wanting to confirm food-intake data with respect to the kinds of fats consumed need only examine the fatty acid composition of the membrane and stored lipids to learn how accurate their food-intake reports are.

Shown in Table 6.9 are some data giving the phospholipid fatty acid composition of livers from rats fed either a 6% corn oil or hydrogenated coconut oil diet. Recall that corn oil is a good source of the unsaturated fatty acids linoleic, oleic and palmitoleic and of the saturated fatty acid, palmitic acid. Note that the corn-oil-fed rats had a phospholipid fatty acid profile that reflected their corn-oil intake. Note, too, that rats fed the hydrogenated coconut oil, which has no linoleic or arachidonic acid, likewise had less of these fatty acids in their profile. These rats tried to compensate for their essential fatty acid-deficient diet by increasing their desaturase and elongase activity. Thus, compared with the corn-oil-fed rats, increases in unsaturated fatty acids (16:1, 18:1, 20:2, 20:3, 22:2, 22:6) were found. Hydrogenated coconut oil contains the medium-chain saturated fatty acids and these account for the fact that hydrogenated coconut oil is a solid at room temperature (20°C). It would be logical to assume that animals consuming this fat would have more rigid (less fluid)

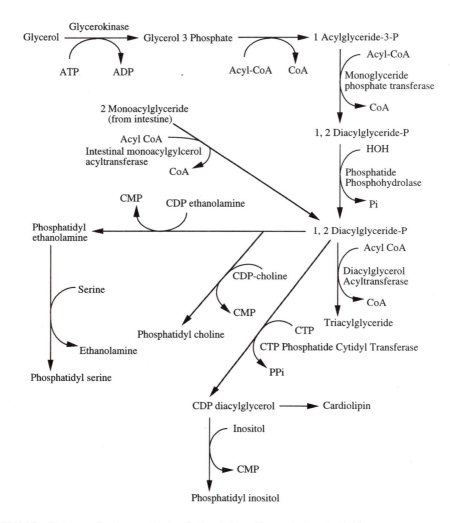

FIGURE 6.17 Pathways for the synthesis of triacylglycerides and phospholipids.

membranes, but Mother Nature has designed a fairly competent compensatory system that can partially overcome the diet fat effect on the membrane. Thus, the increases in the unsaturated fatty acids as noted above.

If the fatty acid unsaturation to saturation ratios (P:S) in these two groups of rats are calculated, it turns out these ratios were nearly the same. Despite this compensation, however, with respect to the phospholipid fatty acid profiles, the consumption of a diet lacking the essential fatty acids results in some profound effects on metabolism and bodily function. Shown in Table 6.10 are some of the features of essential fatty acid deficiency. Detailed studies of cells from deficient rats have revealed diet-induced changes in energetic efficiency that include a partial loss of the ability of mitochondria to trap energy in the high-energy bond of ATP. Myocardial arrhythmias are more frequent in deficient rats and this may be due to the deficiency symptom of dysfunctional mitochondria. Essential fatty acid deficiency also results in an impairment in the glucose transporter activity in selected cells and an alteration in insulin receptor number. Although none of these effects are especially dramatic, collectively they help explain why animals fed such a deficient diet are growth impaired and have poor food efficiency. Some of the effects shown in Table 6.10 can be due to an effect on membranes per se while other effects are attributable to a lack of arachidonic acid to serve as a precursor for eicosanoid synthesis.

TABLE 6.9
Effect of Corn or Coconut Oil Diets on the Phospholipid Fatty Acid Composition of the Livers of Rats

Fatty Acids[1]	Diet	
	Corn Oil	Coconut Oil
	(% of the total)	
14:0	0.09 ± 0.03	0.30 ± 0.03*
14:1	0.10 ± 0.02	0.05 ± 0.01
15:0	0.17 ± 0.03	0.20 ± 0.03
16:0	15.2 ± 0.03	15.4 ± 0.03
16:1	0.70± 0.08	2.26 ± 0.07*
17:0	0.38 ± 0.04	0.13 ± 0.02*
17:1	0.09 ± 0.02	0.11 ± 0.02
18:0	20.8 ± 0.82	2.0 ± 0.4
18:1	7.17 ± 0.61	2.0 ± 0.5*
18:2	14.4 ± 0.4	7.98 ± 0.27*
20:0	0.01 ± 0.01	0.16 ± 0.04*
18:3	0.41 ± 0.06	0.35 ± 0.04
20:1	ND	0.18 ± 0.04
20:2	0.89 ± 0.17	6.44 ± 0.50*
20:3	0.82 ± 0.16	2.20 ± 0.13*
20:4	29.4 ± 0.5	18.0 ± 0.7*
22:1	0.34 ± 0.02	0.35 ± 0.03
22:2	0.14 ± 0.02	0.48 ± 0.03*
24:0	0.96 ± 0.01	0.95 ± 0.03
22:4	1.37 ± 0.09	0.54 ± 0.02*
22:5	2.14 ± 0.25	2.24 ± 0.12
22:6	3.53 ± 0.31	6.64 ± 0.30*
20:5	ND	0.41 ± 0.04

[1] Designations used: number of carbons in chain followed by number of double bonds.

Hydrogenated coconut oil is deficient in essential fatty acid but is a good source for 8, 10, 12, and 14 carbon fatty acids. ND indicates nondetectable; * indicates a significantly different value from that of the corn-oil-fed rats.

EICOSANOIDS

Eicosanoids are 20-carbon molecules having hormone-like activity. In their various forms they are produced and released by many different mammalian cells rather than being produced by highly specialized cells as in the instance of insulin and the β cell in the islets of Langerhans. When each of these compounds is produced, their site of action is local. That is, whereas insulin may be transported from the pancreas to peripheral target cells, the eicosanoids are produced, released, and have as their targets the surrounding cells. For this reason, the eicosanoids are called local hormones. They have a variety of actions. Table 6.11 lists the major eicosanoids and their functions.

The eicosanoids fall into three general groups of compounds:

TABLE 6.10
Major Effects of EFA Deficiency in the Rat

1.	Skin symptoms		Scaly, dry skin
2.	Weight		Decrease
3.	Circulation		Heart enlargement; decreased capillary resistance (lower blood pressure at periphery); increased permeability
4.	Kidney		Enlargement; intertubular hemorrhage
5.	Lung		Cholesterol accumulation
6.	Endocrine glands	(a)	Adrenals: weight decreased in females and increased in males.
		(b)	Thyroid: reduced weight.
7.	Reproduction	(a)	Females: irregular estrus and impaired reproduction and lactation.
		(b)	Males: degeneration of semini-ferrous tubules
8.	Metabolism	(a)	Changes in fatty acid composition of most organs.
		(b)	Increase in cholesterol levels in liver, adrenals, and skin.
		(c)	Decrease in plasma cholesterol.
		(d)	Changes in swelling of heart and liver mitochondria and uncoupling of oxidative phosphorylation.
		(e)	Increased triglyceride synthesis and release by the liver.

From: M.I. Gurr and A.T. James, *Lipid Biochemistry: An Introduction.* Ithaca, Cornell University Press, 1971, p. 56.

TABLE 6.11
Functions of Eicosanoids

Eicosanoids[1-3]	Function
PGG_2	Precursor of PGH_2
PGH_2	Precursor of PGD_2, PGE_2, PGI_2, PGF_2
PGD_2	Promotes sleeping behavior; precursor of PGF_2
PGE_2	Enhances perception of pain when histamine or bradykinin is given. Induces signs of inflammation. Promotes wakefulness. Precursor of $PGF_{2\alpha}$. Reduces gastric acid secretion, induces partuition. Vasoconstrictor in some tissues, vasodilator in others. Maintains the patency of the ductus arteriosis prior to birth.
PGF_2	Bronchial constrictor. Vasoconstrictor, especially in coronary vasculature. Increases sperm motility. Induces partuition; stimulates steroidogenesis corpus luteum; induces luteolysis.
PGI_2	Inhibits platelet aggregation
PGE_1	Inhibits motility of nonpregnant uterus, increases motility of pregnant uterus. Bronchial dilator
TXA_2	Stimulates platelet aggregation. Potent vasoconstrictor
TXB_2	Metabolite of TXA_2
LTA_4	Precursor of LTB_4
LTB_4	Potent chemotaxic agent

[1] the prostaglandins (compounds of the PG series)
[2] the thromboxanes (compounds of the TBX series)
[3] leukotrienes (compounds of the LKT series)

All of these compounds arise from a 20-carbon polyunsaturated fatty acid. This fatty acid is usually arachidonic acid (20 carbons, 4 double bonds at 5, 8, 11, 14). However, in instances where the diet is rich in omega-3 (n-3) fatty acids, the precursor may be a 20-carbon-5 double bond fatty acid, eicosapentaenoic acid (double bonds at 5, 8, 11, 14, 17). Other eicosanoids can be synthesized from a 20-carbon fatty acid, dihomo-γ-linoleic acid, which has 3 double bonds at carbons 8, 11, and 14. Each of these precursors yields a particular set of eicosanoids. During their synthesis they take up oxygen and are cyclized. Dihomo γ linoleic acid is the precursor of prostaglandin E_1 (PGE_1) and prostaglandin $E_{1\alpha}$ ($PGE_{1\alpha}$) and subsequent prostaglandins. Arachidonic acid is the precursor of prostaglandins of the 2 series (PGE_2, $PGF_{2\alpha}$, etc.) and eicosapentaenoic acid is the precursor of prostaglandins of the 3 series (PGE_3, $PGF_{3\alpha}$, etc.).

The cyclization of these 20-carbon fatty acids is accomplished by a complex of enzymes called the prostaglandin synthesis complex. The first step is the cyclooxygenase step, which involves the cyclization of C-9 – C-12 of the precursor to form the cyclic 9-11 endoperoxide 15-hydroperoxide (PGG_2) shown in Figure 6.18. PGG_2 is then used to form prostaglandin H_2 (PGH_2) through the removal of one oxygen from the carbonyl group at carbon 15. Glutathione peroxidase and prostaglandin H synthase catalyze the reaction shown in Figure 6.19. Prostaglandin H synthase is a very unstable, short-lived enzyme with a messenger RNA that is one of the shortest lived species so far found in mammalian cells. The expression of genes for this enzyme is under the control of polypeptide growth factors such as interleukin 1α, and colony stimulating factor 1. Interferon α and β inhibit expression and prostanoid production by the macrophages. Glutathione peroxidase is a selenium-containing enzyme. In animals fed a high-polyunsaturated-fat diet, one might expect to see a higher than normal requirement for selenium in the diet to accommodate the need for this enzyme. However, such an expectation is without merit. Studies of rats fed a high-polyunsaturated-fat diet such as a marine oil-rich diet show a greater need for vitamin E to accommodate the increased need to support the antioxidation system, but not an increased need for selenium. The need to make the eicosanoids is quite low compared with the need to suppress the formation of fatty acid radicals. This probably explains why the selenium requirement is not increased under these dietary conditions.

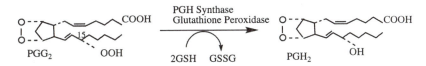

FIGURE 6.18 Cyclization and oxygenation of arachidonic acid.

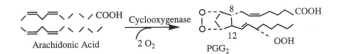

FIGURE 6.19 Oxygen removal to form PGH_2.

PGH_2 is then converted through the action of a variety of isomerases to PGD_2 or PGE_2 or prostacylin I_2 (PGI_2) or prostaglandin $F_{2\alpha}$ ($PGF_{2\alpha}$). These are the primary precursors of the prostaglandins of the D, E, and F series and PGI or thromboxane. The conversion to subsequent prostaglandins is mediated by enzymes that are specific to a certain cell type and tissue. Not all of these subsequent compounds are formed in all tissues. Thus, PGE_2 and $PGF_{2\alpha}$ are produced in the kidney and spleen. $PGF_{2\alpha}$ and PGE are also produced in the uterus only when signals from the pituitary induce their production and so stimulate parturition. PGI_2 is primarily produced by endothelial cells lining the blood vessels. This prostaglandin inhibits platelet aggregation and thus is important to maintaining a blood flow free of clots. It is counteracted by thromboxane A_2 which is produced by the platelets when these cells contact a foreign surface. PGE_2, $PGF_{2\alpha}$, and PGI_2 are formed by the heart in about equal amounts. All of these prostaglandins have a very short half-life. No sooner are they released than they are inactivated. The thromboxanes are highly active metabolites of the prostaglandins. As mentioned above, they are formed when PGH_2 has its cyclopentane ring replaced by a six-membered oxane ring, shown in Figure 6.20. Imidazole is a potent inhibitor of thromboxane A synthase and is used to block TXA_2 production and platelet aggregation.

Thromboxane A_2 has a role in clot formation and the name thromboxane comes from this function (thrombus means clot). The half-life of TXA_2 is less than one minute. TXB_2 is its metabolic end product and has little biological activity. Measuring TXB_2 levels in blood and tissue can give an indication of how much TXA_2 has been produced. PGD_2 and PGE_2 are involved in the regulation of sleep–wake cycles in a variety of species.

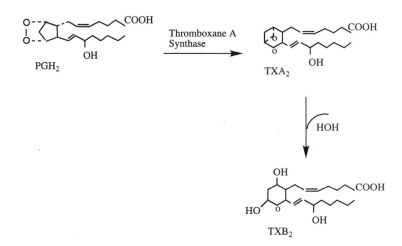

FIGURE 6.20   Reaction sequence that produces TXA_2 and TXB_2.

The cyclooxygenase reaction illustrated in Figure 6.18 can be inhibited by certain anti-inflammatory drugs such as aspirin, indomethacin, and phenylbutazone. These are the nonsteroidal anti-inflammatory drugs that are commonly available in pharmacies. These drugs block the action of cyclooxygenase by acetylating the enzyme. While use of these drugs for the occasional injury or headache is harmless, long-term chronic use can result in untoward effects. Long-term chronic use of aspirin, for example, can affect vascular competence and blood clotting. People consuming large amounts of aspirin over long periods of time may find an increase in bruises (subcutaneous hemorrhages). Small contact injuries that normally would not result in a bruise will do so in these people. Gastric bleeding is another possible complication with long-term chronic aspirin ingestion. Aplastic anemia can result from long-term phenylbutazone therapy. Again, the occasional use of these drugs is not likely to have these effects.

A second group of anti-inflammatory agents are the steroids — hydrocortisone, prednisone, and other similar compounds. These drugs are prescription drugs that act by inhibiting the enzyme phospholipase A_2. Phospholipase A_2 stimulates the release of arachidonic acid from the membrane phospholipids. Hence, inhibition of this reaction will result in a decreased supply of arachidonic acid for prostaglandin synthesis. When the conversion of arachidonic acid to prostaglandins is inhibited as above or when either of the other 20-carbon fatty acids are abundantly available, a different series of prostaglandins and leukotrienes are produced. Eicosapentaenoic acid is not as good a substrate for cyclooxygenation as is arachidonic acid. As a result, less of the arachidonic acid-related prostaglandins (even-numbered PGs and TBXs) are produced and more of the odd-numbered prostaglandins and leukotrienes is produced. Figure 6.21 shows the overall metabolic pathway for eicosanoid synthesis and degradation.

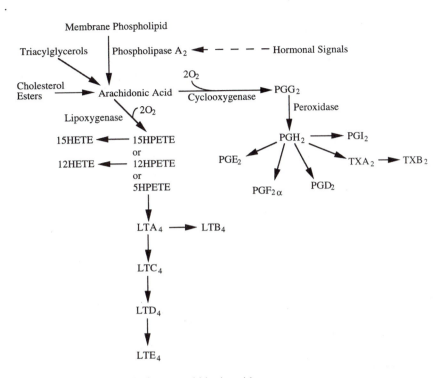

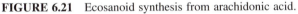

FIGURE 6.21   Ecosanoid synthesis from arachidonic acid.

Although the cyclooxygenase pathway is quite important in the production of prostaglandins, equally important is the lipoxygenase pathway. This pathway is catalyzed by a family of enzymes called the lipoxygenase enzymes. These enzymes differ from the cyclooxygenase enzymes in the catalytic site for oxygen addition to the unsaturated fatty acid. One lipoxygenase is active at the double bond at carbon 5 while a second is active at carbon 11 and a third is active at carbon 15. The products of these reactions are monohydroperoxy-eicosatetraenoic acids (HPETEs) and are numbered according to the location of the double bond to which the oxygen is added. 5HPETE is the major lipoxygenase product in basophils, polymorphonuclear leukocytes, macrophages, mast cells, and any organ undergoing an inflammatory response. 12HPETE is the major product in platelets, pancreatic endocrine cells, vascular smooth muscle, and glomerular cells. 15HPETE predominates in reticulocytes, eosinophils, T-lymphocytes, and tracheal epithelial cells. The HPETEs are not in themselves active hormones; rather, they serve as precursors for the leukotrienes. The leukotrienes are the metabolic end products of the lipoxygenase reaction. These compounds contain at least three conjugated double bonds. The unstable 5HPETE is converted to either an analogous alcohol (hydroxy fatty acid) or is reduced by a peroxide or converted to leukotriene. The peroxidative reduction of 5'HPETE to the stable 5HETE (5 hydroxyeicosatetraenoic acid) is similar to that of 12HPETE to 12HETE and of 15HPETE to 15HETE. In each instance, the carbon–carbon double bonds are unconjugated and the geometry of the double bonds is trans, cis, cis, respectively. In contrast to the active thromboxanes, which have very short half-lives, the leukotrienes can persist as long as 4 hours. These compounds make up a group of substances known as the slow-acting anaphylaxis substances. They cause slowly evolving but protracted contractions of smooth muscles in the airways and gastrointestinal tract. Leukotriene C_4 is rapidly converted to LTD_4, which, in turn, is slowly converted to LTE_4. Enzymes in the plasma are responsible for these conversions.

The products of the lipoxygenase pathway are potent mediators of the response to allergens, tissue damage (inflammation), hormone secretion, cell movement, cell growth, and calcium flux.

Within minutes of stimulation, lipoxygenase products are produced. In an allergy attack, for example, an allergen can instigate the release of leukotrienes, which are the immediate mediators of response. The leukotrienes are more potent than histamine in stimulating the contraction of the bronchial nonvascular smooth muscles. In addition, LTD_4 increases the permeability of the microvasculature. The mono HETEs and LTB_4 stimulate the movement of eosinophils and neutrophils, making them the first line of defense in injury resulting in inflammation.

As mentioned, when dihomo γ linoleic acid or eicosapentaenoic acid serve as substrates for eicosanoid production, the products are either of the 1 series or 3 series. The products they form may be less active than those formed from arachidonic acid and this decrease in activity can be of therapeutic value. Hence, ingestion of omega-3 fatty acids leads to the decreased production of prostaglandin E_2 and its metabolites, a decrease in the production of thromboxane A_2, a potent platelet aggregator and vasoconstrictor; and a decrease in leukotriene B_4, a potent inflammatory hormone and a powerful inducer of leukocyte hemotaxis and adherence. Counteracting these decreases are an increase in thromboxane A_3 (TXA_3), a weak platelet aggregator and vasoconstrictor; an increase in the production of PGI_3 without an increase in PGI_2, which stimulates vasodilation and inhibits platelet aggregation; and an increase in leukotriene B_5, which is a weak inducer of inflammation and a weak chemotoxic agent. Marine oils, rich in omega-3 unsaturated fatty acids, affect (decrease) platelet aggregation because they stimulate the synthesis of thromboxane A_3. Thromboxane A_3 does not have the platelet-aggregating property of the other eicosanoids. In addition, eicosapentaenoic acid is used to make the anti-aggregating prostaglandin PGI_3. Animals fed omega-3-rich oils produce significantly more of the eicosanoids of the LTB_5 series. LTB_4 is an important inflammatory mediator, whereas LTB_5 is not. Fish-oil consumption results in an increased neutrophil LTB_5 production, with a concomitant decrease in LTB_4 production. This diet-influenced change in LTB_4 and LTB_5 production seems to be related to a reduced incidence of autoimmune-inflammatory disorders such as asthma, psoriasis, and rheumatoid arthritis in populations consuming omega-3 fatty acids routinely. Thus, eicosanoid synthesis can be used as an explanation of the beneficial effects of fish-oil ingestion on rheumatoid arthritis. In arthritics, the joints are inflamed and painful. The prostaglandins PGE_2 and leukotriene are both produced from arachidonate. PGE_2 induces the signs of inflammation, which include redness and heat due to arteriolar vasodilation, swelling, and localized edema resulting from increased capillary permeability. Leukotriene prevents platelet aggregation. If there is less arachidonate available for the synthesis of these prostaglandins, then the inflammation is inhibited.

Tumorigenesis likewise can be influenced by the relative amounts of the various eicosanoids. Prostaglandin G of the 2-series acts as a tumor promoter. It down regulates macrophage tumoricidal activities and inhibits interleukin-2 production. Increased PGE_2 levels (from omega-6 fatty acids) have been associated with aggressive growth patterns of both basal and squamous cell skin carcinomas in humans. Vegetable oils are rich in these fatty acids. Products of the lipoxygenase pathway (stimulated by the omega-3 fatty acids) have the reverse effect. While the various eicosanoids have different (and sometimes conflicting) effects on inflammatory processes and on tumor promotion, it might be anticipated that susceptibility to pathogenic organisms would be similarly affected. Studies with mice exposed to a variety of pathogens and fed either a fish-oil or a control diet showed no diet-fat-related differences in susceptibility to these organisms. Other research has suggested that a dietary fat effect on immunological competence might be related to the age of the animal and whether the diet contained sufficient vitamin E to suppress the formation of peroxides, which can facilitate the entry of pathogens into target cells. Both age and vitamin E status apparently affect the disease resistance of animals fed different fats.

All of these observations have prompted nutrition scientists to investigate the possible benefits of consuming foods rich in omega-3 fatty acids. Such foods include ocean fish, marine mammals, and some plant foods. Some vegetable oils such as primrose, canola, wheat germ, linseed, and walnut also contain significant amounts. Small amounts are also found in a number of other foods such as spinach, certain margarines, broccoli, and lettuce. Hens fed omega-3 fatty acid-rich fats will lay eggs containing these fatty acids in the yolks. A number of years ago, a group of Danish scientists compared the food intake and health status of Danes and Greenland Eskimos. Both populations consumed high-protein, high-fat diets; however, where the Danish diet included a variety of milk and meat products, the Eskimo diet included primarily fish and marine creatures such as whale, walrus, seal, and so forth. These marine foods contain fat that is rich in the omega-3 fatty acids such as linolenic, eicosapentanoic, and docosahexanoic acids. The P:S ratio of the Greenland Eskimo diet was 0.84 compared with 0.24 for the Danes. The Eskimo diet contained more fatty acids with a single double bond than did the Danish diet. The Eskimo diet also contained significant amounts of long-chain fatty acids having 5 or 6 double bonds.

The Danish investigators observed these diet differences between Danes and Eskimos and also noticed the differences in blood lipid profiles, as well as differences in the incidence of cardiovascular disease (CVD). While CVD was one of the leading causes of death among the Danes, the leading cause of death in Eskimos was cerebral hemorrhage (stroke). The Eskimos had prolonged bleeding times and a nosebleed was a serious problem. The prolonged clotting time was probably due to the omega-3 fatty acid effect on those eicosanoids involved in clot formation. These death statistics considered age-matched groups, but were not age-adjusted. That is, the investigators compared the two populations using age-matched groups without correcting for total population longevity or for early death due to communicable diseases, malnutrition (in infants particularly), or the hazards of daily life. For the Eskimo, these factors could have been quite important. Furthermore, one must realize that all causes must add up to 100%. Thus, if fewer die of CVD, more may have died from communicable disease or something else. Nonetheless, the findings of the Danes regarding omega-3 fatty-acid intake and cardiovascular disease set off a whole flurry of animal and human studies directed toward understanding how the omega-3 fatty acids affected metabolism.

Consistent with the Danish report of lower levels of blood lipids in the Eskimos, others found that the consumption of marine oils was associated with a significant decline in blood lipid levels. The decrease in serum lipids in man and experimental animals with fish-oil consumption has been demonstrated many times. The reasons for this serum-lipid-lowering effect have been explored. Fish oil in the diet easily oxidizes and forms peroxides. These peroxides are what gives these oils their peculiar and often objectionable odor. Diets containing large amounts of these oils are not as well liked by experimental animals and appetite is suppressed. Food intake may be decreased by as much as 20%. Even when the scientist takes stringent care of the diet by preventing autooxidation, the food intake of fat-rich diets is reduced. Despite a reduction in food intake, animals utilize their diet very well and a marine-oil diet usually is characterized by an increase in feed efficiency. That is, the animal will gain more weight per unit of food consumed than an animal consuming a diet containing some other fat source. This is not always true however. Genetically obese rats and mice gain less weight when fed a marine-oil diet than when fed a corn oil or tallow or safflower oil diet.

At any rate, a decrease in food consumption despite an increase in feed efficiency means that there is less food for the liver to metabolize and convert to VLDL for transport to the peripheral fat depots for storage, and, in part, this explains the effect of the marine oils on serum lipid levels. Dietary marine oils have two other equally important effects that can also explain their serum-lipid-lowering action. The first of these is an inhibition of hepatic fatty acid, phospholipid, and cholesterol synthesis. In part, this attenuation of lipid synthesis by marine oils occurs at the level of specific genes that encode for the lipogenic enzymes. The transcription of genes encoded for enzymes necessary for lipogenesis is suppressed in hepatic tissue from rats fed the marine oils. While we realize that enzymes are never fully active *in vivo* and that the amount of enzyme may not fully predict the amount of product (in this case lipid) produced, these findings do contribute to our understanding of how dietary marine oils can lower serum lipid levels.

Added to the decrease in lipogenic enzyme activity and decreased rates of lipid synthesis observed in animals fed marine oils, is the observation that marine-oil-fed animals also have a reduced hepatic lipid output. This means that lipids formed in the liver are not as readily exported and the liver of the animal fed the marine oils contains more fat than the liver of the rat fed a control diet. Reduced hepatic lipid output by humans consuming fish oil supplements has been reported. This too results in a lowering of serum triglycerides and serum cholesterol. Accumulated lipids in the liver may be an additional reason that lipid synthesis is down regulated. Product inhibition, in this case newly synthesized lipid, is a well recognized metabolic-control mechanism. Consumption of omega-3 fatty acids nonetheless does result in lower blood lipid levels and this effect is presumed to explain the lower incidence of cardiovascular disease in the Eskimos. Whether this presumption is correct cannot be taken for granted. Cardiovascular disease has a complicated pathophysiology that is not well understood. Genetic factors as well as lifestyle choices can influence its development and can determine whether it is a life-threatening condition.

Fatty Acids and Membrane Function

Biological membranes contain a large number of lipids, proteins, lipid-protein complexes, glycolipids, and glycoproteins. The arrangement of these many compounds within the membrane structure has been studied extensively.

The membranes exist as a lipid bilayer because the phospholipids have amphipathic characteristics. They have both polar (the phosphorylated substituent at carbon 3) and nonpolar (the fatty acids) regions. The polar region is hydrophilic and is positioned such that it is in contact with the aqueous media around and within the cells. The nonpolar or fatty acid region is oriented toward the center of the bilayer so that it is protected from contact with the contents of the cell and the fluids that surround it.

The ability of these amphipathic compounds to self-assemble into a bilayer can be demonstrated *in vitro*. Lipid vesicles can be made by the addition of these phospholipids to water. A lipid bilayer will form just as described above. This feature of the phospholipids is consistent with one of the many roles a membrane serves. It is a permeability barrier for the cells and cell compartments. The lipid bilayer forms the matrix into which specific proteins are placed. Each of the individual phospholipids and the cholesterol provide specific regional characteristics that satisfy the insertion requirements of each of the many membrane proteins. The lipid bilayer serves as a seal around these membrane proteins and thus prevents nonspecific leakage. These lipids also serve to maintain the proteins in their most appropriate functional conformations. The polar position of the phospholipids satisfies the requirements for the electrostatic charge that is needed for the surface associations of specific cell surface proteins. All of these characteristics are needed and are critical to normal cell function. For example, an intact permeability barrier to sodium, potassium, calcium, and hydrogen ions is needed so that electrochemical gradients, which in turn drive other membrane transport processes, are maintained.

Cell membranes usually work best when their lipids are in the liquid crystal state. This means that there are regional differences in the physical state of the lipid. Some portions may be fairly fluid whereas others may be fairly solid. The localized difference in physical state or fluidity has to do with the chain length and saturation of the fatty acids attached at carbons 1 and 2 of the phospholipid; it is this portion of the molecule that extends into the center of the bilayer. Membranes whose phospholipid fatty acids are saturated are less fluid than those membranes containing polyunsaturated fatty acids in their phospholipids. Even within a membrane there can be regional differences in fluidity due to the nature of the fatty acids in the phospholipids of that region. Differences in fluidity are due not only to the ratio of saturated fatty acids to unsaturated fatty acids, but also to the ratio of cholesterol to fatty acids. This ratio varies according to the location of the membrane. Plasma membranes, for example, contain more cholesterol than do mitochondrial membranes.

Membrane Phospholipid Composition

There are three major classes of lipids in membranes: glycolipids, cholesterol, and phospholipids. The glycolipids have a role in the cell surface-associated antigens, whereas the cholesterol serves to regulate fluidity. The phospholipids have fatty acids attached at carbons 1 and 2. It is usual to find a saturated fatty acid attached at carbon 1 and an unsaturated fatty acid at carbon 2. In addition, phosphatidylethanolamine and phosphatidylserine usually have fatty acids that are more unsaturated than phosphatidylinositol and phosphatidylcholine. Less than 10% of the membrane phospholipid is phosphatidylinositol. Plasma membranes have no cardiolipin and the mitochondrial membranes have very little phosphatidylserine. Several of these phospholipids have important roles in the signal transduction processes that mediate the action of a variety of hormones. Phosphatidylinositol and its role in the phosphatidylinositol cycle (PIP cycle) is one of the most important. Phosphatidyl-choline and phosphaditylethanolamine also play roles in these systems. Shown in Figure 6.22 is the PIP cycle. Its importance relates to the action of inositol-1, 4, 5-phosphate in moving the calcium ion from its intracellular store to where it can stimulate protein kinase C. Phosphatidylinositol also serves to anchor glycoproteins to the membrane. Glycoproteins are tethered to the external aspect of the plasma membrane and play a role in the cell recognition process. Pathogens and foreign proteins are recognized by these structures.

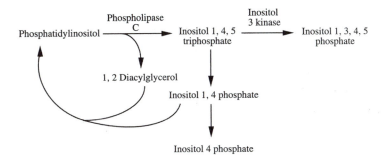

FIGURE 6.22   Phosphatidylinositol (PIP) cycle.

Disease Effects on Membrane Lipids

There are numerous reviews on the effects of diet and disease on the fatty acid content of membrane fatty acids. While the primary focus has been on the abnormalities of the proteins in the membrane lipid bilayer, there is a role for the lipid in some of these disorders. Muscular dystrophy and multiple sclerosis are characterized by changes in the lipid structure of the membrane. In the former, the change consists of an increase in the amount of lysophosphatidylcholine and cardiolipin. In multiple sclerosis there is a degeneration of the myelin of both central and peripheral nerves. The myelin is 75% lipid and 25% protein. Although the disease could be attributed to a specific abnormality in either component, there are reports that the lipid contains about 27% fatty acid (palmitate and oleate) in a covalent linkage and that multiple sclerosis is associated with a derangement in this association and a reduction in the amount of phosphatidylserine. There have been many reports of these lipid changes or a lack of change in myelin; however, it is generally agreed that the disease is not primary to the lipid portion of the membrane. Rather, it is the specific myelin protein that somehow becomes abnormal. Such other diseases as renal disease, hepatic disease, ethanol intoxication, spur cell anemia, and diabetes likewise result in secondary effects on the membrane lipids. These changes can, however, make the disease worse by compromising the functionality of the membrane and its role in metabolic regulation. In humans with cirrhotic liver disease, the erythrocyte membrane fatty acids change. In cirrhotic subjects, the membranes contain less phosphatidylethanolamine and more phosphatidylcholine than membranes from normal subjects. In these subjects, the membrane cholesterol and fatty acid content remains unchanged, but the ratio of cholesterol to phospholipid increases.

Hormonal Effects on Membrane Lipids

The hormone insulin can affect the fatty acid profile of the membrane phospholipids through its effect on glucose conversion to fatty acids and through its effect on the desaturases. Other hormones have an influence on this profile as well. Examples of this influence are shown in Table 6.12. Daily injections of the synthetic glucocorticoid, dexamethasone, resulted in an increase in the mole percent of linoleic (18:2) acid and a decrease in arachidonic acid (20:4). Thyroidectomy resulted in a small increase in rat liver mitochondrial levels of 18:2 and 20:4. This is probably due to the reduction in fatty acid turnover that occurs in the absence of the thyroid gland. Hypophysectomy, which causes a decrease in growth hormone levels, resulted in an increase in 18:2 and a decrease in 20:4 in hepatic mitochondria. Studies on the influence of all the many hormones that affect fatty acid synthesis, phospholipid synthesis, and membrane phospholipid fatty acid levels are not as readily available as are reports on the dietary-fat effects on these parameters. However, they are of interest because these hormones may also have a considerable influence on the function of the protein components that are embedded in the various membranes. These hormones may act directly on the synthesis and activation of these proteins, which in turn may affect their conformation and hence their activity. Thyroxine, for example, negatively affects the activity of the $\Delta 9$ desaturase, which, because it is less active, results in fewer unsaturated fatty acids in the membrane. In turn, microsomal cytochrome b_5 activity is less dependent on the lipid environment. That is, it must be surrounded by a very fluid lipid, and this lipid must have a number of unsaturated fatty acids in it. Just as thyroidectomy results in a decrease in membrane phospholipid fatty acid unsaturation, hyperthyroidism has the reverse effect. The thyroid hormones also affect fatty acid elongation by inducing an increase in the activity of the microsomal fatty acid elongation system, while having little effect on mitochondrial elongation. It has been reported that the incorporation of labeled choline into brain and liver phosphatidylcholine was less in thyrotoxic rats than in normal rats.

TABLE 6.12
Effects of Glucocorticoid or Thyroid Deficiency or Diabetes on Fatty Acid Profiles of Liver or Isolated Liver Mitochondria[a]

	Fatty acids (mol %)						
Treatment	16:0	18:0	18:1	18:2	20:4	22:6	Tissue
1 mg GC/day	14.6	22.7	6.6	28.5	19.0	3.5	Liver
Control	17.0	20.3	7.61	5.12	7.4	1.5	Liver
Thyroidectomy	12.5	21	8.6	19.5	19.0	8.1	RLM
Control	13.0	20	9.0	17.4	15.7	7.0	RLM
Hypophysectomy	27.1	21.5	13.5	17.0	14.5	2.0	RLM
Control	27.4	22	12.2	12.1	17.4	2.8	RLM
Diabetes[b]	24.5	23.3	7.02	2.4	15.2	4.2	RLM
Control	16.9	23.2	9.3	22.7	22.2	3.1	RLM

[a] GC, synthetic glucocorticoid, dexamethasone; RLM, rat liver mitochondria.
[b] Streptozotocin-induced diabetes.

Age Effects on Membrane Lipids

As animals age, their hormonal status changes, as does the lipid component of their membranes. With age, there is a decrease in growth-hormone production, an increase followed by a decrease in the hormones for reproduction, and, as the animal ages, larger fat stores. Larger fat cells are resistant to insulin and insulin levels may rise as a result of increased fat cell size (insulin resistance). As mentioned in the preceding section, these hormones can affect the lipid portion of the membranes within and around the cells and hence affect how these cells regulate their metabolism. With age, the degree of unsaturation of the membrane fatty acids decreases and the cholesterol level rises. There is also an increase in the number of superoxide radicals. This increase may be responsible for the degradation of the membrane lipids, which, in turn, might explain the age-related changes in membrane function. Membranes from aging animals are less fluid and have reduced transport capacities. As animals age, there is a decline in hepatic mitochondrial respiratory rate and a decrease in the respiratory control ratio and the ADP/O ratio. In addition, there are reports of an age-related decrease in membrane fatty acid unsaturation coupled with a decrease in membrane fluidity and a decrease in the exchange of ATP for ADP across the mitochondrial membrane, a decrease in ATP synthesis, and an amelioration of these age-related decreases in mitochondrial function by restricted feeding.

Membrane Function

In the previous section, the importance of diet, age, and hormonal status was described in terms of their influence on the composition of the membrane lipids. Although not emphasized, these compositional differences have important effects on metabolic regulation. This regulation consists of the control of the flux of nutrients, substrates, and/or products into, out of, and between the various compartments of the cell.

The cellular membranes serve as the "gatekeepers" of the cells and their compartments. They regulate the influx and efflux of nutrients, substrates, hormones, and metabolic products produced or used by the cell or compartment in the course of its metabolic activity. For example, the mitochondrial membrane, through its transport of 2- and 4-carbon intermediates and through its exchange of ADP for ATP, regulates the activity of the respiratory chain and ATP synthesis. If too little ADP enters the mitochondria because of decreased ADP transport across the mitochondrial membrane, respiratory chain activity will decrease, less ATP will be synthesized, and there may be a decrease in other mitochondrial reactions that are either driven by ADP influx or dependent on ATP availability. Through its export of citrate from the matrix of the mitochondria, ATP regulates the availability of citrate to the cytosol for cleavage into oxaloacetate and acetyl CoA, the beginning of fatty acid synthesis. If more citrate is exported from the mitochondria than can be split to oxaloacetate and acetyl CoA, this citrate will feed back onto the phosphofructokinase reaction, and glycolysis will be inhibited. Thus, the activity of the mitochondrial membrane tricarboxylate transporter has a role in the control of cytosolic metabolism.

Other transporters such as the dicarboxylate transporter or the adenine nucleotide translocase have similar responsibilities vis-à-vis the control of cytosolic and mitochondrial metabolic activity. In the plasma membrane, receptors embedded in the membrane have a similar function. That is, they control the entry of nutrients or hormones into the cell. Further, the plasma membrane hormone receptor may bind a given hormone and, with binding, elicit a cascade of reactions characteristic of the hormone effect without permitting the entry of the hormone itself into the cystosolic compartment. An example here is the hormone insulin. Insulin binds to its receptor and, in so doing, elicits the cascade of events that include the transport and metabolism of glucose by the cell. The insulin, bound to the receptor site, is inactivated and is brought into the cell by pinocytosis for further degradation. Other hormones, notably the nonprotein steroids and the low-molecular-weight hormones such as epinephrine and thyroxine, pass through the plasma membrane and attach to receptors in the cytosol or nuclear membrane or on the endoplasmic reticulum. Once attached to their respective binding sites, they also elicit a metabolic response.

In the membranes are a variety of closely packed proteins and lipids. The membrane-bound proteins have extensive hydrophobic regions and usually require lipids for the maintenance of their activity. Adenylate cyclase, cytochrome b_5, and cytochrome c oxidase have all been shown to have phospholipid affinities. Cytochrome c oxidase from mitochondria has tightly bound aldehyde lipid that cannot be removed without destroying its activity as the enzyme that transfers electrons to molecular oxygen in the final step of respiration. A number of other membrane proteins have tightly bound fatty acids as part of their structures. These fatty acids are covalently bound to their proteins as a posttranslational event and act to direct, insert, and anchor the proteins in the cell membranes. Other lipids are bound differently to membrane proteins. Some are acylated with fatty acids during their passage from their site of synthesis on the rough endoplasmic reticulum to the membrane, whereas others acquire their lipid component during their placement in the membrane. β-Hydroxybutyrate dehydrogenase, for example, requires the choline head of phosphatidylcholine for its activity. If hepatocytes are caused to increase their synthesis of phosphatidyl-methylethanolamine, which substitutes for phosphatidylcholine in the membrane, β-hydroxybutyrate dehydrogenase activity is reduced.

All of these examples illustrate the importance of the cellular and intracellular membranes in the regulation of metabolism. They illustrate the fact that the gatekeeping property of the membrane is vested in the structure and function of the various transporters and receptors or binding proteins embedded in the membrane. Whereas the genetic heritage of an individual determines the amino acid sequence of the proteins and hence their function, this function can be modified by the lipid milieu in which they exist. Diet, hormonal state, and genetics in turn control the lipid milieu in terms of the kinds and amounts of the different lipids that are synthesized within the cell and incorporated into the membrane.

Fatty Acid Oxidation

While fatty acids are important components of membranes and while certain ones are important precursors of the eicosanoids, the main function of these molecules in the body is to provide energy to sustain life. This provision is accomplished through oxidation. Regardless of whether the fatty acids come from the diet or are mobilized from the tissue triacylglyceride store, the pathway for oxidation is the same once the triacylglyceride has been hydrolyzed.

The hydrolysis of stored lipid is catalyzed in a three-step process by one of the lipases specific to mono, di, or triacylglycerol. Intracellular hormone-sensitive lipase hydrolyzes fatty acids one at a time from all three carbon positions of the glycerol moiety and these fatty acids are then available for oxidation. Interstitial hormone-insensitive lipase has a similar mode of action. The lipases that act on the phospholipids to release arachidonic acid for eicosanoid synthesis or to release inositol-1,3,4-phosphate and diacylglyceride or other components of the phospholipids also provide fatty acids for oxidation — but that is not their primary role.

The lipases in the adipose tissue are the key to the regulated release of fatty acids from the stored triacylglycerides. These fatty acids can be oxidized *in situ* by the adipocyte but usually they are released for transport to other tissues as energy sources. The fatty acids are carried by albumin or by lipoproteins to where they are needed. At the target cell, the fatty acids are liberated from the triacylglycerides carried by the lipoproteins through the action of lipoprotein lipase or liberated from albumin by an (as-yet) undefined mechanism. The liberated fatty acids diffuse through the plasma membrane, bind to the cytosolic fatty acid-binding protein and migrate through the cytoplasm to the outer mitochondrial membrane or to the peroxisomes, microsomes, or the endoplasmic reticulum. At each of these destinations, they are activated by conversion to their CoA thioesters. This activation requires ATP and the enzyme acyl CoA synthase or thiokinase. There are several thiokinases that differ with respect to their specificity for the different fatty acids. The activation step is dependent on the release of energy from two high-energy phosphate bonds. ATP is hydrolyzed to AMP and 2 molecules of inorganic phosphate. Figure 6.23 shows the initial steps in the oxidation of fatty acids. Once the fatty acid is activated, it is bound to carnitine with the release of CoA. The acyl carnitine is then translocated through the mitochondrial membranes into the mitochondrial matrix via the carnitine acylcarnitine translocase. As 1 molecule of acylcarnitine is passed into the matrix, 1 molecule of carnitine is translocated back to the cytosol and the acylcarnitine is converted back to acyl CoA. The acyl CoA can then enter the β oxidation pathway shown in Figure 6.24.

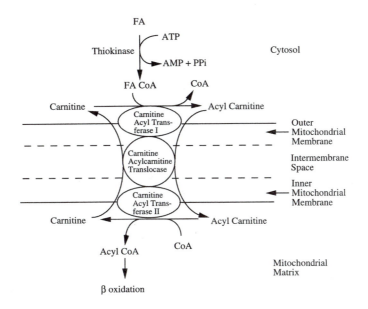

FIGURE 6.23   Mechanism for the entry of fatty acids into the mitochondrial β oxidation pathway.

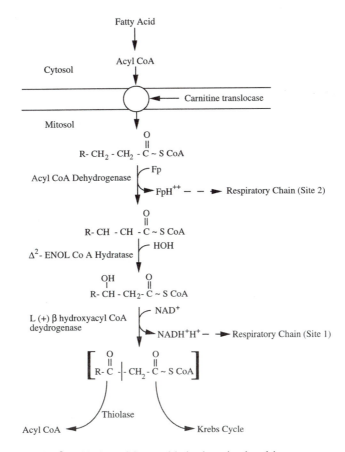

FIGURE 6.24   Pathway for β oxidation of fatty acids in the mitochondria.

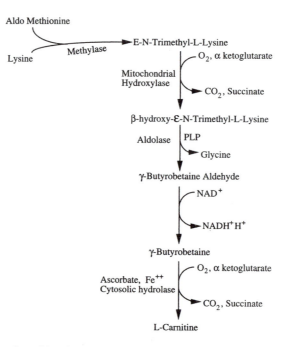

FIGURE 6.25   Synthesis of carnitine from lysine and methionine.

Without carnitine, the oxidation of fatty acids, especially the long-chain fatty acids, cannot proceed. Acyl CoA cannot traverse the membrane into the mitochondria and thus requires a translocase for its entry. The translocase requires carnitine. Carnitine is synthesized from methionine and lysine as shown in Figure 6.25. While most of the fatty acids that enter the β oxidation pathway are completely oxidized via the Krebs cycle and respiratory chain to CO_2 and HOH, some of the acetyl CoA is instead converted to the ketones, acetoacetate, and β hydroxybutyrate. The condensation of 2 molecules of acetyl CoA to acetoacetyl CoA occurs in the mitochondria via the enzyme β-ketothiolase. Acetoacetyl CoA then condenses with another acetyl CoA to form HMG CoA. At last, the HMG CoA is cleaved into acetoacetic acid and acetyl CoA. The acetoacetic acid is reduced to β hydroxybutyrate and this reduction is dependent on the ratio of NAD^+ to $NADH^{++}$. The enzyme for this reduction, β hydroxybutyrate dehydrogenase is tightly bound to the inner aspect of the mitochondrial membrane. Because of its high activity, the product (β hydroxybutyrate) and substrate (acetoacetate) are in equilibrium. Measurements of these two compounds can thus be used to determine the redox state (ratio of oxidized to reduced NAD) of the mitochondrial compartment.

HMG CoA is also synthesized in the cytosol, however, because this compartment lacks the HMG CoA lyase, the ketones are formed only in the mitochondria. In the cytosol, HMG CoA is the beginning substrate for cholesterol synthesis. The ketones can ultimately be used as fuel but may appear in the blood, liver, and other tissues at a level of less than 0.2 mM. In starving individuals, or in people consuming a high-fat diet, blood and tissue ketone levels may rise above normal (3–5 mM). However, unless these levels greatly exceed the body's capacity to use them as fuel (as is the case in uncontrolled diabetes mellitus with levels up to 20 mM) a rise in ketone levels is not a cause for concern. Ketones are choice metabolic fuels for muscle and brain. Although both tissues may prefer to use glucose, the ketones can be used when glucose is in short supply. Ketones are used to spare glucose wherever possible under these conditions. The oxidation of unsaturated fatty acids follows the same pathway as the saturated fatty acids until the double-bonded carbons are reached. At this point, a few side steps must be taken that involve a few additional enzymes. An example of this pathway is shown in Figure 6.26 using linoleate as the fatty acid being oxidized.

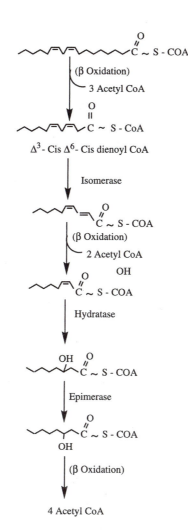

FIGURE 6.26   Modification of β oxidation for unsaturated fatty acid.

Linoleate has two double bonds in the cis configuration. β oxidation removes three acetyl units leaving a CoA attached to the terminal carbon just before the first cis double bond. At this point an isomerase enzyme, Δ^3 cis Δ^6 trans enoyl CoA isomerase, acts to convert the first cis bond to a trans bond. Now this part of the molecule can once again enter the β oxidation sequence and two more acetyl CoA units are released. The second double bond is then opened and a hydroxyl group is inserted. In turn, this hydroxyl group is rotated to the L position and the remaining product can then reenter the β oxidation pathway. Other unsaturated fatty acids can be similarly oxidized. Each time the double bond is approached the isomerization and hydroxyl group addition takes place until all of the fatty acid is oxidized.

While β oxidation is the main pathway for the oxidation of fatty acids, some fatty acids undergo α oxidation so as to provide the substrates for the synthesis of sphingolipids. These reactions occur in the endoplasmic reticulum and mitochondria and involve the mixed function oxidases because they require molecular oxygen, reduced NAD, and specific cytochromes. The fatty acid oxidation that occurs in organelles other than the mitochondria (i.e., peroxisomes) are energy-wasteful reactions because these other organelles do not have the Krebs cycle, nor do they have the respiratory chain that takes the reducing equivalents released by the oxidative steps and combines them with oxygen to make water-releasing energy that is then trapped in the high-energy bonds of the ATP. Peroxisomal oxidation in the kidney and liver is an important aspect of drug metabolism. The peroxisomes are a class of subcellular organelles that are important in the protection against oxygen toxicity. They have a high level of catalase activity, which suggests their importance in the antioxidant system.

The peroxisomal fatty acid oxidation pathway differs in three important ways from the mitochondrial pathway. First, the initial dehydrogenation is accomplished by a cyanide-insensitive oxidase that produces H_2O_2. This H_2O_2 is rapidly extinguished by catalase. Second, the enzymes of the pathway prefer long-chain fatty acids and are slightly different in structure from those (with the same function) of the mitochondrial pathway. Third, β oxidation in the peroxisomes stops at eight carbons rather than proceeding all the way to acetyl CoA. It may be that peroxisomal oxidation helps the body get rid of fatty acids that are in excess of 20 carbons in length. The peroxisomes also serve in the conversion of cholesterol to bile acids and in the formation of ether lipids (plasmalogens). Of interest are the reports of a rare fatal genetic disorder that is characterized by the absence of the peroxisomes. This is called the Zellweger syndrome. Victims of this disorder do not make bile acids or plasmalogens, nor are they able to shorten the very long fatty acids. These biochemical deficiencies are seemingly unrelated to the structural abnormalities observed in liver, kidney, muscle, and brain. Efforts to circumvent the genetic mutation have been unsuccessful. It is possible to detect its presence by the absence of peroxisomal enzymes in amniotic fluid.

DYNAMIC CONSIDERATIONS IN FATTY ACID SYNTHESIS AND USE

The body consists of many different organs and cell types whose fuel needs differ appreciably. Most of the foregoing discussion has focused on the individual reactions that compose fatty acid synthesis and use. However, one must appreciate the complexity of the system that dictates the ebb and flow of these energy-rich molecules. In this, we acknowledge the role of the many hormones that regulate or influence lipogenesis and lipolysis. Fatty acid synthesis in the liver and fat cell is stimulated by insulin and high-carbohydrate diets. Fatty acid release is stimulated by thyroid hormone, growth hormone, epinephrine and norepinephrine, glucocorticoid, glucagon, ACTH, and starvation. Fatty acid oxidation is increased by many of the same hormones that stimulate lipolysis, as well as by high-fat feeding. Communication and transport of fatty acids and glycerides via the blood to tissues that use these lipids from tissues that make them involves the synthesis and degradation of lipoproteins. All of these components are shown in Figure 6.27.

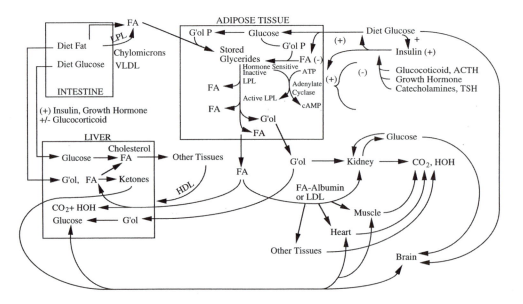

FIGURE 6.27   Integration of diet and hormone effects on fatty acid metabolism.

CHOLESTEROL SYNTHESIS, DEGRADATION, AND USE

Cholesterol is widely distributed in all cells and is an important lipid constituent of membranes. Membranes differ in the amount of cholesterol they contain; mitochondrial membranes contain very little while plasma membranes contain somewhat more. Cholesterol is not very soluble in water but is carried in the blood by the LDL and VLDL. About 70% of the cholesterol carried by these proteins is esterified to a fatty acid while the remaining 30% is unesterified. Cholesterol either from dietary sources or synthesized *de novo*, is the precursor for the synthesis of the bile acids, the adrenal steroids, active vitamin D, and the sex hormones as shown in Figure 6.28. Cholesterol is abundant in bile, where the normal concentration is about 380–400 mg/dl. In bile, 96% of the cholesterol exists in the unesterified form. The bile is the chief route for cholesterol excretion. Any cholesterol that is not reabsorbed by the jejunum and ileum is excreted in the feces. Humans consuming a low-cholesterol (~200 mg/day) diet have approximately 1300 mg/day returned to the liver. Some of this is the reabsorbed cholesterol via the enterohepatic circulation. Some is carried by the HDL from the periphery as lipids are mobilized and used. The bile contains no lipid or cholesterol-carrying protein, but does contain some phospholipid, whose detergent properties keep the cholesterol in solution. If there is a reduction in the amount of phospholipid in the bile, the cholesterol will fall out of solution and form cholesterol aggregates or gall stones. Bile acids also assist in keeping the cholesterol in solution and again, if there is a reduction in bile acid production, cholesterol will precipitate out and collect in the gall bladder.

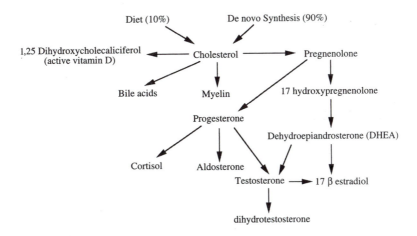

FIGURE 6.28   Overview of cholesterol conversion to biologically important steroids.

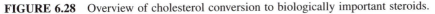

Synthesis

As mentioned, the synthesis of cholesterol begins with acetyl CoA. This synthesis occurs in all cells to varying degrees. The liver, adrenals, gonads and intestine have the greatest cholesterol-synthesizing capacity, for obvious reasons. The pathway for cholesterol synthesis is shown in Figure 6.29.

The total cholesterol pool in the body is carefully regulated. It comes from two sources: the diet and *de novo* synthesis. It is excreted as free cholesterol and as bile acids in the bile. When the amount of cholesterol in the diet is reduced, there is a compensatory increase in *de novo* synthesis by both the liver and the intestine. Once synthesized, it is carried in the blood by lipoprotein B. The liver and intestine are the only tissues that can synthesize apolipoprotein B, hence the cholesterol synthesized in these tissues will be transported primarily by this protein and will be found in the LDL or VLDL lipoprotein class. The LDL is formed when the apolipoprotein C components and triacylglycerides are removed from the VLDL.

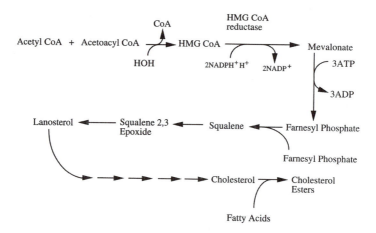

FIGURE 6.29 Cholesterol biosynthesis.

When the diet contains a lot of cholesterol, *de novo* synthesis is almost totally suppressed. Thus, there is an inverse relationship between intake and synthesis. The cholesterol present in the diet is carried in the chylomicrons, not by the VLDL. The high-density lipoproteins (HDL) and the enzyme lecithin: cholesterol acyl transferase (LCAT) are important in the regulation of cholesterol turnover. LCAT catalyzes the transfer of fatty acid in the carbon 2 position of phosphatidylcholine to the 3-hydroxyl group of cholesterol. LCAT is a plasma enzyme and its substrate is the cholesterol carried by HDL. The cholesterol ester generated by the LCAT reaction is carried in the core of the HDL particle, where it is transported to the liver and prepared for excretion as free cholesterol or bile acid in the bile. HDL is thus the vehicle for transporting cholesterol generated in the periphery to the liver for excretion.

Synthesis is controlled primarily at the level of the HMG CoA reductase step. There is feedback inhibition of the enzyme by mevalonate and cholesterol. Mevalonate inactivates the existing enzyme as well as inhibiting the activation of the preexisting enzyme. Blood cholesterol levels rise when the cholesterol biosynthesis is not suppressed. This can occur when the LDL-bound cholesterol fails to enter the cell to suppress the synthesis and activation of HMG CoA reductase. This failure occurs when the LDL receptor fails to bind the LDL and extract the carried cholesterol. The receptor recognizes only the apolipoprotein B (the lipid-carrying protein synthesized in the intestine and liver). It does not recognize any other lipoprotein or any other protein that carries lipid material. All of these have their own receptors. People with a mutation in the gene that encodes the receptors are therefore characterized by high blood levels of cholesterol as well as high rates of endogenous cholesterol synthesis.

The majority of the cholesterol in the circulation is synthesized *de novo* by the body. There are a few people (one in 20,000) who cannot make cholesterol. They have a genetic disorder known as the Smith-Lemli-Opitz syndrome, abbreviated as SLO disease. This disease is sometimes called the RSH syndrome. It is an autosomal recessive disorder characterized by an accumulation of 7-dehydrocholesterol due to a mutation in the gene that encodes $\Delta 7$ cholesterol reductase. This enzyme catalyzes an intermediate step in the synthesis of cholesterol. This metabolite accumulates in many tissues, especially the eye. In doing so, it causes cataracts to form. Children with this disorder fail to grow and develop normally (failure to thrive) because cholesterol is a vital ingredient to so many important biological structures. This is especially true with respect to the cell membranes and the lipids in the central nervous system. Some investigators have tried to provide dietary supplements of cholesterol to these children in an effort to improve their development, however, another feature of these children is their great number of food allergies. Many are allergic to cholesterol-rich foods such as eggs.

HEALTH CONCERNS IN LIPID NUTRITION

CARDIOVASCULAR DISEASE

There are a number of human diseases that are of interest to the lipid nutritionist. In the '50s and '60s, epidemiologists attracted much attention to the association between the incidence of coronary vessel disease and the customary fat intakes of a number of countries throughout the world. Countries with food intakes that were low in saturated fat had low incidences of heart disease and vice versa. These associations neglected all other considerations such as death from communicable disease or malnutrition.

Epidemiologists have not only pointed out an association between saturated-fat intake and CVD, they have also identified an association between CVD and blood cholesterol levels. People with high (greater than 240 mg/dl) serum cholesterol values are at greater risk of having CVD than are people with serum cholesterol levels of less than 200 mg/dl. Regression analysis of the many studies on the effects of dietary fatty acids and cholesterol on serum cholesterol and lipoprotein cholesterol showed that diet can affect the blood lipid levels. However, regression analysis is simply a mathematical array of relating intake to blood lipid levels. It cannot show the next step; that is, that increasing blood lipids are *causal* with respect to CVD. It is not possible, for ethical reasons, to conduct experiments that show causality in humans. As pointed out in the earlier sections on lipid transport and metabolism, the genetics of the consumer is as potent (or perhaps more so) a determinant of blood lipid levels as is the habitual fat intake. Thus, the jury is still out on the question of whether dietary fat is responsible for the high death rate from CVD in developed nations. More than likely, we will find that CVD results from an interaction of genetic factors with lifestyle choices of which the dietary-fat intake is but a part.

MARINE OILS AND DIABETES

The observations on marine oils and CVD have stimulated considerable research on the responses of man and animals to the inclusion of marine oils in the diet. Rats, mice, swine, monkeys, and rabbits have been studied in addition to normal humans and humans having a variety of diseases thought to benefit from the consumption of these oils. Whether the inclusion of omega-3 fatty acids in the diets of hyperlipidemic subjects was of benefit was tested by Phillipson et al. (1985). Twenty hyperlipemic subjects were studied. Ten of these subjects had type IIb lipemia (cholesterol range: 238–411 mg/dl, triglyceride range: 198–720 mg/dl) and 10 had type V lipemia (cholesterol range: 274–840 mg/dl, triglyceride range: 896–5775 mg/dl). The subjects consumed either a corn-oil-based or a fish-oil-based diet or a control diet for 4 weeks each. In the type IIb group, fish-oil consumption resulted in a 27% decrease in plasma cholesterol and a 64% decrease in triglyceride. In the type V group, the reductions were 45% and 79%, respectively. In the type V group, the consumption of the corn-oil diet resulted in a significant rise in plasma triglyceride levels. These and other investigators reported that fish-oil consumption resulted in a decrease in VLDL levels in the blood.

Not only has there been interest in the relationship of dietary omega-3 fatty acids to cardio-vascular disease, there has also been interest in its relationship to diabetes. People with diabetes mellitus have five times the risk of non-diabetics of having cardiovascular disease. Diabetes and heart disease are closely related. With respect to diabetes, Feldman et al. studied two groups of Alaskan Eskimos. One group consumed a typical western diet while the other consumed the traditional Alaskan Eskimo diet which, like the Greenland Eskimo diet, is high in marine foods and low in total carbohydrates as well as sugar. As found in the Greenland Eskimos, serum lipids were very low and glucose tolerance normal, when the traditional diet was consumed. When the Eskimos consumed western diets, which are higher in carbohydrate, particularly sugar, they had significantly higher free fatty acid and triglyceride levels, as well as minor abnormalities in their glucose tolerance. Although Alaskan Eskimos, in general, have a very low prevalence of diabetes, these findings suggest that as these Eskimos begin to include significant amounts of carbohydrate, particularly sweets, in their diet, the prevalence of diabetes may change. In addition, since the Eskimos studied by Feldman consumed significant quantities of marine foods, it might also be inferred that the development of glucose intolerance was genetically controlled and unaffected by the presence of omega-3 fatty acids in the diet.

CANCER AND DIETARY FAT

The many different forms of cancer account for the second-largest number of deaths due to disease in developed nations. It too is probably influenced by the fat intake but in these disorders, it is not the saturated fat that is culpable. Studies on the development of mammary tumors in rats and mice have shown that high intakes of polyunsaturated fat containing the omega-6 fatty acids promote the development of the cancer. Carcinogenesis is thought to occur in two steps. The first is the initiation step. This concerns the conversion of normal DNA to the DNA typical of a cancer cell. Large segments of the gene code are deleted or so changed that the translation products are either not present or are not normal in function. This conversion can be instigated by chemicals such as 7,12-dimethylbenz (α) anthracene (DMBA), by viruses, radiation and perhaps oxidized (free radical) food components. By itself, this initiation step will not progress to the metastatic cell unless the next step, the promotion step, also occurs. Cells whose DNA has been injured will and can repair this DNA. However, if the "right" environment is provided, this does not occur and a metastatic cell is produced *and reproduced*. Dietary corn oil has been shown to be a very good promoter of DMBA-induced breast cancer in rats and mice while dietary beef tallow is not. How corn oil has this effect is not known and, of course, cause-and-effect studies cannot be conducted in humans. Just as epidemiological studies cannot provide definitive proof of the role of diet in CVD development, the same is true for cancer. Both the level of intake and the type of fat have been implicated but strong proof is lacking. As with CVD, the genetic influence is quite strong. Glauert (1993) has recently reviewed the literature on the role of dietary fat in the expression of genes related to cancer development.

OTHER DISEASES

No discussion of the role of dietary fat in human disease would be complete without the mention of obesity. As discussed in the chapter on energy, this disorder has a multiplicity of causes of which the total energy intake is but a part. The excess energy consumed could easily be provided by the dietary fat since it has twice the energy value per gram as does dietary carbohydrate and protein. However, intake alone does not fully explain the obese state. Genetic factors that control energy intake, storage, and use are also important.

Gall bladder disease is frequently associated with excess body fatness (or its loss) and, as explained in the section on absorption, may be attributable to the precipitation of cholesterol from the bile while in the gall bladder. Other genetic diseases involving lipid metabolism are shown in Table 6.13. These diseases are due to mutations in genes for specific enzymes important to the synthesis and degradation of neuronal lipids. Many are associated with mental retardation and early death. None seem to be related to nutrition or dietary fat intake.

Finally, although already described in the section on fatty acid metabolism, mention should be made of the impact on health of essential fatty acid deficiency and of carnitine deficiency. In today's world, these deficiencies are uncommon, except under the special circumstance of long-term sustained intravenous nutritional support of a patient who cannot or will not eat. In both instances, care must be given to provide useful linoleic and linolenic acids in the intravenous nutrient-support solution and to provide these nutrients and carnitine in the formula that supports the premature infant. In both instances, failure to provide these important nutrients can compromise the ability of the individual to survive and thrive. It is generally accepted that 1–2% of the total energy intake

TABLE 6.13
Genetic Diseases in Lipid Metabolism

Disease	Mutation	Characteristics
Tay-Sachs disease	Hexosaminidase A deficiency	Early death, CNS degeneration, ganglioside GM2 accumulates
Gaucher's disease	Glucocerebrosidase deficiency	Enlarged liver and spleen; erosion of long bones and pelvis; mental retardation; glucocerebroside accumulates
Fabry's disease	α Galactosidase A deficiency	Skin rash, kidney failure, pain in legs and feet, ceramide trihexoside accumulates
Niemann-Pick disease	Sphingomyelinase deficiency	Enlarged liver and spleen, mental retardation, sphingomyelin accumulates
Krabbe's disease (Globoid leukodystrophy)	Galactocerebroside deficiency	Mental retardation, absence of myelin
Metachromatic leukodystrophy	Arylsulfatase A deficiency	Mental retardation, sulfatides accumulate
Generalized gangliosidosis	Gmi,Gandioside: β galactosidase deficiency	Mental retardation, enlarged liver
Sandhoff-Jatzkewitz disease	Hexosaminidase A and B deficiency	Same as Tay-Sachs but develops quicker
Fucosidosis	a-L-Fucosidase	Cerebral degeneration, spastic muscles, thick skin
Acetyl CoA carboxylase deficiency	Acetyl CoA carboxylase deficiency	No de novo fatty acid synthesis
Hypercholesterolemia	LDL receptor deficiency	Premature atherosclerosis and death from CVD
Refsum's disease	α hydroxylating enzyme	Neurological problems: deafness, blindness, cerebellar ataxia, phytanic acid accumulates

CPT = Carnitine palmitoyltransferase
ETF = Electron transfer flavoproteins
ETF:QO = ETF = oxidoreductase
LCAD, MCAD, SCAD, VLCAD = long chain, medium chain, short chain, very long chain, 3 hydroxyl-CoA dehydrogenases
LCHAD, SCHAD = long chain and short chain 3 hydroxyacyl-CoA dehydrogenases

from fat should be provided by the essential fatty acids. The usual mixed diet of Americans provides far more than this amount, so the chances of an essential fatty acid deficiency in the normal individual are very slim indeed. With respect to carnitine, intake recommendations for normal humans have not been made because carnitine usually can be synthesized in adequate amounts in the body. There are circumstances where this is not the case and, in these situations, sufficient carnitine must be supplied. The premature infant, the individual consuming a lysine-poor diet, the elderly, and the person being sustained by parenteral nutrition are all suspected to need more carnitine than their bodies can synthesize. While we know that these people probably would benefit from carnitine supplementation, we do not have a sufficiently large database to use in developing an intake recommendation.

SUPPLEMENTARY READINGS

Allred, J.B. and Bowers, D.F. (1993). Regulation of acetyl CoA carboxylase and gene expression. Chapter 12 p. 269-295. In: *Nutrition and Gene Expression* (Berdanier, C.D. and Hargrove, J.L., Eds.). CRC Press, Boca Raton, FL.

Arner, P. (1992). Adrenergic receptor function in fat cells. *Am. J. Clin. Nutr.* 55:228S-236S.

Bartolini, G., Orlandi, M., Chricolo, M., Licastro, F., Zambonelli, P., Minghetti, L., and Tomasi, V. (1990). Interleukins, interferons: Yen-yang modulators of PGH synthase in human macrophages. *Bio Factors* 2:267-270.

Blom, W., DeMunck-Keizer, S.M.P.F., and Scholte, H.R. (1981). Acetyl CoA carboxylase deficiency: An inborn error of *de novo* fatty acid synthesis. *N. Eng. J. Med.* 305:465.

Buettner, G.R. (1993). The pecking order of free radicals and antioxidants: Lipid peroxidation, α tocopherol and ascorbate. *Arch. Biochem. Biophys.* 300:535-543.

Chen, M., Breslow, J.L., Li, W., and Leff, T. (1994). Transcriptional regulation of the apo C-III gene by insulin in diabetic mice: Correlation with changes in plasma triglyceride levels. *J. Lipid Res.* 35:19180-1924.

Clarke, S.D. and Jump, D.B. (1993). Regulation of hepatic gene expression by dietary fats: A unique role for polyunsaturated fatty acids. Chapter 10, pp. 227-246. In: *Nutrition and Gene Expression* (Berdanier, C.D. and Hargrove, J.L., Eds.). CRC Press, Boca Raton, FL.

Coates, P.M. and Tanaka, K. (1992). Molecular basis of mitochondrial fatty acid oxidation defects. *J. Lipid Res.* 33:1099-1110.

Cockcroft, S. and Thoms, G.M.H. (1992). Inositol-lipid-specific phospholipase C isoenzymes and their differential regulation by receptors. *Biochem. J.* 288:1-14.

Duval, D. and Freyss-Beguin, M. (1992). Glucocorticoids and prostaglandin synthesis: We cannot see the wood for the trees. *Prostaglandins, Leukotrienes and Essential Fatty Acids* 45:85-112.

Esterbauer, H. (1993). Cytotoxicity and genotoxicity of lipid oxidation products. *Am. J. Clin. Nutr.* 57:779S-786S.

Field, C.J., Ryan, E.A., Thomson, A.B.R., and Clandinin, M.T. (1990). Diet fat composition alters membrane phospholipid composition, insulin binding and glucose metabolism from control and diabetic animals. *J. Biol. Chem.* 265:11143-11150.

Fisher, M., Levine, P.H., and Leaf, A. (1989). n-3 fatty acids and cellular aspects of atherosclerosis. *Arch. Int. Med.* 149:1726-1728.

Glauert, H.P. (1993). Dietary fat, gene expression and carcinogenesis. Chapter 11. In: *Nutrition and Gene Expression* (Berdanier, C.D. and Hargrove, J.L., Eds.). CRC Press, Boca Raton, FL.

Gimble, J.M., Hua, X., Wanker, F., Morgan, C., Robinson, C., Hill, M.R., and Nadon, N. (1995). *In vivo* and *in vitro* analysis of murine lipoprotein lipase gene promotor: tissue specific expression. *Am. J. Physiol.* 268:E213-218.

Harman, D. (1993). Free radical involvement in aging. *Drugs and Aging* 3:60-80.

Hayaishi, O. (1991). Molecular mechanisms of sleep-wake regulation: Roles of prostaglandins D_2 and E_2. *FASEB J.* 5:2575-2581.

Hegsted, D.M., Ausman, L.M., Johnson, J.A., and Dallal, G.E. (1993). Dietary fat and serum lipids: An evaluation of the experimental data. *Am. J. Clin. Nutr.* 57:875-883.

Horrobin, D.F. (1991). Interactions between n-3 and n-6 essential fatty acids in the regulation of cardiovascular disorders and inflammation. *Prostaglandins, Leukotrienes and Essential Fatty Acids* 44:127-131.

Howard ,B.V., Welty, T.K., Fabsitz, R.R., Cowan, L.D., Oopik, A.J., Lee, N-A., Yeh, J., Savage, P.J., and Lee, L.T. (1992). Risk factors for coronary heart disease in diabetic and nondiabetic native Americans. *Diabetes* 41:4-11.

Irons, M., Elias, R., and Abuelo, D. (1997). Treatment of SLO syndrome: Results of a multicenter trail. *Am. J. Med. Genetics* 68:311-314.

Just, W.W., and Soto, U. (1992). Biogenesis of peroxisomes in mammals. *Cell. Biochem. and Function* 10:159-165.

Leiffert, W.R., Jahangiri, A., and McMurchie, E.J. (1999). Antiarrhythmic fatty acids and antioxidants in animal and cell studies. *J. Nutr. Biochem.* 10.

MacDonald, J.I.S. and Sprechner, H. (1991). Phospholipid remodeling in mammalian cells. *B.B.A.* 1084:105-121.

Mannaerts, G.P. and Van Veldhoven, P.P. (1993). Metabolic pathways in mammalian peroxisomes.

Mayer, R.J. and Marshall, L.A. (1993). New insights on mammalian phospholipase A_2(s); Comparison of arachidonyl-selective and non-selective enzymes *FASEB J.* 7:339-348.

Meldolesi, J. and Magni, M. (1991). Lipid metabolites and growth factor action. *TIBS* 12:362-364.

Milatovich, A., Plattner, R., Heeroma, N.A., Palmer, C.G., Lopez-Casselas, F., and Kim, K-H. (1988). Localization of the gene for acetyl CoA carboxylase to human chromosome 17. *Cytogenet. Cell. Genet.* 48:190-.

Nishina, P.M., Johnson, J.P., Naggert, J.K., and Krauss, R.M. (1992). Linkage of atherogenic lipoprotein phenotype to the low density lipoprotein receptor locus on the short arm of chromosome 19. *Proc. Natl. Acad. Sci. USA* 89:708-712.

Parke, D.V., Ioannides, C., and Lewis, D.F.V. (1991). Role of cytochromes P450 in the detoxification and activation of drugs and other chemicals. *Can. J. Physiol. and Pharmacol.* 69:537-549.

Rebouche, C.J. (1992). Carnitine function and requirements during the life cycle. *FASEB J.* 6:3379-3386.

Rosseneu, M. and Labeur, C. (1995). Physiological significance of apolipoprotein mutants. *FASEB J.* 9:768-774.

Rossouw, J.E. and Rifkind, B.M. (1990). Does lowering serum cholesterol lower coronary heart disease risk? *Endocrinol. Metab. Clinic N.A.* 19:279-297.

Rustan, A.C., Christiansen, E.N., and Drevon, C.A. (1992). Serum lipids, hepatic glycerolipid metabolism and peroxisomal fatty acid oxidation in rats fed ω3 and ω6 fatty acids. *Biochem. J.* 283:333-339.

Smith, W.L. (1992). Prostanoid synthesis and mechanisms of action. *Am. J. Phsiol.* 263:F181-191.

Song, J. and Wander, R.C. (1991). Effects of dietary selenium and fish oil (Max EPA). on arachidonic acid metabolism and hemostatic function in rats. *J. Nutr.* 121:284-292.

Suckling, K.E. and Jackson, B. (1993). Animal models of human lipid metabolism. *Prog. Lipid Res.* 32:1-24.

Vesper, H., Schmelz, E.-M., Nicklova-Karakasian, M.N., Dillehay, D. L., Lynch, D.V., and Merrill, A.H. (1999). Sphingolipids in food and the emerging importance of sphingolipids to nutrition. *J. Nutr.* 129:1239-1250.

Wassif, C.A. , Maslen, C., and Kachelele-Linjewele, S. (1998). Mutations in the human sterol delta-7-reductase gene at 11q 12-13 causes Smith-Lemli-Optiz syndrrome. *Am. J. Human Genetics* 63:55-62.

Wei ,Y-H. and Kao, S-H. (1996). Mitochondrial DNA mutations and lipid peroxidation in human aging. In: *Nutrients and Gene Expression, Clinical Aspects.* CRC Press, pp. 165-188.

Zeisel, S.H. (1993). Choline phospholipids: signal transduction and carcinogenesis. *FASEB J.* 7:551-557.

Books

Vance, D.E. and J.E. Vance, Eds. *Biochemistry of Lipids and Membranes* (1985). Benjamin/Cummings Publishing Co., Menlo Park, CA. 593 pages.

Chow, C.K., Ed., *Fatty Acids in Foods and Their Health Implications* (1992). Marcel Dekker Inc. New York. 890 pages.

Index

Homozygosity 15
Hormones 154–158
  binding 38, 232
  receptors 37–40, 183
    second messenger systems 40
    effect on membrane lipid 302
Hunger, neuronal signals for 119–124
Hyaluronic acid 208
Hydrolysis 33
Hydrocortisone 296
Hydrogen bonding 32, 160
Hydrostatic pressure 36
Hypercortisolism 100
Hyperglycemia 9, 230, 238
Hyperinsulinism 100
Hypermethioninemia 179
Hyperphagia 97, 105
Hypertension 9, 58
Hypophysectomy 302
Hypothalamus 120
  Ventral 120
  Anterolatera 120l

I

Immune system 141–143
Immunoglobulin, protein 39, 142
Indomethacin 296
Infection 93, 240–241
Influenza 241
Insensible water loss 53
Insensible weight loss 53
Insulin 100, 155, 221, 232, 233–248
  deficiency 236
  diabetes 233–248
  resistance 94
Isoleucine 132

K

K⁴⁰, dilution of 50
K^{40}, dilution of 50
Ketose, carbohydrate 198
Kilojoule 64
Krebs cycle 75, 252, 283
Kwashiorkor, protein and 191–192

L

Lactate dehydrogenase 216
Lactate 222
Lactation. 22–25
Lactose 205, 212
  Intolerance 59
Lard 263
Laxatives 12
LDL, *see* low density lipoprotein 272
Lean body mass 46–52
Lecithin:cholesterol acyl transferase (LCAT) 270

Leptin 97
  apoptosis 45–46, 97
  obesity 97
  uncoupling protein 97
Leucine 132, 174
Leukotrienes 297
Life expectancy 7
Lifespan 7–8
Linoleic acid 261–262, 306
Linolenic acid 261–262
Lipase
  inhibitor 103
  lingual 267
  lipoprotein 267
Lipemia 271, 273
Lipid 259–315
  absorption 266–269
  acyl carnitine 304–305
  acylglycerols 289
  adsorption, fiber 211
  allosteric effect 74
  apolipoprotein 266–274
  aspirin 296
  autooxidation 286–288
  autoimmune inflammatory disease 238–240
  bile acids 267–268
  cardiolipin 301
  cardiovascular disease 13, 266–274, 311
  carnitine deficiency 306
  cholecystokinin 155, 211, 267
  cholesterol 309–310
    degradation 309
    ester 264, 309
    synthesis 309
  chylomicron 268–272
  classification 260
  colipase 267
  coronary vessel disease 13, 266–274, 311
  cylcooxygenase 296
  diabetes 233–248, 311
  digestion 266–267
  eicosanoids 293–300
  epinephrine 56, 267
  ethanol intoxication 13, 253–256
  fat 263–265
    cancer correlation 312
  fatty acids 280–308
    autooxidation 286–288
    binding protein 304
  desaturation 285–286
  elongation 285
  essential 292–294
  esterification 289
  membrane function 300
  oxidation 85
    release 304
    saturated 292
    synthesis 282–285
    unsaturated 292
  fish oil 311–312
  gall bladder disease 268, 312

M